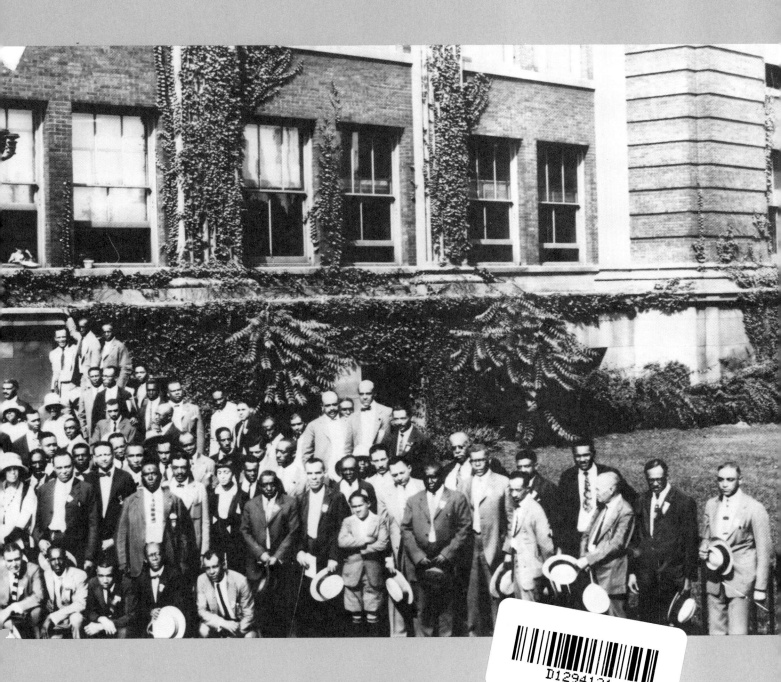

Center for Ethics & Humanities
G-208 East Fee Hall
Michigan State University
East Lansing, MI 48824

D1294121

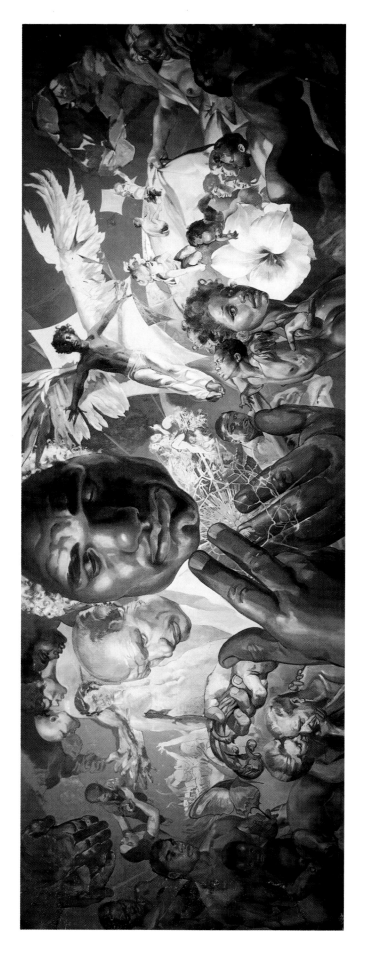

Leroy Foster's magnificent 9' x 28' mural, Kaleidoscope, dominates the lobby of the Southwest Detroit Hospital. The commission for the painting was a joint venture between the medical staff of Boulevard General Hospital and the managers of Southwest Detroit Hospital.

The National Medical Association Demands Equal Opportunity: Nothing More, Nothing Less

BY
CHARLES H. WRIGHT, M.D.

Charro Book Company, Inc.•Southfield, Michigan

The Nation Medical Association Demands Equal Opportunity: Nothing More, Nothing Less

Copyright @ 1995 Charles H. Wright

All rights reserved. This book may not be duplicated in any way without the expressed written consent of the publisher, except in the form of brief excerpts or quotations for the purposes of review. The information contained herein may not be duplicated in other books, databases or any other medium without the written consent of the publisher or author. Making copies of this book, or any portion for any purpose other than your own, is a violation of United States copyright laws.

ISBN: 0962-9468-4-2

Cover design and graphics by Aaron Hightower, making a quiet but eloquent statement: "A man's quest for equal opportunity is an inalienable right that must not be held hostage by anyone."

Desktop publishing production by Charles R. Alexander

First Edition, First Printing

This publication is available at special discounts for bulk purchases for sales promotions, premiums, fund-raising, or educational use. For details, contact the Publisher.

For information address:

Charro Book Company, Inc.

Charro Book Co. Inc.
17344 W. 12 Mile Road
Southfield, MI
48076

PRINTED IN THE UNITED STATES OF AMERICA

Dedication

This book is dedicated to all the women who have directly and indirectly helped to make me who I am. This process began early when a neighbor in Dothan, Ala., asked me "Charles, what do you want to be when you get to be a man?" Without hesitation Laura Wright, my mother, answered "Charles is going to be a doctor.

With that issue all settled, I set about fulfilling my mother's promise the best I could in southern Alabama. Those women in my immediate family who contributed directly to this process, insofar as this book is concern, are my wife, Roberta; daughters Stephanie, Carla, and Barbara; granddaughters Blythe, Christina, and Louisa; and nieces Nadine, Anita, and Danielle.

Those who contributed indirectly (but not limited to) are all the women I have operated on, treated, delivered, or worked with since becoming a doctor in 1943. I thank all of you.

Contents

Preface

Acknowledgements

Introduction 1

Michigan Medical Trailblazers of the 19th Century 11

Joseph Ferguson, Robert Boland,
Henry Fitzbutler, and Sofia Jones

The Founding of the
National Medical Association, 1895 29

Atlanta, The National Medical
Association's Ancestral Home 43

Detroit, The African American
Hospital Capital of the United States 49

The Medical Gospel According to Abraham:
The Flexner Report—1910 87

The National Medical Association
Comes to Detroit (1927) 101

The Hill-Burton Act: (The Hospital Survey
and Construction Act of 1946) 109

Detroit Hosts Her Second NMA Convention (1949) . . . 117

Imhotep Conferences 123

Detroit Hosts Her Third NMA Convention (1959) . . . 129

The NMA—AMA Liaison Committee 131

Detroit Medical Society 139

The Beginning of the Move Toward
Title VI of the Civil Rights Act of 1964 183

A History of the Auxiliary
to the National Medical Association 193

President Leonidas Berry Resumes the
NMA-AMA Liaison Committee 195

The American Medical Association
and the Hungarian Uprising 205

The AMA and the Cuban Doctors 209

Detroit's Fourth NMA Convention, 1979 219

The AMA in South Africa 221

Michigan's African American Medical
Trailblazers of the Twentieth Century 243
Matthew's Disciples 255
African American Firsts in Medicine, in Michigan 269
Detroit's Man and Wife Medical Teams 327
The Medical Progeny of Detroit's
African American Physicians 331
Epilogue 347
Bibliography
Index
About the Author

Preface

The centennial of a person, place or event should mark an occasion to pause and reflect on the past, examine the present and plan for the future. The National Medical Association's (NMA) centenary in 1995 provides thousands of African American physicians an occasion for doing all three.

The publication of the book, *The National Medical Association Demands Equal Opportunity, Nothing More, Nothing Less,* is but one of a series of events that will help celebrate this significant occasion. After 100 years there should be—and is—much to say. Such reporting can help us to avoid many of our prior mistakes. Only then can the challenges of the future be met with the confidence and courage of first-class American citizens who demand, and will accept no less than, equal access to every opportunity this country offers.

The National Medical Association's 100th anniversary is not a moment too soon to begin a more serious quest for freedom and justice wherever they are to be found and at whatever price!

The past that we must consider did not begin when those 12 African American physicians met in Atlanta in 1895 and accepted the fact that because of their color, they had no future in the American Medical Association (AMA). Our past also did not begin in 1847 when the organizers of the AMA chose a racist infrastructure upon which they built an organization that has continuously denied equal recognition to African American physicians.

Our troubles, as a people, began when that first boatload of Europeans landed on the African coast seeking replacements for those "lazy, untrustworthy, red skins" who refused enslavement and died resisting the loss of their freedom and ancestral lands to those same Europeans.

Most, if not all, of our ancestors who survived the "Middle Passage" needed, but were denied, medical care following their abduction to these shores. Instead they were forced into a peculiar American institution, "chattel slavery," which denied their humanity and their need to be respected as human beings.

This denial was inferred in the 1776 Declaration of Independence, as the nation was being born: "All men are created equal and endowed by their Creator with certain inalienable rights." Even then it was clear that the definition of "men" would one day become a top item on some future agenda.

Twelve years later, in 1788, the Founding Fathers sidestepped reality once again by avoiding the use of the word "slavery" in the entire federal Constitution. Instead, they chose to:

1. "Continue that 'Peculiar American Institution chattel slavery,' indefinitely.

2. "Allow the international African slave trade to continue for twenty additional years, giving the slave traders until 1808 to install such profitable alternatives as clandestine shipping routes from Africa to the Sea Islands off the Georgia and South Carolina coasts.

3. "Permit European American enslavers to establish slave-breeding farms within the United States that maintained a steady supply of free African slave labor, despite a constitutional interdiction of such practices.

4. "Deny the ballot to all African Americans—free and enslaved—but increase the political power of the enslavers by awarding to each of them an *additional 3/5 vote* for each African American that the slave owner held in bondage.

5. "Charge any person, in any State, with Treason, Felony, or other Crime, who shall flee from 'Justice,' and be found in another State. Shall on demand of the executive authority of the State from which he fled, be delivered up to be removed to the State having jurisdiction of the 'crime.'"

This article, which gave constitutional sanction to the Fugitive Slave Act of 1773 and its more stringent 1850 Amendment, was a pre-Civil War attempt to avoid secession by the Confederate states. Despite the enormous privation and cost to the enslaved, secession began anyway a decade or so later.

These are but a few examples of the Constitutional rulings, U.S. Supreme Court decisions, congressional acts, Presidential decrees and public policies that led to bitter discussions in the first half of the 19th century that questioned the humanity of African Americans and all other pigmented Americans. Serious questions were raised about their rights to citizenship and their entitlement to respect as human beings by European Americans.

In the early 1840s, an outspoken leader of the pro-slavery faction was Senator John Calhoun, who adamantly proclaimed: "the Equal Rights Doctrine is nonsense." George Fitzhugh, another white supremacist, supported his position as did many others who believed and often declared: "some men are born with saddles, and others are booted and saddled to ride them."

The future Chief Supreme Court Justice Roger Taney, who in 1857 wrote and read the infamous Dred Scott decision, was already spreading the gospel of white supremacy throughout the land. A miasma of racism settled over the land and penetrated every crevice of American society. The Civil War, one of the bloodiest of all times, became inevitable.

At that time, the AMA's early Mission Statement declared: "Resolved that it is expedient for the medical profession of the United States to institute a medical association for the protection of their interests and for the maintenance of their honor and respectability and the advancement of their knowledge and the extension of their usefulness."

Within the Mission Statement, "their" refers only to European American physicians and ignores the presence and aspirations of many non-European American physicians who sought recognition by and acceptance in the AMA as their *Good Housekeeping* seal of approval.

Emphatic denial of membership to African American physicians was the end result of the AMA's initial policy. This was followed by such demeaning concessions as "Provisional" and "Associate" memberships of indefinite length that denied the member the right to vote or hold office. The southern associations offered "Scientific" memberships which allowed African Americans to attend the scientific portions of the membership meetings. However, whenever food and drinks were served or European American women arrived, African Americans were expected to flee.

The medical establishment's powers-that-be have refused to accept the reality that their African American colleagues are human beings too and will no longer accept the biased condescension of the past century. The members of the AMA have demonstrated an unwillingness, or more likely an incapacity, to make fundamental changes in their ways of doing business.

The members of the National Medical Association (NMA) and other victims of the AMA's racist history must not only seek, but find more democratic options elsewhere. The beginning of our second century is not a moment too soon to begin to exercise this respectable option. This book is a clear call to action!

---

1. Article 4, Section 2, Federal Constitution.
2. Dwight Lowell Dumond, *Antislavery*. (Ann Arbor: Univ. of Michigan Press, 1961), p. 305.
3. Benjamin Quarles, *The Negro in the Making of America*. (New York: MacMillan Publishing Co., 1987) p. 67.

Acknowledgments

My interest in producing an Anniversary Statement about the National Medical Association was aroused in 1976, the year after the NMA's 81st anniversary. The Civil Rights movement had run its course, and African American physicians were able to point to some gains therefrom.

I discussed the matter with the editor of the *JNMA* at that time, Dr. Montague Cobb, at his home in Detroit and at his Cosmos Club in Washington, D.C. He told me that he had been working on such a history for some time, but that it was not going well. We discussed a few methods of approaching such a formidable task. Later on, he informed me that he was no longer seriously involved in writing the NMA's history.

The national office of the NMA soon announced that its 1979 annual convention would be held in Detroit. I suggested to them that I would like to write a story about the first 75 years of the NMA, if they would publish it. Since I had just published *Robeson, Labor's Forgotten Champion* and had written several scientific articles for the *National Medical Association Journal,* I assumed that my credentials would be acceptable.

My plan was to complete the story in time to be published in 1979, incidental to the NMA's Detroit convention. The response from NMA was affirmative. Yet, when the manuscript was presented in early 1978, I discovered that my offer had not been taken seriously.

The manuscript remained filed for 15 years until Clarice Lackey, the widow of our illustrious former president of the Detroit Medical Society, Lawrence Lackey, M.D., asked me to write a eulogy to his memory. In the process, I re-read the original manuscript and decided to update and convert it into a Centennial Statement for the NMA. Although the NMA headquarters was notified of my plans, they were not asked to make any commitment to the success of the venture.

In an effort to learn if anyone else was writing the NMA

story, I attended the 1994 session in Orlando, Fla. and heard that someone, apparently not a physician, had been commissioned to write the "authorized" history of the NMA and that all pertinent records and files were to be placed at his disposal. If this person attended the Orlando convention, I was not aware of it.

The convention did provide an opportunity and space for me to mount a poster-display of my book that was visited by many delegates, including president-elect, Dr. Tracy M. Walton, Jr. (see photo). The announcement of my book, *The National Medical Association Demands Equal Opportunity: Nothing More, Nothing Less,* was widely distributed.

The Orlando trip was a disappointment. A "centennial" anniversary is an important event. It was my hope that several books would be in the hopper from many sections of the country, describing the many struggles in which the NMA's members have been engaged during its first century.

Quite sure that no one could write my story, unsure that anyone was writing any story, and absolutely certain that I could not settle for a history of the NMA written by just anybody, I returned home and hunkered down to give my public the benefit (you may choose another word if you like) of my 49 years as a member of the NMA.

Fortunately, I did not have to hunker down alone. When I explained the scope of this once-in-a-lifetime effort, many friends, acquaintances, even strangers wondered about my sanity, but few doubted my commitment. As a general rule, their response was "if you are willing to try it, I'll do what I can to help."

You will meet many of these trusting souls on the following pages. Some will be named in the sections of their involvement. Others may not be named, but will identify themselves as the events unfold, describing their involvement. I am sure that you will recognize the value of each player and how futile my puny efforts would have been without them.

A case in point is the chapter on "Detroit's Medical Progeny." One day, in an expansive mood, I considered including a brief biography of the children of each of Detroit's African American physicians. It soon became apparent that my colleagues had been more productive than even I, an obstetrician, had realized.

Pragmatism forced me to seek the desirable within the obtainable, and the pool of Medical Progeny was reduced with one or two exceptions to those physician's children who became physicians. This decision did not always seem fair to some colleagues whose children did not choose to follow in their wake; but, it did reduce the number to be studied to a more manageable 110.

It is hoped that this study will be repeated elsewhere, and expanded to other professions. The media may not, but should, welcome such difficult-to-find facts about a relatively unknown generation of African Americans.

The chapter on "Hospitals" required getting to know the founders, relatives and/or employees of Detroit's many African American Hospitals, during the 75 years (1918-1993) that the hospitals survived. Although some information may have fallen victim to time and circumstance, the residual riches of what may be this final harvest of history from the remaining founders is a testament to their determination to endure, despite the establishment's "handwriting on the wall" to the contrary.

The most difficult chapter to write, and the one that demanded a "hands-on" relationship with colleagues or their surviving relatives, was "Firsts." The decision on who was "First" became easier when it was defined, insofar as specialty is concerned, as "the first African American physician to be certified in a given specialty, position, etc."

Several questions were raised at this point: Need there be a separate category for men and women? Should the various subspecialties of surgery receive separate recognition? If so, why not medicine? It has not been, as should be apparent, an easy journey.

Having said all that, there remains a central core of constructive critics who read this manuscript and called it the way they saw it. They defended their criticisms with verve, as well as scholarship, for the benefit of us all.

The chairperson of the "Call-It-As-You-See-It" Committee is my wife, **Roberta**. A lawyer with a Ph.D., she is not the easiest person to sway in a contest of wills. Fortunately for me, most of our differences were settled at home and never came to public view.

Roberta's father, Robert I. Greenidge, M.D., was one of the most resourceful persons you will meet on this journey. She knew him well and provided me with a wealth of photographs, a paper trail nine yards long, and a lode of monuments to his memory.

One of these, for instance, was a copy of a birth certificate indicating that Dr. Greenidge had delivered a baby boy for the Charles Diggs family in December 1922, at Woman's Hospital. In the process of verifying this incredible event, I called my old friend, Dr. Frank Bicknell. He remembered Dr. C. Hollister Judd, the staff obstetrician at Woman's Hospital, who had allowed Dr. Greenidge surreptitious entry in the Woman's obstetrical unit to deliver a future congressman.

One thing led to another. While following the Greenidge spoor, I also learned that Dr. Bicknell, former chief of urology at Woman's Hospital, was trained in urology by Dr. Chester Ames, Receiving Hospital's first African American intern, resident, and faculty member. When Dr. Ames was denied a hospital appointment where he could practice his specialty, he abandoned urology and became Joe Louis' first fight physician, a fact verified by Freddie Guinyard, Louis' trainer.

You may begin to realize this has been an incredible journey that has demanded the critical evaluation of a host of trusted advisors that includes, but is not limited to:

1. **David Lawrence**-former publisher of the *Detroit Free Press*, who moved on to the *Miami Herald* where he and Michael Porter supplied unlimited information on the Cuban doctors' invasion of Florida in the 1960s.

2. **Julia Simmons**, of the Wayne State University Medical School, who, among many other things, dug up more than 50 years of medical student's records of that institution.

3. The search was aided and abetted by a visit and several

calls to the University of Michigan Medical School. Although the visits were fewer than to Wayne State Univ., the assistance of the team of **Drs. Linda Gillium** and **Ralph Gibson**, along with **Pam Cupitt, Marcella Rose** and others, helped to level the playing field.

When information was needed about Detroit's first African American medical family, the (Joseph) Fergusons, I turned to **Bert Osterberg**, of whom his wife, **Armaine**, is a descendant, and about whom Bert had already written quite a story.

When information was needed to explain why Robert I. Greenidge migrated from British Guiana (Guyana) to Battle Creek, rather than Detroit, I tapped one of my most reliable resources for Detroit's Museum of African American History and other ventures, **Nurse Ann Flanders**, a longtime resident of Battle Creek.

In this litigious society, one does well to check with a lawyer or two. Ready sources for such caution were **Attorneys William Johnson, Stanley Kirk, Harold Norris** and **William Price**.

It was **Hilanius Phillips**, a Detroit city planner, who first informed us that the old Dunbar Hospital building was to be torn down to expand the Cultural Center. The Detroit Medical Society began salvage operations which led to Dunbar's purchase, restoration and its recycling as a medical museum.

Research assistance was freely given at Shiffman's and Hutzel's medical libraries. Interloaning of data between the two institutions came in handy.

Upon being notified that Woman's Hospital was not eligible for Hill-Burton funds because they practiced racial discrimination, Senator Phil Hart (D-Mich.) initiated such a flurry of inquiries that Hutzel Hospital became integrated, almost overnight, "rather than lose our appropriation."

Gloria Rucker provided valuable information about her father, Dr. Albert W. Dumas, Sr., of Natchez, Miss., who was the NMA's president in 1940, the year the NMA officially severed its title from the dentists and pharmacists.

My former science teacher at Alabama State, **Prof. Henry**

L. Van Dyke, came to my rescue at a crucial time in early 1939. Since my mother had, without consulting me, already announced "Charles is going to be a doctor," I applied to Meharry Medical College during my senior year at Alabama State College. Since ASC's primary goal was to train teachers, the curriculum did not offer courses in such premedical subjects as biology, physiology, physical chemistry, etc.

Meharry's admissions committee took a long gamble on me. Noting that I had nearly all A's in the courses that were taken, I was advised to take summer courses in biology and physical chemistry. They promised to hold a slot for me in the 1939 freshman class, if I passed the final tests.

Prof. Van Dyke, whose laboratory assistant I had been for three years, readily agreed to teach the courses. Not only did I pass them, but I earned an "A" in physical chemistry during my freshman year at Meharry. Without the timely intervention of Prof. Van Dyke, my entire career would have been different. I have been, and will forever be grateful to Dr. Van Dyke and Alabama State's President, H. Council Trenholm.

Another equally significant development occurred in 1975 when my partner, **Dr. William Bentley**, entered into an agreement with **Dr. Tom Batchelor,** medical director of Comprehensive Health Services of Detroit (Detroit's first HMO) that Bentley, **Dr. N.S. Rangarajan** (third partner) and I would take over the Obg. service at CHSD, now The Apple Plan.

This has made many things possible for us that would not have been so, including the publication of this book.

Below is but an abbreviated list of the people I would like to acknowledge for their support of this publication through their informative assistance:

Drs. C. Arnold Curry; Tom Batchelor; James Collins; James Curtis; Gloria Edwards; Linda Gillum, Ph.D.; Herman B. Gray, Jr.; Joel Howell; Ed Littlejohn, attorney and Ph.D.; Wilburn Phillups; Charles Whitten; Delford Williams; Lamont Yeakey, Ph.D. contributed much.

Charles R. Alexander and Paula Bridges (editor) provided hours of time and patience. Photography consultants were John

Williams and Julius Watson. Special thanks to Charles Blockson, Temple University professor.

A word of appreciation is due to Sylvia Ross, D.D.S., who provided the photograph of the 30th NMA Convention in Chicago. Andre Lee returned to Detroit just in time to offer the photographs of Dr. Boyd, the NMA's first president (1895-96) and, what may be, Freedman Hospital's first ambulance (1894). Many such contributions made the job easier and more rewarding.

---

1. Woman's Hospital records reveal that Dr. Judd, a senior attending obstetrician, allowed at least two other African American physicians sporadic and episodic entry into the forbidden territory of Woman's delivery room. The other was Dr. George Bundy, who was originally a priest at St. Matthews Episcopal Church prior to graduating from Wayne Medical School in 1911.

   The record indicates that Dr. Greenidge's first delivery was in 1919 and Dr. Bundy's two were in 1917 and 1919. Dr. Frank Bicknell, a staff associate of Dr. Hollister, was not aware that such practices were going on.

Introduction

It is true, as stated in the Preface, that African American victimization by Europeans did not begin until Europeans went to Africa and seized indigenous Africans to replace those indigenous Native Americans who chose death rather than enslavement.

Native Americans were the first victims of the oppressive genocide that began with Christopher Columbus' invasion of the Caribbean in 1492, and spread to the mainland, thereafter. In October of that year, even before establishing a base in the new world, Columbus confided to his ship's log: "They [the indigenous people of the Caribbean Islands] would make fine servants.... with fifty men, we could subjugate them all and make them do whatever we want."[1] This was the first noted enunciation of white supremacy in the western hemisphere.

In February 1990, I visited Aquadillia, on the northwest coast of Puerto Rico, where Columbus made landfall in 1493, after his second transatlantic voyage. While researching the events of the previous 500 years, I asked some of the local people where were all the Trianos and Arawak Indian tribes who greeted Columbus in Puerto Rico in 1493?

One young man reminded me that they were carnivorous and "ate each other up." I responded with the observation that they all seemed to disappear *after* Columbus' arrival. What did he do to increase their appetite for each other?

They stopped smiling and became defensive. One of them dismissed me and turned to go, saying, "Aw, you know how those Spaniards were."

"Don't go away," I said, "wait and tell me about them." Perhaps they distrusted me because our conversation was in Spanish.

While there, I learned that Juan Ponce de Leon[2] accompanied Columbus on his second voyage to the new world in 1493 and became the first Governor of Puerto Rico in 1507. Following the mandates of white supremacy, he parceled out land and natives to the Europeans. The natives were forced to work in the mines and till the soil to prepare it for farming. The fort at Comparra, built to enforce enslavement of the natives, became the first slave camp in this hemisphere.[3]

The myth of white supremacy was enhanced by the fact that only the natives died from European diseases because they had no immunity. When European corpses were seen after the native uprising, the mystique of the white skin was diminished.

The overworked natives rebelled. The Spanish army was required to quell the 5,000 natives—500 of whom were women. After subjugation, they were forced to work even harder than before. The brutal Ponce de Leon was deposed in 1511. He went northward, searching for the "Fountain of Youth." Instead, he discovered Florida and Seminole Indians, whom he proceeded to drive into the Everglades.

Successive generations of Europeans kept the Seminoles confined there for nearly three centuries. On June 30, 1834, the Bureau of Indian Affairs was established by an act of congress. Four months later, the Bureau ordered the Seminoles and other Native American tribes to evacuate their traditional homelands. The land was confiscated by the U.S. government to accommodate the rapidly expanding European invasion of the new world. The Native Americans were forced to march through wild, unaccommodating country west of the Mississippi River.

Since the evacuation order was issued by General Winfield Scott, under the terms of the fraudulent 1832 Treaty of New Eschota, Seminole Chief Osceola refused to obey it, choosing to fight instead. Unable to conquer the Seminoles in battle, Gen. Scott offered to negotiate and captured Osceola while "negotiating" under a flag of truce. Osceola died while imprisoned on January 30, 1838. His troops continued the struggle although there are no reports of them having been defeated by the U.S. Army.

The fighting continued, however, for four more years until 1842 costing the U.S. 1,500 dead soldiers and an expenditure of $20 million. No one bothered to estimate the price paid by the Seminoles.[4]

It was against the Seminoles that U.S. Army Captain Gabriel J. Raines began to experiment with land mines, a weapon causing major mutilation of the innocent (evidenced most recently with Dr. Jonas Savimbi in Angola, amidst the continuing U.S. support of South Africa.)[5]

The painful expression "Trail of TearsTrail of Tears," dates back to that final, forceful act in December 1838. Seven thousand U.S. soldiers, led by the same Gen. Scott, evicted the last 14,000 Cherokees, Choctaws and other "stubborn red skins" from their 7 million acres of traditional homeland in Georgia and southeastern Tennessee. The land was seized by the U.S. Government and distributed to European Americans.

The evictees were forced to march hundreds of miles to Oklahoma where they were interned under the most primitive conditions imaginable. Enroute, conservative estimates of the death toll exceed 10% and nearly 1,000 escaped. Those who survived the trip did not fare much better.[6]

Native and African Americans have not been the only victims of America's racist, expansionist foreign policy. The first of our southern neighbors to get the boot was Mexico. That experience provides a shameful example of what happens to our neighbors when they attempt to resist the U.S.

Agitation to form the Republic of Texas out of Mexican territory was instigated by the U.S. in the late 1830s. While the Native Americans were being driven westward, African Americans were seeking refuge via the Underground Railroad in the North and eventually Canada.

Texas' sovereignty, as a republic, was soon recognized by the U.S. and friendly governments in Great Britain, Holland and Belgium. On August 23, 1843, Mexican President Antonio Lopez de Sante Anna, hero of The Battle of the Alamo, became suspicious of U.S. intentions and warned the U.S. that any attempt to annex their territory would be considered an "act of war" against the Mexican government.

Ignoring this threat from a "weak" neighbor, the Texas Annexation Treaty was signed by the U.S. and by the Republic

Texas as a territory without the consent of Mexico was voiced by former President Martin VanBuren and Henry Clay of Kentucky. Both men had presidential ambitions and wanted to eliminate Texas as an election issue.

However, on June 8, 1844, the Texas Annexation Treaty failed to win the necessary 2/3 vote for passage in the senate. On March 6, 1845, the annexation of Texas was protested by the Mexican minister and diplomatic relations with Texas were severed three weeks later.

The Bear Flag Revolt was instigated in the San Francisco Bay area when settlers seized the town of Samona and proclaimed it the Republic of California. On June 15, 1845, the U.S. agreed to protect Texas if it would agree to annexation. On November 10, Rep. John Siddell (D-La.) was sent to Mexico by President James K. Polk, as minister plenipotentiary, to restore peaceful relations between the two countries.

Once there, he was denied an audience by the Mexican president. The U.S. had offered $5 million for the purchase of New Mexico and $25 million for California. Both offers were refused. Following a rumor that U.S. forces had been attacked by Mexican forces on April 24, President Polk asked for and was permitted to declare war on Mexico in 1845. Texas was then admitted to the Union as the 28th state on December 29, 1845.

Under the terms of the Texas and New Mexico Act of 1850, Texas' boundaries were established, and a $10 million payment to Texas was authorized for relinquishing its claim to territories beyond the the new state lines. The boundaries of New Mexico were also established.[7]

As a concession to the South, New Mexico would be admitted as a slave or free state according to its constitution upon admission to the Union. This option was part of the Compromise of the Amendment of the Fugitive Slave Law of 1850. The enslaved did not share in the exercise of this option.

The foregoing disclosure is but one narrow segment of the United States' relationship with Mexico, one of its closest neighbors. Even this casual review of the number of acts committed against our neighbors in this hemisphere, and in the Pacific Rim after the Spanish-American War, is mind-boggling.

When the European Americans accepted that Native Americans could not profitably be enslaved, the international African slave trade became an attractive, as well as lucrative, alternative for European capitalists and hastened the outbreak of the Civil War.

Scientific "Proof" of Racial Inferiority

Many European enslavers, trying to find psychological comfort in the buying and selling of human flesh, sought vindication for slavocracy by attempting to prove that African Americans, like the Native Americans, were an inferior breed on the evolutionary scale.

Governor George McDuffie of South Carolina was an outspoken proponent of the "scientific proof of white supremacy." He declared, "slavery is the cornerstone of our Republican edifice."[8]

It was Supreme Court Justice Roger B. Taney's testimony during the Dred Scott trial that told his eager listeners what they wanted to hear:

"The words 'people of the United States' and 'citizens' are synonymous terms and mean the same thing. They both describe the political body which, according to our republican institutions, form the sovereignty and who hold the power and conduct the government through their representatives. They are what we familiarly call the 'sovereign people' and every citizen is one of these people and a constituent member of this sovereignty.

"The question before us is whether that class of persons (the enslaved) described in this abatement compose a portion of this sovereignty. We think they are not, and that they are not included, and were not intended to be included under the word 'citizens' in the Constitution and therefore can claim none of the rights which that instrument provides for and secures to citizens of the United States."

On the contrary, at that time African Americans were considered as a subordinate and inferior class of beings who had been subjugated by the dominant race and "whether emancipated or not, they remain subject to that authority. They have and had no rights nor privileges but such as those who held the power and the Government might choose to grant them."[9]

Some of the most vicious attacks on the humanity of African Americans were delivered by physicians of the 19th century whose prestige and authority went unquestioned by their followers.

The slave owner who spent ten years proving, to the satisfaction of the U.S. Supreme Court, that Dred Scott was not a human being was Dr. John Emerson, an eminent army surgeon.

Dr. Samuel G. Morton of Philadelphia, a teacher of anatomy, was already known for his insights on the germ theory. His works were considered "gospel" in the Southern states. When he died in 1851, the *Charleston Medical Journal* mourned his passing with: "We can only say that we, of the South, should consider him as our benefactor, for aiding most materially, in giving to the Negro his true position as an inferior race."[10]

Dr. Morton, Dr. Charles Caldwell, and their student, Dr. Josiah Nott, became three of the best-known and most often-quoted physician propagandists for the polygenist theory of their time. They declared that African Americans represented a subhuman form of development and therefore, were inferior to the white race.

Dr. Nott was well sought after as a lecturer. In 1854, he joined forces with George R. Glidden, a British adventurer and opportunist, to publish *Types of Mankind*. The publication was designed to present all the anthropological evidence that had been brought forward to support diversity of the races. The publication was one of the most popular of the period, with ten editions in print by the end of the 19th century.[11]

Having served as U.S. vice consul in Egypt, Glidden supplied Morton with human skulls he had collected in his spare time to provide measurements. Glidden made a fortune lecturing on Egyptology, during which he subscribed to the belief that the African

American, with such low cranial capacity, could never have produced the type of civilization that developed in Egypt.[12]

It should be noted that the racial attitudes expressed thus far were not the ranting of a threatened segment of society who were worried about their place at the master's table. No! These are the convictions of European and European American intelligencia who are still seeking, after more than 100 years, or 500 for that matter, to prove that the clock began ticking with Columbus.[13, 14, 15]

In view of these and many other similar conditions that prevailed at the time the American Medical Association (AMA) was established, it is understandable how a group of physicians representing the most learned men of the period, could and did convene a founding session of the AMA in 1847 and created without significant dissent, a medical organization which has continued to deny equal opportunity to qualified African American physicians for nearly 150 years.

It tells us not only how committed the founders were to the policies and practices of white supremacy then, but how much they still are. This narrative will disclose some of the racial prejudices within the medical establishment that are still with us. These prejudices must be eliminated if equal opportunity is to be shared by all.

By allowing its affiliates, county and state, to decide who could join the parent body, the AMA sought to avoid any involvement with racial matters then and in the future. From the outset, it was clear that the founders of AMA did not consider African Americans as potential members.

Dr. Lester B. King, author of *American Medicine Comes of Age 1840-1960,* reminded us, "Many opportunities were available to provide sound, preliminary training for the study of medicine. The medical degree exerted a strong attraction for prestige and an income higher than any other line of endeavor."

This was not true for African Americans. They were denied entry into all Southern university medical schools prior to 1948, and restricted by a quota in all of the other medical schools, except Howard and Meharry; Morehouse and Drew medical schools were opened more recently.

The American Association of Medical Colleges (AAMC) played a key role in establishing the four-year curriculum which met the requirements for adequate medical training. AMA President Dr. Frank Billings told his 1903 inaugural audience, "The status of medical college education is very much improved in the last 20 years, more than in all preceding time."

Dr. Billings was not addressing the status of medical education for African Americans. Within those 20 years that were included in his remarks, several medical schools were established by African American doctors in an attempt to improve their opportunities to obtain a medical education. Three years after Dr. Billings' address, the AMA hired Abraham Flexner to investigate these schools. Consequently, they were all closed. (See "The Medical Gospel According to Abraham").

In 1906, the AMA's Council on Medical Education advised that the nurturing benefit of hospital affiliation was essential for medical training. Internships became mandatory, thereafter, for all physicians except African Americans. The first and second African American interns in Detroit were appointed in 1926 and 1943, 20 and 37 years later, respectively.

Proposals have been made on several occasions that the AMA change its constitution and allow direct memberships; the centenary celebration in 1947 was one such occasion. Twenty-four years later, the AMA's House of Delegates finally agreed to consider making such a change. I could find no evidence of the passage of any enabling legislation to such an end, nor tangible results therefrom.

It seems apparent that the survival of a medical establishment that can, and will, serve the best interests of all the people will require more fundamental changes than the words on a written document.

Today, we, the members of the NMA, are on the threshold of our second century of service to our fellow men and women. This is the moment for critical decisions. Do we continue seeking alms from those who are only capable of criticism and contempt? Or do we see ourselves, as Dr. James McCune Smith did 150 years ago, as victors rather than victims? Take heed of his advice below and not only read it now, but daily, until it forces you to action.

James McCune Smith, M.D. (Univ. of Glasgow), said, "The time has come when our people must assume the rank of a first-rate power in the battle against caste and slavery. It is, emphatically, our battle. No one can fight it for us, and with God's help, we must fight it ourselves."

1. *Native American Rights Fund* (Boulder, Colo., 1992).

2. Richard N. Current, Alexander DeConde, and Harris L. Dante, *United States History.* (Cott Foresman and Co., 1967) p. 25.

3. Charles H. Wright, M.D., "Was Columbus an Explorer or an Invader?" Lecture at Midwest Labor Institute for Social Studies (Detroit: October 20, 1992).

4. Gorton Garutte, *The Encyclopedia of American Facts and Dates*, 8th Ed. (New York: Harper and Row, 1817) p. 190.

5. Garutte, p. 196.

6. Ibid.

7. Garutte., p. 200-203.

8. Dwight Lowell Dumond, *Antislavery*. (Univ. of Mich. Press, 1961) p. 288.

9. Leon Higginbotham, Jr., *In the Matter of Color Race and the American Legal Process*. (New York: Oxford University Press, 1978) p. 5.

10. Audrey Smedley, *Race in North America*. (Boulder: West View Press, 1993) p. 236.

11. Ibid.

12. Smedley, p. 238.

13. *Facts and Dates,* (December 1839) p. 208. "In the end 7,000 U.S. soldiers seized 7,000,000 acres of Cherokee land and distributed it to the European American settlers."

14. *Facts and Dates,* (June 30, 1834) p. 198. The resulting cost to the U.S. to quell the Seminole resistance against the U.S. conquest was *1,500 dead and $20 million. The cost to the Seminole nation was not given.*

15. *Facts and Dates,* (January, 1845) p. 224. Exploration and settlement: wars. The annexation of Texas finally became a reality after long, political bickering. Anti-slavery forces were opposed to annexation because Texas was certain to become a slave state. Others wanted to act lest Great Britain or France developed a relationship with the Republic of Texas, whose independence from Mexico, from whom it was seized, went unrecognized. In April 1844, although preoccupied with enslavement and rebellious Native Americans, President John Tyler found time to submit to the senate a treaty of annexation. But it was rejected in June.

In December, President Tyler offered a joint resolution to cover annexation that required a simple majority for ratification, instead of the previously agreed 2/3, much to the displeasure of the Mexican majority still living in Texas. This altered Annexation Treaty was completed and accepted by the U.S. Congress on February 28, 1845 and by the Congress of Texas, five months later, on June 23rd. Mexico, like many of her neighbors before and especially since, never forgave nor forgot.

Michigan Medical Trailblazers of the 19th Century

The following text highlights four of Michigan's African American, medical trailblazers of the 19th century: Joseph Ferguson, Robert Boland, Henry Fitzbutler and Sophia Jones. Two were early graduates of the Detroit medical schools. The other two graduated from the University of Michigan and were born in the same country, Canada.

Although all of them struggled to earn their degrees in the new field of medicine, they were saddled with the added problems of race and in one case, sex. Despite incredible handicaps, each of them went on to enjoy relatively successful careers in medicine and to fight for first-class privileges as U.S. citizens.

While this presentation is limited to partial reports of only four of the trailblazers, their stories represent thousands of their African American colleagues who have followed in their wake and gained from their experiences. At the same time, they are sufficiently varied to provide some appreciation of the difficulties they overcame in their early quests for equality of medical opportunity in a most hostile society.

We must also remember that many of the early antagonists of the African American physicians were the European politicians, professionals, and other intellectuals of that period. Their attitudes and actions legitimized, and later supported, such organizations as the Ku Klux Klan, which did not spring up, root and vine, until the end of the Civil War in 1866.[1]

Joseph Ferguson, M.D. (1822-1877)

Dr. Joseph Ferguson was reputed to be Detroit's, and most likely Michigan's, first African American physician. He began his medical career as a "free Negro" barber in Richmond, Va. Like many other barbers, he had become quite skilled in leeching and cupping, an accepted practice of treating patients by scarifying and bleeding them to relieve their inflammations and swellings.

In an effort to abandon such primitive techniques and become more scientific in his medical practice, Ferguson took his wife and two children, Laura and John, north to Pittsburgh where he served as an apprentice to Dr. George McCook, a European American physician.

During his six years in Pittsburgh, Ferguson's wife died and he re-married Martha Ann Webb, the daughter of William and Agnes Webb. Martha, Joseph and their three children, William, Charles and Florence moved to Cleveland, Ohio, in 1855, where the doctor furthered his medical studies at the Cleveland Medical College for one year and continued his practice in the surrounding community.

In 1857, the Fergusons, and Martha's family, the Webbs, moved to Detroit, which was one of the largest towns in the midwest. Although the Continental Congress by its Ordinance of 1787 forbade slavery in the Northwest Territory, enslavement of Native and African Americans was still prevalent among the British and French settlers.

Under a treaty arrangement with their respective governments these settlers were allowed to keep their enslaved people under the jurisdiction of the U.S. Likewise, some African Americans were held in bondage by European Americans despite the law.[2]

But despite the Ordinance of the Continental Congress and the 1834 admission of Michigan to the Union as a free state, Detroit was under the control of a Democratic, pro-slavery administration with a hostile media calling most of the shots, especially the *Detroit Free Press.*

Despite an undertow of racial hostility, the Fergusons and the Webbs settled in the eastern part of downtown Detroit, a region that was already being treated as a "black ghetto." They began family lineages that have written much of the history of Detroit since that time.

Webb established and operated a grocery store in his home at 185 East Congress Street. Nearby, Dr. Ferguson had resumed his medical practice, still, without a medical degree or license.

The absence of a medical degree and license was not unusual at that time. The AMA, founded in 1847, was still so preoccupied with establishing its own infrastructure that it had not taken time to lay the foundations for a national organization as it exists today. Such developments as the selection of educational curriculum, the licensing of practitioners after graduation, and the standardization of medical care were all in their infancy and left much to be desired.

Although the nation was already rushing headlong toward a civil war, open hostilities did not begin until 1861, four years later. It was during this period that the Ferguson and Webb families became aligned with other members of Detroit's African American community to unite their meager resources for an all-out fight for equality of opportunity that would continue for the rest of their lives.[3]

Both Webb and Ferguson became actively involved in the African American's struggles for freedom and justice, especially in the operation of the Underground Railroad. The cruel 1850 Amendment of the original Fugitive Slave Act of 1793, and Detroit's proximity to Canada separated by the Detroit river, made it a vital staging area for enslaved fugitives' desperate dash across the river to freedom's "Canaan Land."

The unlimited authority given to the enslavers by the 1850 Amendment of the fugitive slave law, and its threat of fines and imprisonment to the Underground Railroad's station masters, made their work more dangerous than ever. But they never faltered at their tasks.

A bitter and typical protest against the amendment was delivered by Dr. Martin R. Delaney, once described by W.E.B. Dubois as "the most distinguished Northern Negro in South Carolina," Delaney stated:

"Honorable Mayor, whatever ideas of liberty I may have, have been received from reading the lives of your revolutionary fathers. I have, therein, learned that a man has a right to defend his castle with his life, even to the taking of a life. Sir, my house is my castle; in that castle are none but my wife and my children, as free as the angels in heaven and whose liberty is as sacred as the pillars of God.

"If any man approaches that house in search of a slave—I care not who he may be, whether constable or sheriff, magistrate or even judge of the Supreme Court—Nay, let it be he who sanctioned this act to become law [President Milliard Fillmore], surrounded by his cabinet as his body guard, with the Declaration [of Independence] waving about his head as his banner and the constitution of his country on his breast as his shield—if he crosses the threshold of my door, and I do not lay him a lifeless corpse at my feet, I hope the grave may refuse my body a resting place, and righteous Heaven my spirit a home. Oh, no, he cannot enter that house and we both live!"

These brave and fearless African American citizens were responsible for hiding and protecting the frightened, destitute and bewildered victims of slavery until it was safe to smuggle them across the river to Canada, usually under the cover of darkness. The 1850 Fugitive Slave Act made any effort to assist the enslaved a punishable, criminal offense. These "station masters" were not seriously intimidated by the threat of police and klan action. [4]

Some of the best remembered station masters were Rev. William Monroe, founder of Second Baptist and St. Matthews Episcopal Churches; John D. Richards; William Wilson; Joseph Ferguson and John deBaptiste. They attended a secret meeting at Webb's home with abolitionist Frederick Douglass and John Brown, the European-American and anti-slavery zealot on March 12, 1859. [5]

Douglass, one the greatest orators of that period, had been invited to come to Detroit to deliver another passionate plea for the end of enslavement. Brown's mission was to deliver a group of 14 "contraband" persons from Kansas to "Caananland," across the Detroit River. After the "merchandise" was delivered, he made his way to the Webb home.

Although the true agenda for this illegal gathering was never divulged, the *Detroit Free Press* speculated, for nearly a full page, that Brown's other mission was to recruit volunteers, especially

Douglass, for his ill-fated raid on the Harpers Ferry (Va.) arsenal seven months later.

None of the African Americans who attended that Douglass/Brown meeting participated in the raid. Yet when the raid failed and Brown and his men were captured and hung, many of Detroit's attendees went "underground" or like Douglass, left the country. Douglass, more vulnerable than his Detroit colleagues, met Brown later in a Chambersburg, Va. quarry in August, just two months before the raid.

When the federal government disclosed that some of Douglass' papers were found among Brown's confiscated effects, Douglass decided that England was a safer site from which to monitor the post-raid events back home. Dr. Ferguson, unfazed by these developments, continued his medical practice in Detroit.

Although Dr. Ferguson was not an active participant in the Civil War, he continued to provide community leadership and health care to African Americans throughout the period and beyond. It was in 1863, for instance, that an African American named William Faulkner was falsely accused of attacking two nine year-old girls, one black and the other white. Despite the lack of supporting evidence, Faulkner was brought to trial.

Tension reached such a peak that, as it was later proved, a guard fired into a white mob that threatened Faulkner. White artist Charles Lander was killed and Faulkner became the scapegoat for Lander's death. Detroit's first race riot ensued, venting years of pent-up racial hostility.

Before order was restored, fires had destroyed 35 buildings owned by African Americans. There were scores of injuries and wide-spread homelessness in the African American neighborhoods. As in Detroit's later riots, the militia came from Fort Wayne to restore order.

Dr. Ferguson entered the riot-torn area to administer aid and help find shelter for the homeless. Despite threats of harm and danger, he continued his ministry to the injured until the danger was over. The jury found Faulkner guilty and he served seven years in Michigan's Jackson Prison before the girls confessed that they had made the entire story up to avoid punishment for coming home late.[6]

Not very long after the riot, Dr. Theodore McGraw, a surgeon in the Union Army, headed a team which organized the Detroit College of Medicine (DCM) in 1868. Following a reorganization of the school in 1885, Dr. McGraw became its president and served until his retirement in 1915.[7]

Ferguson applied, and was admitted, to the first class of DCM. For many years, he had sought the opportunity to attend a proper medical school, earn an M.D. degree, and legitimize his title. He was the *only* African American in a class of thirty males in 1868.[8]

At first the medical school was located in a group of temporary buildings that later became Harper Hospital. After a temporary move to the old YMCA building on Farmer Street, the medical school occupied its own building in 1932 on St. Antoine, adjacent to St. Mary's Hospital. During the mid-1960s, expansion of the Medical Center moved the Medical School northward to Canfield at Brush, to join other medical institutions that, now, make up the Medical Center.

The pursuit of a medical degree did not interfere with Dr. Ferguson's fight against racism in society and in the public school system in particular. As a student in 1868, he joined a community petition drive to integrate Detroit's public schools which were already legislated under the authority of the Civil Rights Act of 1866.

Following its passage, the first of several such post-Civil War measures, the Michigan Legislature amended the primary school law to provide, "That all students, of any district, should have an equal right to attend any school in that district." The Detroit School Board demurred and claimed a special exemption. They ignored the mandate and continued their pre-war policy of racial segregation.

The issue was renewed in April 1868, when Joseph Workman's child was denied admission to the all-white Duffield School because he was black. The Michigan legislators demanded that the City show cause why Workman's child should be denied the right to attend the public school.

The school board's attorneys claimed that not only was it well within the school's jurisdiction to maintain school segregation, but the regulation was reasonable "for the good government and prosperity of the free schools."

Their position was further supported by adding: "Among a large majority of Detroit's white population, a strong prejudice or animosity exists against colored people, which is largely transmitted to the children within the school. This feeling would engender quarrels and contention if colored children were admitted to white schools."[9]

Opposition from Workman's counsel and a community petition drive led Chief Justice Tom Cooley to rule: "The general law is complementary to the special legislation and is necessary to give it complete operation. The conclusion is inevitable that the legislature designed the impartial rule and they established it to be of universal application."

This decision forced the admission of the first African American students to Detroit's public schools on October 11, 1869. William W. Ferguson, Dr. Ferguson's second son, was the first African American male student to enter Detroit's integrated classrooms.

Although passage of the Fifteenth Amendment in 1870 promised freed men the vote with hope that they could help make the promise of racial integration a reality, it never happened. Through the use of grandfather clauses, literacy tests, white primaries, poll taxes, and other racist ruses, the Fifteenth Amendment was defanged for 95 years. The Selma-Montgomery March forced the U.S. government to pass the Voting Rights Act of 1965 which restored teeth to the 15th Amendment.

Following President Andrew Johnson's withdrawal of Union troops from the South in 1877, all seven of the prior Civil Rights Acts were promptly declared unconstitutional by the pro-segregationist U.S. Supreme Court. The Republican effort at Reconstruction was declared a dismal failure, and civil rights for African Americans were put on hold for the next 80 years. All subsequent civil rights legislation suffered defeat until 1957.

In 1880, Frederick Douglass laid Reconstruction to rest with the following obituary:

"Our Reconstruction measures were radically defective... To the freedmen was given machinery of liberty, but they were denied the freedom to put them into motion. They were given the uniform of soldiers, but no arms; they were called citizens, but left subjects; they were called free, but left almost slaves. The old master class... retained the power to starve them to death, and wherever this power is held, there is the power of slavery."[10]

It wasn't until 1954 when the U.S. Supreme Court in *Brown v. Board of Educ.* reversed its own "separate but equal" *Plessy v. Ferguson* decision that a new awareness and a new search for identity on the part of African Americans became manifest.

The drive toward independence by many African countries and the need to demonstrate the validity of democracy to meet the rising challenges of international communism were some of the imperatives that led the U.S. Congress to pass, and President Eisenhower to sign, the first Civil Rights Act to be adopted in 82 years on September 9, 1957.

Although feeble in its initial steps, the eventual broad sweep of the civil rights movement propelled thousands of civil rights activists, many of them physicians, to protest in the streets. Many were arrested; but they finally did force some improvement in this biased medical establishment.

The foregoing report fails to do justice to Dr. Ferguson's tireless and courageous efforts to bring justice and freedom to his African American brothers and sisters during his entire lifetime. He did set a fine example, however, for the thousands who followed in his wake.

One example that comes to mind was Dr. Ferguson's implementation of the Civil Rights Act of 1866. It was the opening battle of the same war that Dr. Remus Robinson, another African American physician, waged against the same evil, racial segregation in Detroit's public schools, one hundred years later.

Dr. Ferguson was active in the Bethel A.M.E. Church, as well as other community endeavors. Following his death at the age of 55, a grateful community overflowed Bethel to pay their last respects to a true leader. His burial in the Elmwood cemetery (Lot 25, Section P), was noted in three newspapers:

"Physician, community leader and abolitionist. One of Michigan's first black doctors. He was a practicing, licensed physician as a freed man in Richmond, Virginia, before coming to Detroit.

Dr. Ferguson, Michigan's earliest African American medical trailblazer, set high standards of courage, commitment and scholarship for hundreds, even thousands, of physicians since that time. While this narrative does not permit adequate time and space to deal with all of them, it is hoped that this feeble effort will spur others to step forward, briskly, to continue, if not complete, this unfinished symphony of service and sacrifice in the unending search for Freedom and Justice, wherever they are to be found.

Robert J. Boland, M.D. 1850-1918

The fact that Robert J. Boland was the illegitimate son of an enslaved, teen-aged mother and her owner's son, propels some historians to excuse such predatory behavior among enslavers as a benefit bestowed on the slaves. Undue emphasis was placed on the issue of Robert being mulatto as a probable explanation for his rise to prominence.

Robert was born in 1850, the year the Fugitive Slave Law was more rigidly amended to satisfy the critics of the earlier version's "laxity."[11] This restrictive measure, making the fugitive subject to recapture and re-enslavement anywhere in the U.S., was a testament to the ingenuity of the abolitionists and the courage of the escapees.

Robert was 13 years-old when the pro-slavery segregationists of the Confederacy refused to be intimidated by President Lincoln's threat to issue an Emancipation Proclamation to free the slaves, if the enslavers did not comply voluntarily.

They ignored the President's threat, forcing him to issue the Emancipation Proclamation on January 1, 1863 which finally gave purpose to the Civil War. Unable to wait for the 13th

Amendment to legitimize his freedom, Robert escaped from his grandfather's La Grange, Ga, plantation and fled to Atlanta in 1865.

During his three-year pause in Atlanta, his thirst for knowledge was quenched by employment at the American Missionary Association. Later, he became the janitor at the Storr School for Colored Children. Robert's next move northward was to Detroit where he found employment at the Russell House, a popular downtown hotel. While in Atlanta, Robert had shown evidence of being a bright and aggressive student, anxious to acquire an education.

He enrolled in Detroit's Bishop and Barstow schools to complete his elementary training at age 26. He continued his education at Capital High School, located on Griswold in downtown Detroit.

During this period, he lived and worked as a waiter at the William Downey Ice Cream and Oyster House on Woodward and Adams. Later, he got a room nearby on Monroe Street.

Robert joined the Bethel A.M.E. church, then located downtown on Lafayette and was asked to serve as superintendent of the Sunday School. Dr. Ferguson's family, one of Detroit's most respected, also worshipped there.

It is most likely that contact with Dr. Ferguson and his son, John Cyrus, who followed his father into medicine, was an early incentive for Robert to consider medicine as a profession. A two-year apprenticeship with Dr. Pratt, a white physician, increased Boland's eligibility and confirmed his decision to study medicine.

At that time, Detroit had two medical schools. The older, Detroit College of Med. (DCM) and the Michigan College of Medicine (MCM), a rival institution located on St. Antoine which was incorporated in 1879. The MCM's two-year curriculum offered the same classes as the DCM. The MCM group did not, however, have access to the area hospitals, so they converted the second floor of their medical school into a hospital.

Dr. Boland graduated in 1883, the only African American in a class of 28. With no internship available to him, he opened an office in his home on the corner of Brady and Hastings, an area not so sharply segregated as the more southeasterly downtown region.

Dr. Boland never quite became a permanent fixture in the professional society of Detroit. When he left Detroit is uncertain, but records of the period indicate that sometime in 1886, Dr. Boland married Perdita Golden and secured a medical license to practice in Virginia. He continued his practice for 27 years and died on November 16, 1918, at the age of 68. His death was mourned by his third wife, Kate Taliafero, a music teacher in Roanoke, Va., and three sons, Charles, Robert H. and Jesse L.

Detroit's African American connection with the MCM was through Dr. Boland. Insofar as I was able to determine, no other African American attended MCM. Its rivalry with the Detroit College of Med. was brief and of no lasting consequence.

The other two medical trailblazers, chosen to represent the African American medical community in the 19th century, were both Canadians and alumni of the older Univ. of Mich. Medical School.

Henry Fitzbutler, M.D. (1842-1901)

Henry Fitzbutler was the first African American to receive an M.D. degree from the Univ. of Mich. in 1872. He had attended DCM the year before, but transferred to Ann Arbor for his final year.

His father was William Henry Butler, an escaped, enslaved coachman, who fled to Canada and became a farmer. His mother had been an English immigrant of the indentured servant class. Originally named after his father, William Henry, Jr. dropped his first name and added "Fitz" to his last name.

Widespread hostility, aroused by his parents' interracial marriage, forced the Butlers to flee to Amherstburg, Canada, before their son was born. After completing his secondary school work in Amherstburg, Henry registered for a medical preparatory course at Michigan's Adrian College in 1864.

In 1866, Henry returned to Canada and married Sarah McCurdy, the daughter of a prosperous Canadian farmer. She became his life-long companion and helpmate and, eventually, a fellow physician.

After completing his preparatory training at Adrian, Henry began studying medicine at DCM in 1871. Although some journals reported that he was DMC's first African American medical student, the record will show that Joseph Ferguson was indeed enrolled in DMC's first class in 1868.

One of the earliest medical influences on this young African Canadian was exerted by Daniel Pearson, another African Canadian. Although he had neither a medical degree nor a medical license, Pearson did treat some illnesses. He encouraged young Henry to become a doctor and gave him free access to his 900-book, private library.

A second source of inspiration was Dr. William C. Lundy, a young, European Canadian physician who had graduated in 1867 from Victoria University in Toronto. Since the medical school would not accept the name of an unlicensed doctor as his mentor, Dr. Lundy's name, alone, appears on Dr. Fitzbutler's medical file as his mentor.

During his first year at the DCM, Fitzbutler studied chemistry and toxicology; anatomy; materia medica and therapeutics; physiology and microscopy; gynecology; principles and practices of medicine; and surgery.

In the fall of 1871, he transferred to the Univ. of Mich. Med. School and graduated in 1872, becoming the university's first African American medical school graduate and the state of Michigan's second.

After graduation, Dr. Fitzbutler and his wife settled in Louisville, Ky., becoming the first African American physician in the state. From a pamphlet that published sketches of "colored men in Kentucky," I learned that Dr. Fitzbutler caused considerable anxiety in both communities by ignoring the established order of doing things and failing to pay proper homage to the primacy of white supremacy.

He also had the annoying habit of ignoring Louisville's "colored intermediators" and doing things his own way. He organized, for instance, African American groups that discussed methods of improving the education of their children. These "colored intermediators" predicted that Dr. Fitzbutler had a short fuse and waited for his implosion. He outlasted many of them.

Early in his medical career, Dr. Fitzbutler began publishing *The Planet* and *The Ohio Falls Express* which served as "fearless advocates of equal rights" and were devoted to the educational interests of colored people.

Among the many things that worried Dr. Fitzbutler was the racially-induced shortage of African American physicians being trained in the U.S., despite the vast medical needs of the African American communities nationwide.

The only medical schools to which African Americans had easy access were Meharry Medical College in Nashville, Tenn. and Howard University, in Washington, D.C. Dr. Fitzbutler established the Louisville National Medical College (LNMC) in 1888 and was named dean.

Since Kentucky's lone medical school did not accept African Americans, Dr. Fitzbutler made it clear that LNMC was "established to aid Meharry Medical College and Howard University in training Negro doctors." With the approval, endorsement, and financial support of Kentucky's state legislature, including the Governor, LNMC was able to open the doors of its rented hall to six students.[12]

So grateful were the members of Kentucky's Medical Licensing Board, that LNMC's alumni were encouraged to set up practices in the state and serve the dire needs of the African American communities until the school was forced to close in 1912, after the Flexner Commission's Report was released.

Initially, with the help of a grateful public, LNMC acquired its own building, and later, a hospital that was maintained chiefly with Dr. Fitzbutler's own funds. Over the 24-year life of the college, the number of faculty members fluctuated from 12 to 43. Enrollment averaged 30 students per year and an average of six graduating annually.

The faculty members used their own private practices and public clinics to provide clinical material for teaching; hospital experiences were episodic and left much to be desired. There was no evidence of any contact between LNMC and Kentucky's one, regular medical school.

Although Sarah, Dr. Fitzbutler's wife, was the mother of six children, she graduated from LNMC in 1892, nine years before her husband's death in 1901. After his death, she, and close associate Dr. W.A. Burney, took over the management and maintenance of the medical school. One of Fitzbutler's daughters also graduated from LNMC

Sarah devoted much of her time toward establishing a nursing school in an effort to improve the woefully pitiful supply of African American nurses available to various hospitals and clinics throughout the state.

During LNMC's 24 years of operation, 75 physicians received their medical degrees and provided much-needed medical care to African American communities that had none previously. The racial impediments that Dr. Fitzbutler faced in 1888 worsened with the U.S. Supreme Court's passage of the *Plessy v. Ferguson.* Nine years later, life was made even more difficult for African Americans by the racists within his own state government.

In 1906, the Kentucky legislature successfully challenged the authority of the U.S. Supreme Court to enforce the "equal" part of the "separate but equal " clause of the *Plessy v. Ferguson* decision.[13]

When the Supreme Court capitulated to Kentucky, the segregationists were in full control until the Supreme Court reasserted its authority 48 years later in *Brown v. Board of Educ.*, on May 17, 1954.[14]

The LNMC was closed in 1912, two years after the Flexner Report was issued in 1910. At that time, Kentucky's only other medical school still did not accept African American medical students.

A second medical school was not opened in Kentucky until 1960. One African American medical student was accepted, Carl Webber Watson of Lexington.[15] He went on to become certified in obg. and is now practicing in Berkeley, Calif.

Sophia Bethena Jones, M.D. (1857-1932)

Sophia Bethena Jones, M.D., not only attended the same medical school as did Fitzbutler, but they were also both born in

Canada. John Hope Franklin often referred to the frequency of Canadians becoming U.S. physicians.[16]

Upon graduating in 1885, she launched a 47-year career that was almost entirely devoted to the practice of a then unknown specialty of medicine, Public Health.

Atlanta Georgia's Spelman College was the first, post-graduate stop on her nation-wide journeys to teach the recently freed victims of enslavement the principles of hygiene and preventative medicine. By 1887, she had established a nurse's training class at Spelman. Later she taught at other colleges in such places as St. Louis, Philadelphia and Kansas City. She became a resident physician for a while at Wilberforce College, where an older sister worked as a teacher and was a leader in the woman's movement.

Dr. Jones' practice of public health was so celebrated that she was the only physician, and only woman, asked to present a paper during the 50th Anniversary of the Emancipation Proclamation in Philadelphia in 1913.

Among the other 23 speakers on that auspicious occasion were Kelly Miller, L.L.D., dean of Howard Univ.; Monroe Work, editor of *Journal Statistics on Lynching;* Booker T. Washington, L.L.D. founder of Tuskegee Institute; and W.E.B. DuBois, Ph.D., editor, *The Crisis,* New York.

Dr. Jones, then resident physician at The Agricultural and Mechanical College, Greensboro, N.C., held her mostly male audience mesmerized with her brilliant, half-hour lectures on the "Abnormally High Death Rates From Tuberculosis" and "The Grave Problem of Infant Mortality." Both discussions were timely and provocative.

She described health clubs that were being set up on every campus where she had served as resident physician. Sanitation, public health and the risks of "extra conjugal sex" were discussed with students and teachers alike.

Dr. Jones' final charge to that blue-ribbon audience was: "Let the teaching of general, elementary physiology, including sex physiology, and sanitation be placed on a rational basis in all colored schools and colleges, in the hands of men and women thoroughly trained and with full knowledge of the health problems named above.

"There can be little doubt that the issue of the conflict will be such a rapidly declining death rate and reduced morbidity as will astonish the civilized world."[17]

Although not generally credited with being a founder of Public Health as a specialty, Dr. Jones spent nearly a half century doing nothing else. She was the first African American female to earn an M.D. degree at any predominately white medical school.

If it is true that Dr. Marjorie Meyers was the first African American woman to graduate from Wayne Univ.'s Medical College in 1943, it happened much earlier at the Univ. of Mich., where Dr. Jones had graduated some 42 years earlier.

Dr. Jones died in Monrovia, Calif., at age 75, on September 8, 1932. Although unmarried and childless, she was mourned by thousands who claimed her as their own.

This brief summary, like many others in this series, fails to do justice to Dr. Sophia Jones. Let us hope that a reader of these notes, perhaps a Spelmanite, will help to recover this remarkable woman from the trash-heap of historical obscurity and give her the belated recognition that she so richly deserves.

1. Jessie P. Guzman, *The Negro Yearbook.* (Alabama: The department of records and research, Tuskegee Institute, 1938) p. 215. "It is probable that the original Ku Klux Klan began in 1866, as a club of young men in Pulaski, Tenn. Bed sheets worn by horsemen at night proved terrifying to superstitious Negroes, but soon, the Klan grew into an "order" for "keeping the Negro in his place."

   Also see: W.E.B. Dubois, *Black Reconstruction in America.* (New York: Antheneum, 1985) p. 440.

2. Snow Grigsby, *Brainwashed* (Detroit: 1976) p. 1. "The early history of Michigan is replete with hardships suffered by its people, but the Negro indentured servant encountered difficulties much more varied and fought with graver consequences. Michigan's first slaves were Indians. In 1782, the Michigan territory was given to the United States, at the conclusion of the Revolutionary War. The land donation included 179 Africans, who became Michigan's first African American citizens."

3. London Hargrave, *Getting Into the Fight*, Vol. 75, No. 1. (Michigan History, Jan./Feb. 1991) p. 26.

4. William Loren Katz, *Eyewitness: The Negro in American History.* (New York: Pittman Publishing, 1967) p. 194.

    Hubert Delaney, well-remembered for calling it the way he saw it, offered advice to President Andrew Johnson during Reconstruction: "What becomes necessary to secure and perpetuate the Union is simply the enfranchisement and recognition of the political equality of the power that saved the nation from destruction-a recognition of the political equality of the blacks, with the whites, in all their relations as American citizens."

5. The site is now occupied by the Blue Cross building and displays a historic marker to prove its historic significance. Second Baptist Church on Monroe Street, was a former Underground Railroad station and still has a cell in its basement where fugitives were protected until the coast was clear for their final night flight to "Canaan Land."

6. Wilma Wood Henrickson, *Detroit Perspectives.* (Detroit: Wayne State University Press, 1991) p. 157-162.

7. Note: *Medical History of Michigan.* Published under the auspices of the Michigan State Medical Society. (Minneapolis-St. Paul: Bruce Publishing Co., 1930) p. 825.

8. George B. Catlin, *The Story of Detroit.* (Detroit: The Detroit News, 1926) p. 692.

9. Lewis G. Vander Velde, *The Michigan Supreme Court Defines Negro Rights, 1866-69,* LXIII, No. 21. (Michigan Quarterly Review: August 1957) p. 277-294.

10. G. B. Nash, John R. Howe, Julie Roy Jeffrey, P.J. Frederick, A. F. Davis, and A. M. Winkler, *The American People.* (New York: Harper & Row, 1990) p. 567.

11. Weinberg, Meyer, *W.E.B. Dubois: A Reader.* (New York: Harper & Row, Publishers, 1970) p. 72. "The Fugitive Slave Law of 1850 made personal freedom difficult, and in 1857 the Supreme Court declared that African Americans were not citizens and had always been considered as having 'no rights which a white man was bound to respect."

12. *African American Editors,* p. 317. "The legislature of Kentucky, at the 1888 session, granted a charter to Doctors H. Fitzbutler, W.A. Burney and R. Conrad to conduct, in Kentucky, the Louisville National Medical College; and that charter was signed by the

Governor, April 22, 1888. This school is now in operation with some of the best talent to be found in the country, as students."

13. Loren Miller, *The Petitioners*. (New York: Pantheon Books Random House, 1966) p. 197. A little band of Christians established Berea College in the Kentucky hill country in 1854; touting their religious beliefs—"God hath made of one blood all nations that dwell upon the face of the earth." The practice of this principle produced a student body of 753 European American and 174 African American students in 1904.

In that same year, the Kentucky legislature enacted a statute forbidding the maintenance of any school, college or institution where the races were taught at the same time within 25 miles of each other. The U.S. Supreme Court concurred, and the African American students were driven away from the school, with no pretense to offer separate but equal accommodations.

14. In 1905, the Kentucky Government informed the officials of its Berea College, midterm, that integration of the students was in violation of a state statute that "forbids teaching of white and black students at the same school, at the same time. If the two groups were taught at the same time, they must be separated by, at least, 25 miles. The law levied a fine of $1,000 on a violating institution, $100 for each day's violation and a fine of $50 on its students.

The case was heard by the U.S. Supreme Court and only Justice John Harlan, the lone dissenter in the *Plessy v. Ferguson* case, supported the right of choice for African Americans.

As a result of the official beginning of the recognition of states rights over human rights, Berea College was forcibly segregated during a class period. This action left no doubt in the minds of the officials of LNMC that their situation was not likely to improve in the foreseeable future.

15. Miller, p. 197.

16. John H. Franklin, *From Slavery to Freedom*. (New York: Vantage Books, 1969) p. 294.

17. S. B. Jones, M.D., *Fifty Years of Negro Public Health*, Vol. XLIX. (The American Academy of Political and Social Science: September 1913) pp. 138-146.

The Founding of the National Medical Association, 1895

The continuing acceptance of racial bias from the nation's health care establishment, without serious questioning, has resulted in the denial of equal access to available medical resources for thousands of African American physicians and millions of their patients for more than one hundred years.

Several attempts were made prior to 1895 to organize a national medical association to serve the best interest of these groups. One of the earliest, and best remembered, was the Medico Chirrurigical Society of Washington, D.C. To a large extent, its membership was made up of discharged physician-veterans of the Union Army who joined the newly-formed faculty of Howard University's Medical School. These and other efforts were made in the latter half of the 1880s; yet their scope was too limited to allow expansion into national organizations.

At the end of 1892, Dr. Miles V. Lynk, a Meharry Medical School graduate at age 20, became the first African American publisher of an African American medical journal. He used the pages of his *Medical and Surgical Observer,* to propose, again, the formation of a national organization of African American physicians.

Apparently this was an idea whose time had come. Many African American physicians were facing a future with mounting despair, resignation, and anger. They were forced to accept the built-in racism of the AMA, which denied them membership and equal access to medical resources which their European American colleagues took for granted.

The responses to his call for a meeting were favorable and spurred Dr. Lynk to action. In close cooperation with several of his colleagues, he sought a time and place that seemed likely to attract the largest representative group of African American doctors.

They discovered that a group of Southern politicians and businessmen had scheduled a meeting of the Cotton States International Exposition on September 18, 1895, in Atlanta, Ga. The guest speaker for the Exposition was to be Booker T. Washington. Although he was born enslaved in 1859, Washington graduated from Hampton Institute in Virginia in 1875 and founded the Tuskegee Institute in Alabama in 1881. Already he was beginning to attract public attention.

After several prior failures to organize a national medical group, Dr. Lynk and his colleagues studied this opportunity very carefully before sending out invitations for a meeting to coincide with the Exposition. Although there were some late cancellations, they refused to be deterred and hoped that all twelve of the African American physicians who agreed to come would do so.

This International Exposition was a significant event for those citizens of the secessionist Confederacy. Despite that earlier loss, they were now more determined than ever to win the peace on their terms.

Slave Codes of the antebellum period had been replaced with a facsimile "black codes" in the reconstruction era. All of the civil rights legislation enacted throughout slavery had been declared unconstitutional by a reactionary U.S. Supreme Court.

The promise of the ballot to the freed men, via passage of the 15th Amendment in 1870, was thwarted by grandfather clauses, white primaries, literacy tests, and lynching parties of Ku Klux Klansmen.

The Exposition was equally important for the citizens of Atlanta whose town had been left in shambles by General William T. Sherman before that Union Commander departed for the open sea. They wanted everyone to come and see that Atlanta was in full recovery from "Sherman's Folly."

It was no accident that Booker T. Washington was chosen to deliver the main address. Of course it would provide visible proof that the South was willing to let "bygones be bygones." While Washington's philosophy was not entirely to their liking, it was closer than that of the celebrated and provocative abolitionist, Frederick Douglass, who had died earlier that year.[1]

More importantly, the choice of the speaker provided the Southern oligarchy with a golden opportunity to help choose Douglass' successor, as the "Voice of the Negro." Washington and W.E.B. Dubois, the Harvard-trained African American scholar, had already begun to voice publicly their often acrimonious disagreements on whether the best post-reconstruction course for the next African American leader was to challenge racism or make accommodations for white supremacy.

By that time white Southerners and Northern capitalists had begun to pay increasing attention to Washington. His comments at the 1893 Atlanta Conference of Christian Workers in the United States and Canada encouraged the exposition sponsors to ask Washington to join them in the nation's capital to seek funds for the next exposition.

In the spring of 1895, Washington accompanied a 28-man (twenty-five were white) committee to Washington to seek congressional funds to underwrite the Exposition. The last to speak, Washington made a profound impression on the congressmen as well as his committee. The Exposition received its funding and Washington was chosen as the keynote speaker, "The first time that an African American had been asked to speak from the same platform with white Southern men and women on any important national occasion."[2]

Washington was an excellent choice for the role they expected him to play. He accepted the assignment and spent several days writing what Dubois later referred to as "The Atlanta Compromise." On the other hand, another African American scholar, Rayford Logan, referred to the Washington speech as, "One of the most effective pieces of political oratory in the history of the United States."[3]

Concurrently, the U.S. Supreme Court's *Plessy v. Ferguson* hearings had been in litigation for three years and their decision to legalize racial segregation was less than a year away. The European American Southerners were overjoyed by what they interpreted as Washington's endorsement of their pro-segregationist position.

Dubois and other liberals denounced and were saddened by the speech. He went even further to reject it bitterly as "the trading of black political activity and integration for black economic progress."

A brief look at the political and social climate of the time and a study of the organizational infrastructure of the medical establishment may provide some idea of the formidable impediments faced by African American physicians in our quest for equal opportunity in the medical marketplaces of the U.S.

Racial segregation was legitimized by the U.S. Supreme Court's *Plessy v. Ferguson* decision just one year after the NMA was formed. Thus, racial segregation has been a millstone around the necks of NMA members since it was organized.

With the passage of time, it had become increasingly apparent that the rulers of the "New South" convened the Exposition to serve their personal agenda. It is unlikely that they knew, or cared, about the mission of the twelve African American physicians who sat in the segregated section of the auditorium to hear Booker T. Washington's most remembered speech of all times.

Reconstruction, insofar as the rulers of the secessionist states were concerned, was dead and buried. Although passage of the 13th (1865) and 14th Amendments (1867) prevented the outright return to slavocracy, the enslavers never stopped searching for loop holes.

The major impediment to the restoration of the antebellum autonomy of the "New South" was the unsettled question of racial segregation. The members of the Southern oligarchy knew that this issue had already been in litigation in the U.S. Supreme Court for three years and was heading toward a decision. The future of white supremacy as the "American Way of Life" hung in the balance.

The events that led to one of the most important decisions in U.S. Supreme Court history, *Plessy v. Ferguson*, began quietly on June 7, 1892, like the Montgomery Bus Boycott more than a half

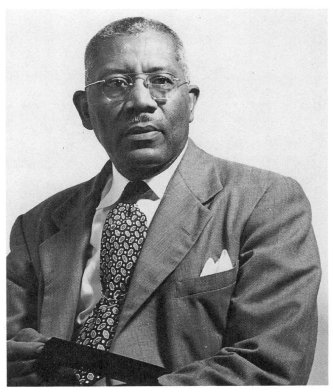

Robert I. Greenidge, M.D., Wayne, 1915; cert. X-ray, 1941. A founder of: (1) Detroit Memorial Park Cemetery, (2) Home Federal Savings and Loan Assoc., (3) Great Lakes Mutual Ins. Co., (4) East Side Medical Laboratory, and (5) the Fairview Hospital with Drs. J.J. McClendon and Rupert Markoe as co-founders.

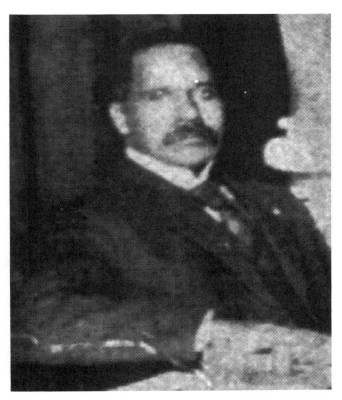

Robert S. Boyd, M.D., Meharry, 1886; D.D.S., Meharry, 1887; P.H.C., 1890 was NMA's first president and served two terms (1895-1897).

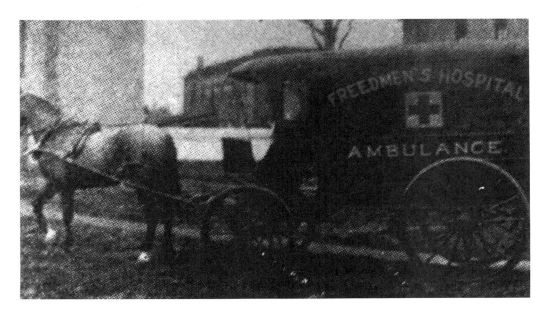

This horse-drawn ambulance served Freedmen's Washington, D.C. hospital. (circa 1894)

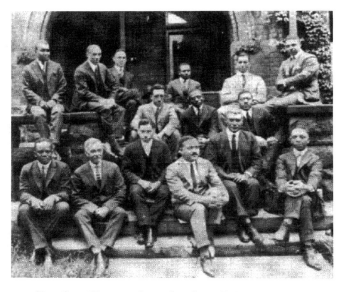

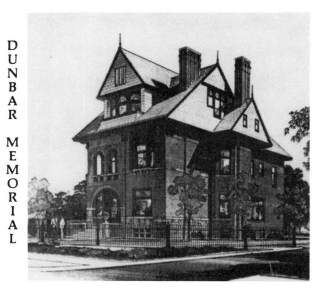

Dunbar Hospital medical staff, 1922 (left to right): Row 1; Joseph Wills, M.D.; James Ames, M.D.; James Young, M.D.; Parker G. Gamble, M.D.; George Bundy, M.D.; Henry Cleage, M.D.; Row 2; Lloyd Bailer, M.D.; Ed Carter, M.D.; Robert Greenidge, M.D.; Row 3; John Miller, M.D.; Leo Welker, M.D.; Charles Greene, M.D.; Frank Raiford, M.D.; Emmill Morton, M.D.; Herbert Sims, M.D.

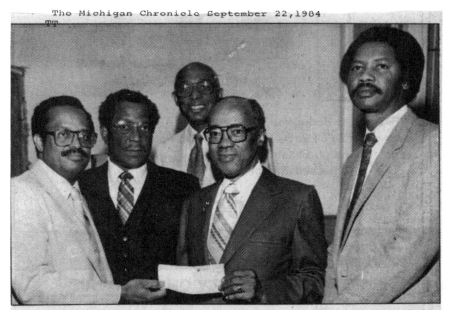

The Michigan Chronicle September 22, 1984

FOR DUNBAR MUSEUM — After 24 years of providing financial support for African medical students, the African Medical Education Fund's board of trustees voted to dissolve the organization and turn its assets over to two other tax-exempt organizations. And so, on Sept. 7, a check for $10,000 was turned over by Dr. Robyn Arrington Sr. (third from left), of the education fund, to Dr. George Lightbourn, executive director, Dunbar Memorial Hospital Museum (DMHM) and immediate past president of the Detroit Medical Society. The funds are earmarked for completion of the Detroit Medical Society office in the Dunbar Building and will be dedicated to the memory of Dr. Ethelene Crockett, a founder of the education fund. Others taking part in the ceremony were (from left) George Crockett III, Dr. Crockett's son; Dr. Charles Wright, member, Detroit Medical Society, and Dr. Harold Tubbs, board chairman, DMHM. Dunbar Hospital served for more than a century as the city's first Black non-profit community hospital and nursing school and the museum will trace the struggle of Black doctors in Detroit.

Trustees of the African Medical Education Fund make a final payout to the Dunbar Memorial Hospital Museum as it goes out of business, after 24 years of assistance to 50 African medical students from 13 African nations.

DETROIT DEPARTMENT OF HEALTH
VITAL STATISTICS DIVISION

PLACE OF BIRTH
County of.... WAYNE

Corr. Suppl.
Father
8-21-45,

STATE OF MICHIGAN
Department of State—Division of Vital Statistics.

RECORD OF BIRTH 25007

Township of ....
or
Village of DETROIT
or
City of....................

(No. *Woman's Hosp.* ....St., ...Ward)
(If birth occurs in a hospital or other institution, give name of same instead of street and number.)

Registered No. ....

FULL NAME
OF CHILD.... *Charles Coleo Diggs Jr*

{ If child is not yet named, make supplemental report, as directed.

| Sex of child *M.* | Twin, triplet, or other? | and | Number in order of birth | Legitimate? *Yes* | Date of Birth *12 – 2*, 19*22* (Month) (Day) (Year) |

FATHER
Full Name *Charles C. Diggs*

MOTHER
Full Maiden Name *Mamie Ethel Jones*

Residence (P. O. Address) *1371 Mullett*

Residence (P. O. Address) *Same.*

| Color or Race *Col.* | Age at Last Birthday *27.* (Years) | Color or Race *Col.* | Age at Last Birthday *22.* (Years) |

Birthplace *Miss.*

Birthplace *Tenn.*

Occupation (And Industry) *Undertaker*

Occupation (And Industry) *H. wife*

Number of child of this mother.... *1*   Number of children, of this mother, now living.... *1*

CERTIFICATE OF ATTENDING PHYSICIAN OR MIDWIFE.

I hereby certify that I attended the birth of this child, who was.................... at *8 05 a* M, on the date above stated.
(Born alive or stillborn.)

Have eyes of child been treated with a prophylaxis solution? *Yes*

(Signature) *Dr. R. Greenidge*
Dated *12-5* 19*22*   *614 Columbia*
(Attending physician, midwife, father, etc.)

Given or christian name added from a supplemental report.................... 19....

Address....................

Filed *12-5 1922*

Registrar.

I hereby certify that the foregoing is a true copy of the record on file in the Detroit Department of Health; attested by the raised seal of the City of Detroit.

Irene Rendz

IRENE RENDZ
Division Head, Vital Statistics

Dated   JUL 1 8 1974

century later. Homer A. Plessy, a mulatto African American, purchased a first-class train ticket to travel 50 miles from Covington to New Orleans, La. He took his seat in the first class coach but never went anywhere.

The European American train conductor, well-schooled in racial matters, informed Plessy that his presence in the coach violated Louisiana's anti-trespassing law and that he would have to move. When informed that the train did not provide first-class seats to second-class citizens, Plessy elected to keep his seat.

Like that Montgomery bus driver in 1955, the train conductor summoned a policeman who arrested Plessy and immediately brought him before Judge Ferguson.

Thus began a bitter battle that culminated in one of the most regrettable Supreme Court decisions in the history of all American jurisprudence (*Plessy v. Ferguson*, 163 U.S. 537.) The trial had just entered its fourth year of litigation when the Cotton States Exposition was held.

With the death of abolitionist Frederick Douglass, there were two highly visible candidates for his mantle as African America's foremost spokesman. One was W.E.B. Dubois, a brilliant academician who had earned his Ph.D. at Harvard University that year and the other, Booker T. Washington, founder and head of the 14 year-old Tuskegee Institute in Alabama.

Dubois, a disciple of Frederick Douglass, was frowned upon by the Southern establishment. He often differed with them uncompromisingly. On the other hand, the establishment found favor with the more conciliatory assertions and actions of Booker T. Washington. The differences between the two leaders were widened by comments from the media.

In a well-calculated move to tip the scales of public opinion toward racial segregation, Washington was chosen to address the Exposition, which was filled to capacity. As he spoke, his sponsors were reassured that their money was on the right horse.

"To those of the white race ... were I permitted, I would say what I say to my own race; Cast down your bucket where you are.

Cast it down among the 8 million Negroes whose habits you know, whose fidelity and love you have tested in days when to have proved treacherous meant the ruin of your firesides.

"Cast down your buckets among these people who have, without strikes and labor wars, tilled your fields, cleared your forests, built your railroads and cities and brought forth treasures from the bowels of the earth.

"As we have proved our loyalty to you, in the past, in nursing your children, watching by the sick beds of your mothers and fathers, and often following them with tear-dimmed eyes to their graves, so in the future in our humble way, we will stand by you with a devotion that no foreigner can approach, ready to lay down our lives, if need be, in defense of yours in a way that shall make the interests of both races one.

"In all things that are purely social, we can be as separate as the fingers, yet one as the hand in all things essential to mutual progress."[4]

The European Americans cheered Washington to the rafters. They found acceptance of segregation in his statement "as to the fingers and the hand." Many African Americans rebuked the speech and the speaker. Dubois forever referred to it disapprovingly as the "Atlanta Compromise."

Life was never the same for Washington after his Atlanta speech. Crowds met his train to present him with flowers and other gifts. He dined at the White House with the President of the United States. Tuskegee Institute prospered to become one of the leading African American colleges of the country. The Carnegie Foundation alone appropriated $600,000 to Tuskegee after the speech, accompanied by words of high praise from the philanthropist.

Washington's influence became so dominant between his speech in 1895 and his death in 1915, that some historians have referred to the period as the "Age of Booker T. Washington." Very few newspapers in the country ignored the eloquence of Booker T. Washington's first major speech, which lasted only 20 minutes. One or two newspapers reminded the public that Washington was the first African American to share the podium with a white man.

It is regrettable that neither the media nor the public listened to what Judge Emory Speer, "the orator of the day," had to say following Washington's speech. His principal and undeniable theme was: "In the United States, the old Anglo-Saxon stock has ever predominated." For more than an hour, he championed the cause of Anglo-Saxons or white supremacists and assured his listeners that Anglo Saxons could and would take care of everything and everybody because of their "imperious and commanding nature" and their large percentage of "old Southern Stock."

By the time Judge Speer reached the podium, I. Garland Penn, the African American Commissioner of the Exposition had no doubt gathered the twelve African American doctors for their organizational meeting in Atlanta's First Congregational Church.[5]

Only somewhat mindful of the full magnitude of the political games being played out in the main auditorium of the Exposition Hall and how their lives would be affected by them, henceforth, the 12 physicians under the leadership of Drs. Myles V. Lynk and Robert F. Boyd, proceeded to complete their mission.

Following the plans of their host, Atlanta's R. Butler, M.D., the group met in the church to organize The National Association of Colored Physicians, Dentists and Pharmacists.

Among the physicians who attended the first meeting were; Robert F. Boyd, M.D., (1858-1912) chosen president, National Association of Colored Physicians Dentists and Pharmacists. (Although rarely used, this was the proper name of the organization until 1940. During the presidency of Dr. Albert Dumas, Sr., of Natchez, Miss., the dentists and pharmacists were formally disaffiliated.)

Dr. Boyd attended Central State College and Fisk Univ. graduated from Meharry Medical College, M.D.(1886), D.D.S. (1887); and Certificate of Pharmacy (1890); he was superintendent and chief surgeon, Mercy Hospital and founder of Boyd's Infirmary, both in Nashville and Meharry's primary teaching hospital for many years.

D.L. Martin, M.D., secretary, Nashville, Tenn.

D.N.C., Scott, M.D. treasurer, Montgomery, Ala.

Vice-president: Daniel Hale Williams, M.D. (1856-1931), attended premedical school at Hare's Academy in Hollidaysburg, Pa. and earned his M.D. at Chicago Medical College in 1883. He divided Freedmen's Hospital into departments to improve its efficiency; was the co-founder of Provident Hospital (Chicago); and was the only African American among the 100 charter members of the American College of Surgeons.

Chr. Ex. Comm. and host R. Butler, M.D., had been elected president of the Colored Physicians of Georgia, in 1893.

Miles Vandahurst Lynk, M.D., one of the principle organizers of the Atlanta meeting, graduated from Meharry Medical College in 1891 at the age of 20. He was the publisher of *Medical and Surgical Conserver* in 1892, the first medical journal published by a black man in the U.S., and several books followed.

The last decade of the 19th century was not the most ideal time for any African American group to try to launch a new national organization, despite the imperatives to do so. They all had to deal with a resurgent, secessionist, Southern oligarchy which was determined to replace the outlawed institution of slavery with a reasonable facsimile.

The Southerners rewrote their state constitutions, making some effort to avoid a frontal attack on the 15th Amendment. Their two main thrusts for power were:

1. African Americans not be given the ballot, but it must not be denied because of their color. The guardians of status quo devised difficult literacy tests, white primaries, grandfather clauses and other guises to deny the ballot to eligible African Americans.

2. When all else failed, terrorist attacks by the Ku Klux Klan were launched against prospective African American voters, especially after passage of the 15th Amendment in 1870.[6] Lynchings reached a new high during that period. Their methods were so effective that Atlanta newspaperman Henry Grady observed: "The Negro as a political force has dropped out of consideration."[7]

3. Segregation. Many former slave owners felt that if slavery could not be reimposed, the complete segregation of the African American was a reasonable alternative. The *Plessy v. Ferguson* decision was, to them, like manna from heaven.

Among the minority of African Americans who violently opposed this trend toward total segregation and boldly tested its constitutionality was Homer Plessy. Although he knew that the train seat he chose in 1892 was reserved for European Americans, Plessy sat down anyway. This simple act by one man led to four years of litigation by some of the best legal minds of the period. The decision was opposed by only one justice, John Harlan, a liberal Kentuckian.

The Supreme Court's decision, announced a year after the NMA was organized, was easily predictable: six of the seven Justices, who ruled on the *Plessy v. Ferguson* decision, had served as lawyers for railroads or corporations closely related thereto (Justice John Harlan dissented and Justice David Brewer did not participate in the case). Justice David Field of California, for instance, "had had a long, judicial love affair with the Southern Pacific Railroad."

Yet the highest tribunal in the U.S. spent four years deciding that Plessy, an African American, was sub-human. Moreover, in similar cases already litigated in Louisiana in 1869-1877, and in Mississippi in 1888, some of those same justices had already come to that conclusion.

Several years after its founding, the NMA's fifth president and first editor of its journal, Dr. Charles V. Roman, expressed in his first editorial the spirit that had propelled the members of this new organization to form a separate body—A Mission Statement:

"Conceived in no spirit of racial exclusiveness, fostering no ethnic antagonisms, but born of the exigencies of the American environment, the National Medical Association has for its object the banding together for mutual cooperation and helpfulness, the men and women of African descent who are legally and

37

honorably engaged in the practice of the cognate profession of medicine, surgery, pharmacy, and dentistry."

For many years I wondered why the first NMA membership included pharmacists and dentists, as well as physicians, when no mention was made of dentists nor pharmacists being present at the beginning. An obvious reply was there were so few physicians, dentists or pharmacists, that all three groups met together to ensure a quorum.

While doing research for this book, I learned that the NMA's first president, Dr. Robert F. Boyd, held degrees and practiced in all three fields, pharmacy, dentistry, and medicine. Joint meetings of all three groups flourished in the small towns, especially in the South.

Most of the early African American physicians, including many in Detroit, entered the practice of medicine with little or no hospital experience except that which they received as students in their segregated medical schools, hospitals, and clinics.

If hospitals were available to them, they were usually poorly operated, inadequately staffed and hardly equipped for proper training. They did not provide libraries, regular teaching rounds, lectures or the fruitful exchanges of ideas so essential in a rapidly changing field like medicine.

The growth and development of the NMA, although slow and sporadic, frequently served as the only source of light in a professional world dimmed by disfranchisement and discrimination. Eventually, the NMA began to fulfill the promise to some of its constituents by encouraging the establishment of local affiliates in those areas where the number of physicians was sufficient to support it.

The NMA's 1896 meeting was held in Nashville, Tenn., with Dr. Boyd presiding. He reported that the membership of the Association embraced "about two-thirds of the colored physicians of the South." Many registrants were unable to attend because of a yellow fever epidemic that swept through the South that year.

The *New York Post* reported that at one of the NMA's early meetings in August that the NMA delegates had, "Gathered at the Lincoln Hospital (Bronx) to watch extremely delicate and masterful operations by Dr. Austin Curtis, of Washington, D.C.; Dr. Daniel Hale Williams, of Chicago; and John E. Hunter, of Lexington, Ky." In the afternoon, the delegates convened at the nearby Plaza assembly rooms to hear a number of solid, scientific papers.

The Journal of the National Medical Association

Although the NMA was organized in 1895, the Journal did not begin publication until 1909. The Journal's first editor was Dr. Charles V. Roman, M.D. (Meharry, 1890), a man of considerable talents. By 1905, he had become known as the "Sage" of the association. Thus it is not surprising that he became the founding editor of the *Journal,* whose first editorial has also become known as the NMA's "Mission Statement."

Dr. Roman, the NMA's fifth president, was the editor for 10 years. He was assisted by then managing and future editor, Dr. John Andrew Kenny, Sr., M.D., founder of the John A. Andrews Medical Clinic, in Tuskegee, Ala.

Dr. Kenny was a graduate of Leonard Medical School Class of 1901 at Raleigh, N.C.'s Shaw University. After ten years of apprenticeship with Dr. Roman (which included his 1913 term as NMA president, he became NMA's most durable editor—1916 through 1948) In his spare time he was the director of Tuskegee's John A. Andrews Medical Clinic, physician to Tuskegee's students and faculty, and personal friend and private physician to its founder, Booker T. Washington. Despite such credentials and connections, Dr. Kenny was run out of Tuskegee by a mob of irate klansmen. They held him responsible for the federal government's decision to admit African American patients to the then new Tuskegee's Veteran's Hospital rather than to admit European Americans.

The Klan threat was so serious that a guard was assigned to Dr. Kenny while he terminated his affairs at Tuskegee. Mrs. Kenny, with the assistance of Dr. Peter Marshall Murray, found refuge for herself and her sons in Newark, N.J. As quickly and as quietly as possible, Kenny closed down his Southern operation and rejoined his family in the East.[8]

Although these events took place some seventy years earlier, Dr. Kenney, Jr. recalled them with sudden clarity as if they had just occurred, when I interviewed him during the NMA's 1994 convention in Orlando, Fla. Since the elder Kenney's problem was color and not geography, it should not be surprising to learn that he continued to be hounded by members of the New Jersey Klan for the rest of his days.

The third editor of the Journal was Ulysses Grant Dailey, M.D. (Northwestern, 1906). He was attending surgeon at Chicago's Provident Hospital and instructor of surgery at Chicago Medical College. He served as editor of the Journal for one year before departing for post-graduate surgical training in Paris and Berlin.

W. Montague Cobb, M.D. (Howard, 1929), succeeded Dr. Dailey and held the post until 1978. Prior to coming to the Journal Dr. Cobb served as editor of the *Bulletin of the Medico-Chirurgical Society* of the District of Columbia. The bulletin started by him ran for 39 issues, inconsistently, during the 1940s. In 1939, Dr. Cobb authored, *The First Negro Medical Society.*

During Cobb's term as editor, he was also a national trustee and a presiding officer of the Executive Board of the NAACP. The influence of this exposure to and the opportunity to participation in the civil rights agenda in the mid-20th century were unique for anyone, especially physicians. The issues that he dealt with are still with us, demanding our attention.

Dr. Cobb provided leadership in such struggles as the Imhotep Committee meetings, NMA-AMA Liaison conferences, the defeat of the AMA's opposition to Medicare and passage of the Omnibus Civil Rights Act of 1964 that "purportedly" removed the degrading "separate but equal" clause from the Hill-Burton Survey and Hospital Construction Act.

Posthumous homage was paid to Dr. Cobb during the residents' session on writing papers during the NMA's 99th session in Orlando, Fl; in 1994. One of the presenters reminded us how valuable a source of information on African American medical history Dr. Cobb's journals are and that they must be preserved for posterity.

As teacher of anatomy at Howard's Medical School and Trustee of the NAACP for many years, Dr. Cobb's influence was felt far beyond the pages of the *Journal* and this book. Since you will meet him so many times and under such a variety of circumstances on the road ahead, I will allow those events to continue his remarkable story.

Calvin Sampson, M.D. (Meharry, 1971), succeeded Dr. Cobb as the journal's fourth editor. His pre-journal career was also very fruitful. A brilliant student, he graduated from Meharry with honors. He chose pathology as his specialty and was one the first African Americans to be certified as a clinical pathologist.

Before accepting the appointment of editor of the *Journal*, Dr. Sampson had already distinguished himself academically as director of Laboratories and pathologist at Freedman's Hospital and at Howard University's School of Medicine.

He went on to be named the first director of Howard's School of Medical Technology in 1971, and later, the first acting chairman of its newly-established department of allied health professions. Before moving to the position of full-time editor of the *Journal*, Dr. Sampson had become a full professor and vice chairman of the department of pathology. With more than 100 publications credited to him, and the high esteem of his colleagues clearly evident, he gathered up the reins of editorial authority in 1977 and headed into the 21st century.

From 1909 to 1938, the *Journal* was produced quarterly. In 1939, it began appearing bi-monthly and since 1977 it has been published monthly. The *Journal* has an internal circulation and is exchanged with many other medical journals, at home and abroad. It is indexed in the National Library of Medicine and the *Index Medicus.*

1. Katz, William L. (1967). *Eyewitness: The Negro in American History.* New York: Pittman Publishing Corporation, 348-349.

2. Washington, Booker T. (1900). *Up From Slavery.* New York: Bantam Books, 147-152.

3. Logan, Rayford W. (1965). *The Betrayal of the Negro.* New York: Collier Books, 276-312.

4. Katz, William L. (1967). *Eyewitness: The Negro in American History.* New York: Pittman Publishing Corporation, 357-358.

5. Logan, 303.

6. Grady, (1890). *The New South.* 244.

7. Grady, 166.

8. Dr. Kenny, Jr., and his father, the only father and son team to share the presidency of the NMA, informed me that Tuskegee's European American community was infuriated that the Veterans Administration chose to build a veterans hospital for African Americans in Tuskegee, instead of one for them. Washington, who had dined at the White House with Theodore Roosevelt after his "Lay Down Your Bucket" speech in Atlanta, was considered untouchable; so the Klan went after Dr. Kenny, Sr. The senior Kenny was placed in protective custody while he closed out his medical affairs.

9. Yenser, Thomas. (1933). *Who's Who in Colored America.* Brooklyn, 145.

Atlanta, The National Medical Association's Ancestral Home

The birthplace of the NMA, Atlanta, should be considered our ancestral home, where its members are welcomed with open arms. This has not always been the case. The year following the organization of the NMA in 1896, a race riot broke out in Atlanta that overshadowed the memory of Booker T. Washington's speech the year before. A more serious reincarnation of racial violence occurred in 1906 in Brownsville, a suburb of Atlanta. The rioting lasted several days and members of both races fell victim.

These and similar events sullied Atlanta's start into the new century, causing it to fare poorly in Georgia. The later experiences of two of our 20th Century Trailblazers suggest how endemic violence was borne through their personal accounts which will be discussed under that heading.

A rather disturbing report by the Atlanta Branch of the Urban League disclosed that in 1947, the year after the first Hill-Burton Act was passed, African American patients became the most neglected group in the entire community. Rather than open up the existing hospitals to them, the Fulton Dekalb Hospital Authority, which dispensed Hill-Burton funds throughout Georgia, approved a grant of $1,439,609 to build a segregated hospital for African Americans who could pay.

To ensure the eternal gratitude of the African American community, this "separate but equal" hospital was named for the chairman of the Hospital Authority, Hugh Spaulding. The Hugh Spaulding Pavilion opened in 1950 and was expected to divert the attention of the integrationist, which it did for a while.[10]

While some of the Southern states were preparing to accept African Americans as full members of their medical societies, the Georgia State Medical Society passed a resolution that delineated "scientific" memberships for African Americans which allowed them to attend only scientific portions of the membership meeting. They were denied voting privileges as well as the right to be present during social gatherings. [11]

Many Southern states ignored and insulted their African American colleagues. Georgia's officials went even further in underscoring their antipathy toward African American physicians—they added abuse.

The most shocking crime against an African American physician in the 1950s was the murder of Dr. Thomas Brewer, Sr., of Columbus, Ga. Dr. Brewer was a fearless freedom fighter who dared to invade the inner sanctum of white supremacy, the white primary. His unflagging leadership cost him his life and precipitated the flight of his family to Columbus, Ohio. [12]

On February 28, 1961, eight members of the NMA, Drs. F. Earle McClendon, Louis F. Reese, John T. Gill, Jr.; Albert M. Davis; George C. Lawrence; James P. Ellison: Roosevelt P. Jackson; and Clinton P. Warner were registered delegates at the annual meeting of the Atlanta Graduate Assembly, held under the auspices of the Fulton County Medical Society.

A spokesman for the medical assembly announced to the public that, "The African Americans were welcome to attend the business functions of the assembly, but the matter of eating is a hotel management problem."

Although the police brought paddy wagons to transfer those African American doctors, who attempted to eat, to police headquarters, the actual transfers took place in cars, where they were booked and finger-printed and taken directly to the city courtroom where they were given a hearing and permitted to sign their own $100 bonds. Judge James Webb bound them over to the Fulton County Criminal Court.

On January 11, 1964, twenty-three sit-in demonstrators arrested at the Heart of Atlanta Hotel, including Dr. C. Miles Smith, a dentist and president of the Atlanta branch of the NAACP and Dr. Clinton Warner, local surgeon and NAACP vice president. The hotel allegedly refused to join 14 other hotels and motels that had agreed earlier to drop the color bar.

Evidence that Georgia's officials were violence-prone seemed incontrovertible upon first inspection of the experiences of Drs. William Anderson and Joshua Williams (see 20th Century Trailblazers) who were both victims of racial harassment. Dr. Williams argued against this theory. It was his contention that a more militant breed of African American in Georgia excited a more repressive response from the white oppressors than would have been the case.

Aside from the "Heart of Atlanta" incident, Georgia's African American physicians also participated in litigation for justice in medical institutions. Clinton Warner, M.D., was a complainant in the case of *Bell et al v. The Georgia Dental Association* and *The Northern District Dental Society et al*, a case that produced a major breakthrough in desegregating professional societies.

In the summer of 1962, the following individuals filed a civil suit against the Georgia Dental Association, the Northern Dental Society, Grady Hospital, the Fulton County Medical Society and the Medical Association of Georgia: R.E. Bell, D.D.S.; Clinton Warner, M.D.; Ruby Smith, a Spelman student seeking to enter Grady's School of Nursing on a non-segregated basis; Edwina Smith; John Middleton; Dorothy F. Cotton; and Septima Clark, who'd sought emergency care at Grady Hospital and was refused.

The Fulton County Medical Society was charged with denying membership to African American physicians and Grady Hospital for allegedly discriminating against African American nurses and patients. It was further charged that the defendants had violated the Defendants' constitutional rights under the 5th, 14th and 15th Amendments by discriminating against African American professionals and technicians and by segregating African American patients and nurses.[13]

This omnibus trial took advantage of the experiences that the NAACP had gained in earlier cases. Dental, medical, nursing and patients' complaints were presented in a single court action, reducing the chances for summary dismissal.

In earlier cases, European American professional societies had claimed that they were private institutions and, therefore, not subject to the Constitutional provisions against racial discrimination.

To counter this claim by the Dental Societies (Northern District Dental Society and the Georgia Dental Association) the plaintiffs' lawyers disclosed that the Georgia Dental Association nominated practicing dentists from the Georgia Board of Dental Examiners to the Board of Health and appointed their members to the Georgia State Hospital Advisory Committee.

The plaintiffs held that this relationship with the government made the professional societies subject to the constitutional constraints against racial discrimination.

The Georgia Dental Association and the Northern Dental Association moved to dismiss the case against them stating the findings were insufficient to change their private status. U.S. District Judge Frank Hopper rejected their argument and denied the motion. He agreed that the dental societies were, to the extent described, agencies of the state.

This preliminary decision was hailed as a breakthrough, insofar as the effort to integrate professional societies was concerned. The conclusion was supported by developments in the county and state medical societies. Long before the final decision in this case was rendered, the two medical societies accepted African Americans as members. Soon after, Emory University's Medical School accepted an African American intern to Grady Hospital.

On June 19, 1962, an African American physician, a dentist and five citizens filed suit against several health institutions in Atlanta, charging racial discrimination. That very same day, the U.S. Justice Department filed supporting briefs in Atlanta and Greensboro, N.C.

As a direct result of the pressure exerted by the Atlanta suit, Drs. William Stewart and James Palmer were admitted to the staff of Grady Hospital in August 1962. On October 5, 1962, Dr. Asa Yancey was admitted to "full" membership in the Fulton

County Medical Society, with the demeaning "scientific" classification omitted.

These cases are but a small sample of the protests by African American professionals that spread across the nation during the civil rights movement between 1945 and 1965. They provide insight into the problems that were faced and solved by African American doctors, nurses, and patients during that turbulent time.

Although we have made some progress since our founders sought recognition in this city one hundred years ago, we must constantly remind ourselves that it's more difficult to catch up than it is to keep up. We still have a long, long way to go.

10. *JNMA*, (1950). Vol. 42, 118.

11. *JNMA*, (1952). Vol. 44, 316.

12. *JNMA*, (1956). Vol. 48, 190-193.

13. *JNMA*, (1964). Vol. 56, 204.

Detroit, The African American Hospital Capital of the United States

As mentioned earlier, in 1913 Dr. Arthur Dean Bevan, chairman of the AMA's Council of Medical Education, declared: "The development of hospital teaching is the most important, active question before the medical educators at this time."[1] Without that exposure to the maturing process, which is acquired only by hospital affiliation, the education of the physician is forever inadequate. The importance of that question has grown exponentially since that time.

The blame for this denial of access to hospital affiliation was placed on "unqualified" African American physicians. Under such circumstances they were denied the best training and their patients the best medical care available. After nearly a half century of shameful rejections (1847-1895), African American physicians were forced to accept the fact that they were invisible and inaudible to the members of the AMA and that a mutually respectable relationship was not possible.

Forced to seek solutions to the problems thrust upon them, Detroit's African American physicians, like those in other cities, followed the example already set by the NMA and created their own hospitals despite the fact that many adequate hospitals were already available to European American physicians and their patients.

The Sisters of Charity in Detroit led the way by building St. Mary's Hospital on Clinton St. near St. Antoine in 1838. By 1917, Detroit's African American physicians had finally accepted the futility of attempts to gain admitting privileges in the existing hospitals. They opened the 20-bed Mercy General Hospital. By this time Harper, Grace, Ford, Providence, Herman Kiefer and Receiving Hospitals were already in full, but racially restrictive, operation.[2]

Thus the victims of racial oppression began what proved to be a 75-year effort to survive its ill effects at a time when they were sick and most vulnerable. While seeking survival, Detroit was given the ubiquitous title "The Black Hospital Capital of the U.S.A.," by many who were disposed to be unkind.

The project began when 25-30 of Detroit's African American physicians met in 1917 to form the Allied Medical Society. They sought to maximize their meager resources by becoming affiliated with the NMA, which was organized 22 years earlier for the same reason.

The physicians immediate goal was to establish their own hospital. A husband and wife physician team, Drs. Daisy and David Northcross, were members of the group and had just fled from the Ku Klux Klan in Montgomery, Alabama, where they had practiced together in their own "Northcross" sanitarium.

This couple brought with them much-needed medical and administrative experiences that were helpful in the preliminary discussions about hospitals. It soon became apparent, however, that a joint venture between the Northcrosses and the other African American physicians was not possible, so the Northcrosses chose to go it alone. They established Detroit's first African American "hospital," **Mercy Hospital**, at 73 Russell St. near the Detroit River.

Ophelia Northcross, a nurse and their daughter-in-law, cautioned against too literal use of the word "hospital" at that time. She was told "it all began when office patients were too ill to go home after treatment. Some were allowed to spend the night in the back of the office; and somebody would stay on to watch over them and administer the medicine."

In due course, the patient load soon exceeded the available space and Mercy Hospital was moved to a larger house at 688 Winder St., between St. Antoine and Hastings. It remained there for several years until the Winder property was condemned by the city to clear the way for the proposed I-75 expressway.

It was at this time in the late 1950s that the Northcrosses and representatives of the other private, independent hospitals were summoned to a meeting of Medical Center planners, Blue Cross

BOULEVARD

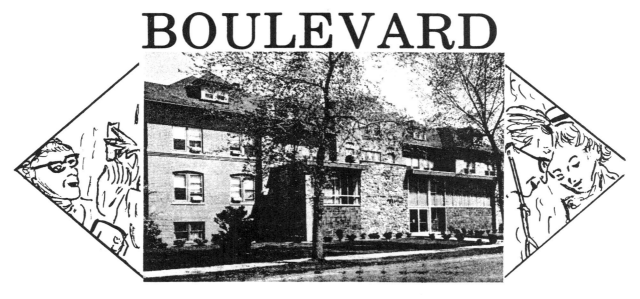

Boulevard General Hospital, the successor to Trinity Hospital, D.G. Williams, chief of staff, 1969-1984.

SOUTHWEST DETROIT HOSPITAL CORPORATION

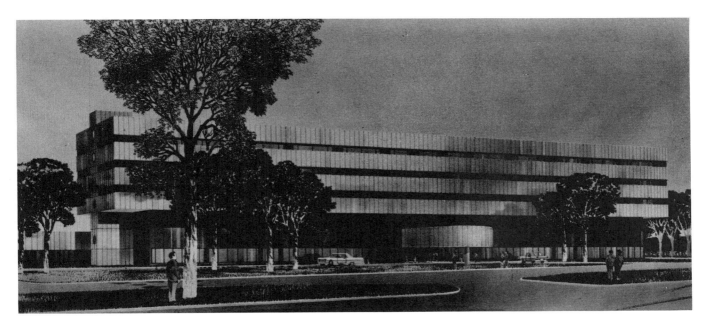

Ground-Breaking Ceremonies / Sunday, November 28, 1971 — 3:00 p.m.

Southwest Detroit Hospital was the product of the merging of: Boulevard General, Delray, Trumbull General and Burton Mercy hospitals, 1974-1993. Detroit's reign as the African American hospital capitol came to an end during its 75th year, 1918-1993.

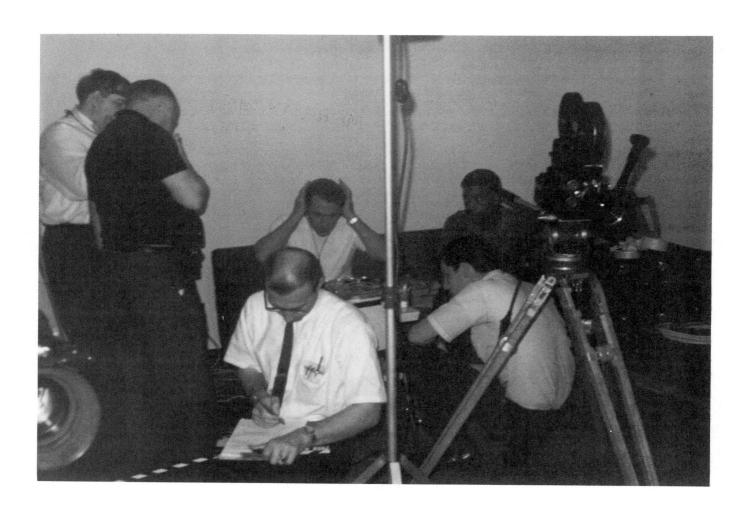

The Carl Balduf Crew is shooting the medical recruitment film: *You Can Be A Doctor,* at the Kirwood Hospital, 1967. The project was sponsored by the Detroit Medical Society and the Museum of African American History. The film was distributed by the McGraw-Hill Book Company.

officials and city representatives at the Book Cadillac Hotel to learn that the days of their institutions were numbered.

The long-range plans, according to the establishment's spokesmen, were to close all of the small hospitals and direct patient flow toward the Medical Center in the interest of Wayne State Univ. Medical School and its affiliated corridor hospitals. When it became clear that Blue Cross and other third-party payers were supporting this decision, the representatives of the small hospitals were not only speechless, but helpless as well.

The first casualty of this African American hospital consolidation plan was Mercy Hospital. Dr. David Northcross, Jr. and his wife, Ophelia, had become the second generation of Mercy's owners. They were now caught between the highway commissioners on the one hand (who needed their Winder St. property for expressway expansion and the medical establishment's move toward hospital consolidation and patient redistribution), and the Northcross' desire to remain in the hospital business on the other.

Instead of selling the hospital and calling it quits, as the Hospital Authority had hoped, the Northcross' sold the Winder St. property for more than $400,000 and added enough of their own money to build another Mercy Hospital at 2929 W. Boston Blvd. In less than a year, the new 50-bed structure was completed. In one day, all 35 Mercy patients were transferred to the new Boston Boulevard facility.

Mrs. Northcross remembered that the members of the medical establishment never forgot nor forgave them for building another small hospital. Their participation with Blue Cross was reduced from a cost plus arrangement that permitted survival, to a flat-rate reimbursement that eventually forced foreclosure.

In a desperate bid to protect his half-million dollar investment, Dr. Northcross converted the economically unsound facility into a methadone clinic that operated despite neighbors protests for two or three years. The next bid for more profits, but one that attracted even more protests, was the establishment of an abortion clinic. Unfortunately, after two to three years of lucrative, yet unpopular operation, a patient died incident to an abortion.

To the neighborhood's relief, the hospital was closed by the Board of Health. Two years later, just as plans were being finalized to reopen Mercy General as a mental hospital, someone threw a firebomb through a hospital window and it was burned beyond repair. This brought a fiery finish to Detroit's first African American hospital after more than forty years of survival.

After Mercy General Hospital was launched in 1917, the remaining members of the Allied Medical Society met with a bi-racial committee of community leaders and formed a subsidiary group to seek health care provisions for Detroit's expanding African American population that already exceeded 20,000. Instead of attacking the racism of the hospitals, the group elected to form the Dunbar Hospital organizing board of trustees and worked hard to create an acceptable, segregated alternative—the **Dunbar Hospital**.

Dunbar Hospital's first board of trustees included John Dancy, Executive Director of the Urban League; John Lyle; William C. Osby (who in addition to leadership roles in the NAACP and Urban League, served as general manager of the Dunbar Hospital through the mid-1920s); Alice Stone; and Charles Webb. As president, Osby led the board's first, city-wide financial campaign.

Dr. Babcock, a Grace Hospital administrator and a national authority on hospital building and management, spent many helpful hours with Dunbar's and, later, Parkside Hospital's management team. Fred Butzel, one of Detroit's most generous contributors to African American causes, often came to the hospital's rescue in times of need. Aided by Trustee John Dancy, who was a member of Senator James Couzens Community Affairs committee, the Dunbar Trustees were able to gain the congressman's attention when hospital matters became urgent.

The trustees and staff acquired a three-story dwelling at 580 Frederick St. which had been built in 1892 by Detroit jeweler Charles W. Warren. They occupied it in 1918 and converted it into

Detroit's first non-profit, African American, general hospital. When fully operational, Dunbar could accommodate 30 patients. Although the administrators did boast of a "well-run" operating room, no facilities for obstetrical deliveries were mentioned.[3]

The trustees chose two of Detroit's most prestigious African American physicians to direct the medical affairs of Dunbar Hospital, Dr. James Ames and Dr. Alexander Turner:

James Ames, M.D. (Howard Univ., 1894)—began his private practice in Detroit soon after graduation. Dr. Ames and Florence Cole, the daughter of wealthy businessman James H. Cole, were married near the turn of the century. Their son, Chester, followed his father into the field of medicine and went on to become Detroit's first African American intern, resident and member of the Wayne Univ. medical faculty.

Dr. Ames' long and interesting public career included a variety of professional, political and business interests. Aside from his appointment as the Medical Director (Supt.) of Dunbar Hospital, he was appointed Diagnostician of Detroit's Board of Health (1901-1915) and served several terms as a city physician.[4] On July 23, 1915, at the end of his term as superintendent on the Detroit Board of Health, Dr. Ames issued a perceptive observation on "Negro Mortality in Detroit."[5]

Dr. Ames was listed as a member of the Wayne County and State Medical Societies and of the AMA—the first, known African American member in Michigan. Dr. Ames became active in Wayne County's Republican politics and served as a delegate to many Republican state and county conventions. In 1900, he was elected to Michigan's House of Representatives for one term.

Other civic duties included: Director of the Phyllis Wheatley House for Indigent Colored Women; Board of Supervisors, Wayne County (beginning in 1918); and organizer of the Florence Ames Temple. He was awarded a Certificate of Appreciation by President Franklin D. Roosevelt in recognition of "uncompensated services, patriotically rendered to his country, in the administration of the Selective Service System during the Second World War." He was a member of Gamma

Lambda Chapter of the Alpha Phi Alpha Fraternity, 1919; and also past Exalted Ruler of Wolverine Lodge No. 72.

Alexander L. Turner M.D. (Univ. of Mich., 1912)—was appointed chief of surgery at Dunbar Hospital. In lieu of an internship, Turner did post-graduate work in surgery at Howard Univ. Medical School before opening a private office at Gratiot and St. Antoine. Later, he moved to W. Warren Ave. to a predominantly Polish community. Due to his surgical skill, his growing European American patient clientele, and his frequent use of European doctors as consultants, the medical establishment recognized Dr. Turner's economic potential as a source of patient referrals. He alone, among African American physicians, was accepted on the staffs of Grace and Woman's hospitals, primarily Woman's.[6]

While the 1922 roster of the early Dunbar Hospital lists Dr. Turner as chief of surgery, there is little evidence of his presence at that institution. Having practiced at Grace and Woman's Hospitals before Dunbar Hospital was organized, he would have found very little to attract him to the smaller, poorly equipped institution.

Dr. Turner does not appear in the Dunbar Hospital photo taken in 1922 and is not well-remembered by many of those physicians who survived his period. Other physicians shown in the photo were:

Lloyd Bailer, M.D. (Univ. of Nebraska)—practiced Eye, Ear, Nose, Throat, briefly. He was the first African American doctor to limit his practice to a specialty. Eventually, he abandoned medicine altogether in deference to his wife's strong belief in and practice of Christian Science.

George Bundy, M.D. (Det. College of Medicine and later, Wayne Univ.)—formerly served as priest of St. Matthew's Episcopal Parish before earning an M.D. at Wayne Univ. Medical School. Known as "the baby doctor," he was one of the few African American physicians allowed to perform an occasional, clandestine delivery at Woman's Hospital in the early 1920s.

Albert B. Cleage, M.D. (Univ. of Indiana, 1910)—scored second highest in a competitive examination for internships at the Indianapolis Dispensary. He went on to serve as an ambulance physician and surgeon. He began practicing medicine in Kalamazoo in 1912 before moving to Detroit. Dr. Cleage may have been the only Dunbar physician to serve an internship before it opened.

Parker G. Gamble, M.D. (Univ. of Mich., 1912)—became chief of staff of Parkside Hospital in the 1930s.

Robert Greenidge, M.D. (Det. College of Medicine, 1915)—was the first of Michigan's African American physicians to become a certified specialist in X-ray in 1941. He served as chairman of the board and chief of X-ray at Dunbar and Parkside Hospitals for many years.

Frank Raiford, Sr., M.D. (Univ. of Mich., 1917)—was a co-founder of Trinity Hospital (along with Drs. Chester Ames and Harold Johnson) which was a primary source for post graduate training of African American physicians when internships and residencies were not made available elsewhere.

James Young, M.D. (Wayne Univ., 1915)—was well remembered as having been appointed a city physician by one of Detroit's most illustrious citizens, Mayor Frank Murphy.

Dunbar Hospital Expands its Operation

By 1924, Dunbar Hospital had outgrown its space at 580 Frederick. The members of Allied Medical Society and trustees of Dunbar Hospital acquired an adjacent building, adding space for offices, a reception room, a medical library, nurses quarters and boosting the bed capacity from twenty-seven to forty.

Dr. Ames continued as medical director of Dunbar Hospital for several years, but the position was shared by other staff doctors as well. His many political and social obligations were demanding on his time, but medicine remained his highest priority.

Dr. Turner's reputation as a skilled surgeon, and his ability to hospitalize and treat his patients in Woman's Hospital were parlayed into a lifestyle that included fine homes in Detroit and Mt. Clemens; chauffeur-driven, expensive cars; and pedigreed pets, for which he is remembered most. It is entirely possible that Turner was connected to Dunbar Hospital in name only.

Upon first glance it appeared that all of Detroit's hospital doors were completely closed to African American physicians. However, Dr. Greenidge's archives revealed a lone birth certificate which stated he had delivered a male child to Charles and Mayme Diggs in Woman's Hospital on December 2, 1922.

When confronted with this finding, some of Woman's (currently Hutzel) senior obstetricians were highly skeptical that such an event would take place in 1922 at that facility. Others dismissed the rumor as a Greenidge fabrication. Spurred to further study, Dr. Greenidge's great granddaughter, and my early editor, Blythe Allen, discovered that:

Dr. Charles Hollister Judd, a European American, had been a generous, brave, and exceptional member of Woman's Hospital's Ob-gyn staff. He had allowed Drs. Greenidge and Bundy (the former St. Matthews Episcopal priest) to enter the "back door" of Woman's obstetrical unit and deliver babies on several occasions. Although only Dr. Greenidges name appears on the Diggs' child's birth certificate, Judd/Greenidge does appear on the delivery room sheet, for the date of the delivery.

Insofar as the hospital was concerned, aside from the delivery room sheet, this clandestine delivery of Charles Diggs, Jr., who later became a U.S. Congressman, was a non-event. It is not too difficult to imagine two young, enterprising African Americans—one a doctor (Greenidge) and the other an undertaker (Diggs)—putting their heads together to plan a proper hospital delivery for the businessman's first born.

It is also understandable how a former priest of one of Detroit's most prestigious Episcopal Churches, now a physician, 'would have sufficient ecclesiastical connections to exploit the same source for an occasional obstetrical bed in a reputable hospital. But what about the source of that unusual benevolence, Dr. Judd?

Dr. Judd was an influential member of the Woman's obstetrical staff who served somewhat like a house doctor in the early part of the 20th century. He is well-remembered by Dr. Frank Bicknell, retired former Hutzel Chief of Urology, who recalled:

"Judd was a studious, kind-hearted physician, who went out of his way to be helpful." While Judd had never divulged the "back-door" obstetrical activities to his friend, Dr. Bicknell did not seem surprised when questioned about the episode.

Aside from these few crumbs of obstetrical opportunity that fell periodically from the master's table, the perils to pregnant African American women and their progenies during home deliveries were great and ever-present.

Primitive home deliveries performed by physicians who had not had internships nor other hospital experiences, and the absence of a nurse or hospital back-up for emergencies, made every delivery a potential disaster. The high maternal and infant morbidity and mortality rates among African Americans provided grim evidence of how often these potential disasters became real for all involved.

While this denial of hospital privileges weighed heavily on Dunbar's doctors, the wide-spread racism which permeated the fabric of their professional lives was constant. They had to make degrading and often fatal accommodations with this reality quite regularly.

By 1925, during the 10th year of his medical practice, Dr. Greenidge made many such accommodations which led him to take matters into his own hands. Since Dr. Greenidge's role is so prominent in much of the remainder of this very human drama, I will pause for a detailed introduction.

Robert I. Greenidge was born in British Guiana, South America in 1888, and was a British subject until he migrated to Battle Creek, Mich. in 1909. At that time, British Guiana was still one of the few outposts of the British Empire still maintaining its presence in the Americas; and the only one in South America. Guiana, the size of Idaho, occupies 83,000 square miles on the north coast of South America and is bounded by Venezuela on the west, Surinam on the east, Brazil on the south and the Atlantic Ocean on the north.

It was a Dutch possession in the 17th century; however, the British became its defacto rulers in 1796 when they colonized the country. They remained in control until May 26,

1966, when British Guiana ceased to be a British colony and became Guyana, a member of the British Commonwealth. Prior to the ending of enslavement in 1834, ships loaded with their human cargo made regular stops at the capital of Georgetown. Their main purpose was to replace the enslaved who had been worked to death on sugarcane plantations and to export cargoes of highly prized brown sugar to the rum manufacturers in New England.

When the international slave trade ended in 1807, formerly enslaved Guianeas fled from the plantations into the towns and villages to take advantage of all of the educational opportunities available to them. They anticipated receiving jobs as civil servants, clerks, teachers and skilled tradesmen.

At a time when U.S. slave codes were enforced and reconstructionist black codes made it a crime to teach African Americans how to read and write, Guiana had one of the best school systems in the region. Contrary to their Northern U.S. counterparts, the former slaves were encouraged to study.

Just as they'd done elsewhere in their far-flung colonial empire, the British survived the abolishment of African enslavement by hiring indentured servants, chiefly East Indians. Unlike their treatment of Africans, the British offered the Asians a five-year plan that enabled them to pay off the obligations of servitude and purchase a stake in the land. Today, East Indians own most of the land and constitute more than half of the population in Guyana.

Between 1838 and 1917, some 240,000 indentured workers were recruited as laborers for the plantations and by 1949, only 75,000 East Indians had returned home. The others remain as the most unassimilated groups in the entire country.

When Queen Victoria declared an end to British slavery in 1834, there was great rejoicing and thanksgiving among the 831,000 freedmen. Despite the anger and frustration among the plantation owners, there was no period of vindictive persecution or bloody violence as occurred during the U.S. Emancipation and Reconstruction periods thirty years later.

It was during the final period of enslavement that the first record of a Greenidge appeared on the Guiana scene. Isaac

Theophilus Greenidge was a white shipowner who operated a brisk business between Barbados and British Guiana, including slave trading. His son, Isaac I. Greenidge, abandoned the sea and became a mason and bricklayer in British Guiana.

The next descendant in the Guiana chain of Greenidges was Isaac I. Greenidge III, an engineer, who was chiefly employed at sugar estates. While at Plantation Industry, one of the estates located on the eastern coast about 16 miles from Georgetown, young Isaac became enamored with Angelina Greaves. She was described as a short, black woman hailing from nearby Buxton. Her forebearers had been imported and enslaved to toil on Guianas sugarcane plantations.

Following a brief courtship, Angelina bore a son for Isaac III on October 27, 1888, whom they named Robert Isaac Greenidge. Angelina never fully recovered from the delivery and died while Robert was still an infant. Fortunately the Seears family, Angelina's sister and brother-in-law, adopted young Robert and maintained custody over him throughout his youth. They discovered their young charge was bright and industrious and could read the *Bible* at the age of five. His first formal training was at the Christ Church School in Georgetown.

In 1897, he was transferred to Mrs. Sarples School for more advanced training. In October, 1900, Edward Blackman began teaching Robert privately at the Hand of Justice Hall. Blackman was so impressed with the aptitude of his student that he awarded him four English Certificates during his period of study.

Robert climbed the next rung of his academic ladder at the Stanislau School and College where he excelled in English, typing, and shorthand. Although St. Stanislau was not a true college, it did offer two years of study following high school which would have been considered the equivalent of junior college.

It was during this period that Robert took up the piano, organ and violin. He attended church regularly and sang in the choir. His violin was always close at hand. His daughter,

Roberta, recalled how the family often "suffered" through his impromptu, unsolicited violin solos at inopportune times.

Robert's high school work was interrupted by the death of his uncle, Robert Seears (his main source of support), on February 14, 1905. His aunt died soon afterwards, depressed by the death of her husband. In his diary, Robert described himself as being "relativeless" since he had not heard from his father in many years. He started thinking seriously about his future.

His job search took him to Kerr's Photo Studio where he found employment for $2 a month. This began his life-long romance with the camera and may have influenced his later decision to become an X-ray specialist. He soon left the photographic studio for a job at an auction house which paid a $1 more per month. Because business was often slow, he took to writing humorous articles to entertain his fellow employees.

One of these articles was entered in a local literary contest and won a prize. The sponsors of the contest published the winning essay in the *Argosy,* a Georgetown newspaper. The editor of the paper read the essay and immediately offered Robert a position as the manager's stenographer at a starting salary of 60 cents-per-week. When the full extent of Robert's writing skills and knowledge of grammar became obvious, his salary was increased steadily to $20 a month.

His aunt's death was a cause of great sadness for young Robert. His aunt and uncle had been the only maternal relatives. Robert soon became depressed and sought relief by going on binges that included "late hours, card playing, smoking and girls," a deviation from the straight and narrow path that his aunt had insisted he follow.

By nature, Robert made no real effort to cultivate close friends. He had a natural air of aloofness and preoccupation that discouraged intimacy. Thus his "binge" was short-lived and was followed by a period on meditation and introspection. In 1908 at age 20, he began to worry about his future and his responsibility for extending the family name into the next generation, in Guiana or elsewhere.

When he looked around at his peers in Georgetown, he saw laborers, small shopkeepers and petty politicians. Fortunately, he aspired to something more. With no family or close friends, his dependency on the Seventh Day Adventist Church, for help, increased; and he found solace in the form of a Christian conversion:

"As a child, I knew the Holy Scriptures. Those principles will never depart from me. They are in my innermost parts and are a part of my make up. If I am ever privileged to have a family, by the grace of God, the Christian influence shall and must be the prevailing scene in my home. May the Golden Rule sink more deeply, day by day, into my ego."

The supplicant underwent a renewing confirmatory, Christian experience, two years later: "One Sunday evening I visited the Adventist meeting in Georgetown and was in some way, I do not quite understand yet, practically transformed into a new man.

"My spirit was turned against women, although my flesh was weak. Yet, despite all the weakness of my flesh, I have miraculously kept from contact with such temptations until this day of September 18, 1910, for over two years. This was not a part of my own weak will. I, resolutely, decided to abide by the principles of the church."

The same divine inspiration that compelled Robert to embrace the Christian life led him to a decision to come to the U.S. It was no accident that he decided to come to Michigan and work in the Battle Creek Sanitarium. That health emporium was owned and controlled by the Kellogg family, one of the best-known Seventh Day Adventist families in the U.S.

Once the decision to leave Guiana was made, Robert moved quickly to close out that phase of his life. He requested a letter of recommendation from his employer at the Argosy. When efforts to dissuade Robert from departing failed, his employer bade him farewell with a very supportive letter to his next employer.

When Robert told the church officials of his decision to go to the U.S. to seek his fortune, they were certain that he

61

should go to their church in Battle Creek and work at the world famous Battle Creek Sanitarium. Like the management of the *Argosy,* the Church officials had learned to respect and trust Robert and they sent an equally glowing letter of recommendation.

The Argosy Co., Ltd.
Booksellers, Stationers,
Printers and Publishers
Georgetown

July 13, 1909

This serves to introduce Mr. Robert I. Greenidge, who goes to the United States to find his way in the world. He has been employed by this company for some time as a typist and correspondence clerk and has always given the utmost satisfaction. Polite, industrious and ambitious, he is almost certain to do well in any situation he obtains.

He has our best wishes for his future success.

J.R. Sennett, Manager

When Robert reached Battle Creek in July 1909, his arrival was anticipated by several people at "The San," as the Kellogg Sanitarium was referred to by nearly everyone. Armed with referrals from a reputable business firm and an influential religious body, plus a creative, inquiring mind, Robert departed his native land for the first time. He did not have much money, but his self-confident stride, knowing smile and no-nonsense approach to life portrayed sufficient self-esteem to make up for the shortfall.

Having undergone a Christian conversion as an Adventist before migrating to the U.S., Guiana church officials had made plans for Greenidge to live and work at the "San."

In addition to being one of the most well-known Adventists in the country, Dr. Henry Kellogg was also a celebrated surgeon and a great humanitarian. He attracted patients from across the nation and his apparent lack of racial prejudice set him apart from most of his contemporaries.

It was fortuitous that Robert spent his first two years in close, if not direct, contact with Dr. Kellogg. Before his arrival in Battle Creek, he had manifested, neither by word nor deed, even a latent interest in medicine as a career. Yet, upon leaving Battle Creek, two years later, he seemed drawn toward medical school, from which he obtained a M.D. degree in 1915.

When his bubble of hope, the Florence Crittenton Home, burst in his face years later, he entered into a phase of community entrepreneurship that was reflective of Dr. Kellogg's Battle Creek activities. These acts helped in part to save his sanity.

During his first 10 years in the U.S. (two with the Kellogg Sanitarium; four in Wayne Univ. Medical School; and four years practicing medicine), Dr. Greenidge had never come face-to-face with the brutal American residue of chattel slavery. Always quiet, reserved and dignified, he couldnt remember ever having been called a "nigger," not even in jest.

Without seeking the advice of his colleagues, Dr. Greenidge decided to try his own hand to strike a blow for freedom and justice for African American womanhood and her off-spring. He sought and kept his own counsel for a venture into unknown and dangerous territory.

Fortunately, Dr. Greenidge left a paper trail that describes his most embarrassing, painful, and unforgettable 30-minute journey to "niggerhood," a voyage all African Americans are forced to take, sooner or later.

This narrative is preserved in a series of revealing letters that expose the soul of one of the world's worst evils, the illusion of white supremacy. The letters were all authenticated by the signatures of their authors: M. Louise Hood, superintendent and Wayland D. Stearns, vice president of the Florence Crittenton Home; Percival Dodge, assistant secretary of the Detroit Community Union; and John Dancy, the executive secretary of the Detroit Urban League.

A careful reading of these letters and other pertinent data, provides a brief glance of racism at work, protecting the prerogatives of white supremacy. In preparation for what proved to be one of the most memorable series of events of his life, Dr. Greenidge did what he thought was careful, preliminary research which revealed that:

1. The Administrators of Detroit's Florence Crittenton Home, an obstetrical hospital, had never granted staff privileges to an African American physician.

2. The Hospital received a portion of its operating funds from the Detroit Community Union, a public fund.

3. Miss Hood had sent invitations to all the European American physicians in the vicinity, soliciting their obstetrical patronage. In strict conformity with the racist policies of the Crittenton Home, Hood went out of her way to make sure that no African American physician was solicited.

Dr. Greenidge made a handsome contribution to the Detroit Community Union, selected a test case, and bided his time. On the morning of February 28, 1925, the chosen patient called to inform Dr. Greenidge that she was in labor. Although not acquainted with the hospital's layout, he directed the patient to the Florence Crittenton Home without notifying the hospital staff. He arrived at the hospital soon after the patient did and somehow found his way to the Obstetrical area without being accosted.

Before he could completely disrobe and don his cap, mask, and delivery gown, Supt. Hood was notified that an unidentified black man had invaded their space. She sped to the scene and, undeterred by Dr. Greenidge's medical credentials, ordered him out of the hospital. The patient, having arrived earlier, had already been examined by the resident. She was found to be in early labor, therefore delivery was not anticipated for several hours.

Supt. Hood, now playing before a full house, pressed home her two demands while pretending that Dr. Greenidge was not in the room:

1. "Dr. Greenidge must leave, the hospital, forthwith! If he elects to do so, he can take his patient with him.

2. If she remains for delivery, it will be done by the resident who will take charge of and manage the delivery and provide post-partum care."

The prospect of discharging the patient from the hospital for a home delivery did not seem a very attractive option to the doctor nor the patient. Greenidge was aware that all eyes of his expanding European American audience were on him, expecting a reply. The few African American employees present were speechless and obviously embarrassed and uncomfortable.

Fortunately, the patient's husband intervened and transferred his wife to the resident's care. As quickly as possible, Dr. Greenidge gathered up his possessions, glanced at his watch and departed, a far different person than he had been upon arrival, 30 minutes earlier.

For the rest of his life, wherever he went, Dr. Greenidge was able to tell his audiences not just the hour but the minute when he was finally forced from the status of South American immigrant to that of "North American nigger." Whenever Dr. Greenidge relived that scene, he could never recall the exact details of how he escaped from that hostile event, though he did remember that the time was 11 a.m., and the date, February 25, 1925.

Down, but not out, Dr. Greenidge fought back. His first quest for relief was a letter to his friend, John Dancy, recounting the events and charging the hospital with racial discrimination. Dancy sent a letter of inquiry and a copy of Dr. Greenidges' letter to Percival Dodge, at Detroit Community Union, the funding source.

Dodge wrote to Stearns, who asked Hood for the details. Her reply was clear, straightforward and devoid of any hint of embarrassment or guilt:

Whenever a colored patient has made application for admittance, she has been informed that it will be necessary for her to enter under a white physician, usually our resident physician.

In August, we notified a large number of Wayne County physicians that we would be glad to have them bring patients to our hospital. A very careful check was made that no colored physicians were in the list.

Whenever a physician desires to make reservation for a patient, and the supervisor of the hospital or the superintendent receives the call, it is understood, and has been the custom, that any physician not known is asked the question if he or his patient is colored and answered accordingly.

Mrs. Matthews entered the hospital at 7:05 a.m. Her baby was delivered at 12:05. You note there were five hours for her to be removed from the hospital.

Upon returning to my office, I called Mr. Norton and discussed the matter with him, being assured by him that, inasmuch as it is not the policy of the

65

Home to permit colored physicians to bring in patients, I was told that I was justified in maintaining that policy and not to worry!

I do not feel that it is in good taste to accuse Dr. Greenidge of trying to put something over, but I must confess that it is significant that he was too wise to call either the supervisor of nurses or the superintendent.

To my knowledge, only the Woman's Hospital receives and permits colored physicians to bring in and attend patients, aside from the two hospitals for colored people—the Dunbar and the Mercy.

Yours very truly,

M. Louise Hood
Superintendent

Stearns sent Dodge a copy of Hood's letter, with this closing statement:

Miss Hood, in my opinion, explains the matter satisfactorily, and I trust that after reading her letter you will consider the matter closed.

Mr. Dodge passed the ball back to Dancy, whose letter had initiated the exchange, for final disposition:

Dear Mr. Dancy:

Enclosed is a letter from Mr. W.D. Stearns of the Florence Crittenton Home and a long explanation by Miss Hood. I am passing this correspondence on to you to take up with Dr. Greenidge, if you feel that advisable, or handle in any way you see fit. My only hope is that you will be able to satisfy Dr. Greenidge so that he will still remain a friend of the Community Fund.

Yours very truly,

Percival Dodge
Assistant Secretary

The only one who showed any remorse was Supt. Hood who wondered how well she had served the hospital's interest during this racial crisis. She was congratulated on her performance as the hospital's enforcer of its racist policy. When reassured that she was "justified" and need not worry, the matter, for her, was closed.

Whether Dancy transmitted the "Guardians of Status Quo" dismissal message to Dr. Greenidge or not, is unknown. I could not find that any of the other principals ever gave this matter a second thought. Even Mr. Dancy failed to mention this face-off in his book "Sands Against the Wind." On the other hand, it was one of Dr. Greenidge's most unforgettable and painful experiences and is recounted in many of his written speeches.

Since only Dancy expresses any sensitivity about Dr. Greenidge's mistreatment, the establishment left it up to him to apologize "only if you think it advisable."

Even to the end, Dodge reminded Dancy that he was in charge by issuing to him the final directive: "My only hope is that you will be able to satisfy Dr. Greenidge so that he will **still remain a friend of the Common Fund**!"

Dodge's final statement in this incredible exchange is highlighted to signify its importance as a technique used by white supremacists to retain absolute control. They must induce losers to continue to play their game; because they are convinced that theirs "is the only game in town." The fact that this assignment was passed on to Dancy informed both Greenidge and Dancy that the matter was closed.

It is understandable that Dr. Greenidge was never the same following that traumatic episode. His enduring feeling of vulnerability never allowed him to confront, head-on, the European American establishment again. Instead, he picked his self-esteem up from the floor, dusted it off, checked himself in the mirror of public opinion and took off in another direction.

It was at this time that Dr. Greenidge's creative entrepreneurship was aroused, forcing him to concentrate on developing those latent resources already existing in the African American community. He wasted no time weeping about the past.

It was at this time that his community interests broadened and took on characteristics similar to those which had been manifested by Dr. Kellogg in Battle Creek, who showed a strong interest in helping people that extended well beyond the field of medicine.

After the embarrassment at the Crittenton Home, a different Robert emerged.

In June 1925, just four months after the Crittenton episode, Dr. Greenidge attended the first meeting that led to the establishment of Detroit Memorial Park Cemetery which is still one of Michigan's oldest and most profitable African American businesses. He went on to help create Great Lakes Mutual Insurance Company; Victory Loan Association and Home Federal Savings and Loan Association. The East Side Medical Laboratory at 4839 Beaubien was his own, private creation.[7]

Like Detroit Memorial Park, Home Federal Savings and Loan Association still serves the community after 50 years and from several locations. The continuing success of these ventures is a tribute to a medical pioneer from Guyana who saw racism at its worse and dealt with it under his own terms.

Following Florence Crittenton's unchallenged ejection of Dr. Greenidge from its premises, it became abundantly clear that the African American physicians had no alternative but to meet this challenge themselves. Their most viable option was to try to improve the quality of care being provided at the 35-bed Dunbar Hospital.

Unfortunately, events at the hospital took a downward turn that eventually led to its transfer to a new site at Brush and Illinois streets and a name change to Parkside Hospital. It was their forlorn hope that a new name and a few cosmetic improvements in the hospital's amenities would bolster the public's sagging perspective of it.

Soon after it opened, Dunbar Hospital's administrators had entered into an agreement with the officials of Receiving Hospital to accept the city's overflow patients for hospital care at a per diem rate less than Receiving's—an arrangement that served the best interest of the hospitals, but not the patients.

Insofar as I have been able to determine, only African American patients were transferred from Receiving's new, efficiently operated facilities to the rather primitive facilities at the understaffed Dunbar. There was no follow-up by the Receiving Hospital staff after patients were transferred to Dunbar.

During my four years as a general practitioner, with Parkside as my main hospital, I don't recall that any patients were ever returned to Receiving Hospital because of deterioration in their conditions. Nor did I ever encounter a European American patient who was transferred from Receiving to Parkside. Many of the acutely ill patients died soon after being transferred, earning Dunbar/Parkside a bad reputation in the community.

For a brief time, Dunbar/Parkside Hospital officials were reported to have convinced an accrediting agency that the hospital was qualified to train interns. Dr. Joseph Dancy, John Dancy's brother, is said to have been its first intern.[8] However, the accreditation of Parkside Hospital for internship training was never officially recognized.

The hospital remained a source of contention throughout the nearly forty years of its existence. Instead of being rebuilt for African American management, as proposed by one faction of the Medical Center Authority, it was torn down in 1962 to allow the Medical Center Authority to build Receiving Hospital, on that site, as originally planned.

Thus, Dunbar/Parkside Hospital, Detroit's African American community's second venture into hospital administration, bowed out ungracefully as did Mercy General.

By mid-century, the stubborn refusal of the medical establishment to abandon its policy of racial segregation caused many African American physicians to seek their own private solutions to this thorny hospital problem. They built and operated more small, private hospitals in Detroit, than elsewhere in the country.

The best remembered of these later institutions were: **Bethesda** and **Edith K. Thomas Hospitals**, at 535 E. Garfield and **Haynes Memorial Hospital**, at 73 Palmer, which were all owned by the Drs. Alfred Thomas, Sr. and his son, Alfred, Jr.

Fairview, **Bethesda** and **Good Samaritan Hospitals** were the African American community's response to pleas for help from Dr. Chadwick, and other members of Detroit's Board of Health. A raging TB epidemic had overwhelmed the limited, segregated facilities at Herman Kiefer Hospital, causing the Department of Health to seek segregated alternatives elsewhere.

Rather than sit tight and force the Department of Health to abandon its policy of segregation at Herman Kiefer, the

69

Fairview TB Sanitarium was established in two apartment buildings at Ferry and Brush by Drs. Greenidge, Rupert Markoe and James McClendon.[9] This development is presented in considerable detail, later on.

Kirwood Hospital, then located at 301 E. Kirby, was founded in 1943 by Guy O. Saulsberry M.D. (Howard Univ., 1927). The building's first phase of reconstruction as a hospital yielded a facility of 27 beds. Two additional expansions provided a total of 50 beds at Kirwood's first site. The next move to Davison and Petoskey allowed the Hospital to expand to nearly 84 beds.

Early in his Detroit medical career, Dr. Saulsberry aspired to provide comprehensive care to his patients. Since his first affiliation was with the small, distant Delray Hospital in southwest Detroit, he tried to gain admission to the staff of, nearer by, Woman's Hospital, but his acceptance was less than cordial.

From that moment, Dr. Saulsberry worked night and day to establish his own hospital. His first purchase was the palatial home of two sisters at 301 E. Kirby. At first, they refused to sell it to him; however, they did sell the building, located only six blocks from Woman's Hospital, to his wife.

The first expansion was to an adjacent building which provided increased medical, surgical, and obstetrical care. Later, he purchased a third building, nearby, that was renovated to serve as a convalescent hospital.

Some of Dr. Charles Whitten's initial Sickle Cell research was done at Kirwood Hospital. In the spring of 1978, **Family Health Center**, an ambulatory care facility, became operational. It provided preventative care and offered advice on nutrition, hypertension and other maladies of major concern to the African American community.

For more than 25 years, Saulsberry worked diligently to prove to the medical establishment that he was a person who merited their attention and respect. His quest for a proper staff for his expanded hospital caused him to dispatch a trusted colleague, Dr. Tom Green, to the Philippines to recruit physicians to serve on Kirwood's staff.

Dr. Saulsberry's widow, Essell, recalled the pressures applied by the city and the medical establishment to force the hospital to move from its prime location. Medical Center developers, having met the minimum demands of the federal government for funding, were going full steam ahead. Cultural Center developers received authorization to demolish Kirwood Hospital and replace it with the Center for Creative Studies. [10]

This pressure forced Kirwood Hospital to close and move several miles northwest to Davison and Petoskey. By the time of Dr. Saulsberry's death in 1978, the diversionary effects on patient flow from the smaller hospitals—caused by the Medical Center—were well underway. Blue Cross and Blue Shield were disallowing hospital reimbursements at an alarming rate and competition from HMOs were on the rise. More African American medical specialists were being admitted to the university-affiliated general hospitals for training and staff affiliation, at the expense of the smaller, private, segregated institutions.

When Kirwood Hospital reopened at Davison and Petoskey for a second beginning, the administrative and medical staffs worked diligently to make the new hospital a profitable venture. Dr. Alma Rose George and Wilburn Phillips were named chief of staff and hospital director, respectively. Their medical acumen and foresight were essential in keeping the hospital going.

For several years, the Kirwood staff created a fund that was designated to assist in financing various hospital improvements. It was scrapped when they discovered that weather and age had rendered most of the building irreparable. The hospital was closed and partially demolished. The remainder was converted into a drug store.

The staff fund, accumulated to finance the proposed renovation, was comprised, in part, of tuition paid by podiatry students being trained at Kirwood Hospital. These funds were deposited in Home Federal Savings and Loan Association in Dr. George's custody.

With the approval of her former Kirwood colleagues, Dr. George added these funds to contributions from the Detroit Medical Society and the Society's Woman's Auxiliary to pay off the Dunbar Medical Museum's final mortgage of $34,934 on December 22, 1993. Words of appreciation were sent out to all of the contributors in these three organizations. Christmas, 1993 was celebrated with a mortgage-free Dunbar Memorial Museum for the first time since the historic landmark was purchased in 1977.

Neither Kirwood, nor any of the other small, private hospitals in Detroit's African American community, ever achieved full certification as first-rate, well-run institutions. Yet many provided unique opportunities that proximated what was denied them elsewhere due to racial bias. Reference is often made to the use of Kirwood Hospital for Dr. Whitten's sickle cell screening and training programs and also in Podiatry during Dr. George's tour of duty as medical director.

In 1967, the members of the board of trustees of Detroit's Museum of African American History realized that none of the available recruitment films for medical schools addressed potential African American medical students. The Museum's trustees entered into an agreement with the Detroit Medical Society to make a relevant film at Kirwood Hospital which provided an African American setting, cast of characters, etc.

A team of cinematographers, led by Carl Balduf, a member of the museum's staff, produced a film that was beautifully done in record time and at minimum cost. The very successful, 15-minute recruitment film was distributed nationally by the McGraw-Hill Book Co. and all of the profits flowed back to the Museum.

In his discourse on establishing Detroit's first HMO, Dr. Thomas Batchelor informed us that through his direct contact with the American Board of Regents of the American College of Physicians, "I became involved with the establishment of internship and residency programs through closer contact with the Joint Commission. This was the agency through which I was able to establish an approved residency for six people at Kirwood Hospital until 1969, when I moved to the Model Neighborhood Program."

The NMA celebrated its 100th Anniversary during the Atlanta meeting in July of 1995. The DMS and its Woman's Auxiliary are discussing plans to make the restored Dunbar Memorial Museum the jewel of Detroit's Medical Center as a follow-up to the historic event. Since Dunbar is our only remaining link to our eventful past, it deserves, and should become, the beneficiary of our best efforts.[11]

The members of the Detroit Medical Society were grateful for the triple play by the Auxiliary, DMS and Kirwood Hospital when they presented the Society a free and clear Christmas present in 1993.

Mt. Lebanon Hospital, at 2610 14th St., was founded by general practitioner Dr. C.W. Preston, who was the principal staff member. He was still practicing at the time of his death and his widow operated the hospital for a short while thereafter.

The founders of **Trinity Hospital**, Chester Ames, M.D. (Wayne Medical School); Harold Johnson, M.D. (Detroit College of Medicine); and Frank Raiford, Sr., M.D. (Univ. of Michigan) established their first hospital in a building on E. Congress and Dubois Streets in 1936. According to Frank Raiford, Jr., M.D., it was moved to 681 East Vernor Highway in 1942.

Trinity Hospital was the major source of post-graduate, surgical training for African American physicians prior to the availability of such appointments to certified residency programs elsewhere. Drs. Walter Mack, Johnny Green, and Robyn Arrington were among the early beneficiaries of this program. Many of those physicians resided in and dined at Trinity as residents during their training.

Starting in the late 1950s, pressure from the African American community, led by members of the DMS, forced the large, general hospitals to integrate their training programs. Only then did certified residencies become available to African Americans physicians within Detroit.

The community owes a debt of gratitude to those hospitals, especially Trinity, for continuing the struggle for good medical care until public and governmental pressures forced the medical establishment to abandon some of its racist prerogatives.

As inferred earlier, during the first half of the 1960s, several events served notice that the days of the small, proprietary hospitals—African and European American—were numbered. Among those events were:

1. Soaring maintenance costs and limited reimbursement from third party payers, especially Blue Cross, when major economic factors contributed to the decline and eventual fall of the independent proprietary hospitals.

2. According to Dr. Frank Raiford, Jr., son of one of its founders, Trinity Hospital, like Mercy, Dunbar, Parkside and Kirwood was also condemned and razed to clear the right-of-way for developments of a higher priority:

"We were paid $200,000 for the Trinity property and invested it in the rehabilitation of Resthaven Hospital at 1852 West Grand Boulevard." Resthaven had been a TB hospital until the introduction of antibiotics made such institutions obsolete.

Resthaven was in such a state of disrepair that renovation costs exceeded the estimate, and the project went into bankruptcy. Blue Cross added to Trinity's woes by reducing its reimbursement rate to $15 per day. Unable to continue, Trinity's officials turned their interest over to an independent group of physicians who sought legal advice on removing themselves from bankruptcy. Upon the advice of counsel, this new group formed the Crestwood Corporation, assessed themselves $1,000 each to raise operational funds, and resumed "normal" operations.

The new facility, reborn as **Boulevard General Hospital**, attracted a staff of more than 40 physicians. With assistance from Detroit's fiscal guru, Alfred Pelham, and under the administration of George Allen, Blue Cross was sufficiently impressed with a pledge of $5,000 from each member of the Crestwood Group to restore Boulevard General Hospital's full affiliation, enabling it to seek and find relief from the burdens of bankruptcy.

These emergency measures only delayed temporarily, Boulevard General Hospital's eventual merger with Burton Mercy, Delray and Trumbull General Hospitals to create **Southwest Detroit Hospital**.

Two additional hospitals that served the community well for a number of years were located on Eliott St., between John R and Brush. Wayne Diagnostic Hospital was a joint venture between Drs. Chester Ames and D.T. Burton.

DeWitt T. Burton, M.D. (1892-1970), graduated from Meharry Medical College in 1921 and immediately began his private practice in Detroit on McGraw St. Responding to the racially discriminatory practices of the period, Burton formed a medical partnership with Dr. Ames. They established the 50-bed Wayne Diagnostic Hospital on the north side of Eliott St. and Wayne Diagnostic (No.2) for mental patients, diagonally across the street, adjacent to the offices of the *Michigan Chronicle.*

Dr. Ames served an internship, a residency in urological surgery and for a brief period, was a member of Wayne State Univ. Urology medical faculty. He brought to the partnership more experience in hospital development than was available elsewhere in the African American community.

The Wayne Diagnostic Hospital proved to be very popular and attracted the support of many of Detroit's newly-arrived physicians during the late 1930s and early 1940s. Just before the 50-bed Wayne Diagnostic Hospital was expanded into the 96-bed Burton Mercy Hospital, Dr. Ames suffered an acute heart attack and died. D.T. Burton's (D.T.) wife and helpmate since 1922, Alice, stepped forward to assist him in bringing the hospital's expansion project to full fruition.

When the NMA held its 1949 convention in Detroit, the hospitals transition from Wayne Diagnostic to Burton Mercy was all but complete.

The delegates found that the training opportunities at Trinity and Burton Mercy Hospitals were increasing and the quality of medical care at the African American owned hospitals significantly improved. The number of residents in training elsewhere, but headed toward Detroit, was also encouraging.

During the last two decades of his life, D.T. was in the thick of Detroit's struggle for freedom of choice and racial justice. Aside from direct medical involvement through hospitals and the DMS, board trusteeships in the Boy Scouts of America, NAACP, the United Negro College Fund, the Urban League, Wayne State University and the YMCA, all helped to maximize his influence many times over. In 1956, for instance, his quiet diplomacy, during a financial crisis helped produce a million-dollar grant for his alma mater, Meharry Medical College.

D.T.'s death in February 1970 was a great loss for Detroit and the medical community, in particular. The recognition of that event by his 72 "Honorary" pallbearers from all segments of the community symbolized the highest regard and respect for a true medical entrepreneur. For a brief moment, the moguls and minions mingled at his bier to pay their final respects to our dearly, beloved D.T.

Dr. Burton's youngest child, Gail, M.D. (New York Univ.), carried on the family's medical tradition as a psychiatrist in the first generation of the Burton progeny. The second generation of medical Burtons include:

1. Alicia Heron, M.D. (Univ. of Mich., 1974)
2. Alva Heron, M.D. (Meharry, 1976)
3. Cal Dudley, M.D. (Meharry, 1980)

Alice Burton's on-the-job training began long before Dr. Ames' death. It prepared her to steer the Burton Mercy Hospital ship with a steady, but questioning hand until it merged with Boulevard General, Delray and Trumbull General Hospitals to form the 246-bed, $21 million Southwest Detroit Hospital in 1979. Although it was not obvious at the time, this move became the end stage of Detroit's 75-year reign as the "African American Hospital Capital of the United States."

The closure of the above hospitals and their merger to form Southwest Detroit Hospital were proof positive that the establishments earlier prediction of the fate of the small hospitals was coming to pass.

Among the assets accumulated by the Boulevard General staff, prior to the merger, was a fund of approximately $25,000. Upon hearing of their plans for a huge "going away party," I approached the doctors with a proposal for a joint venture with Detroit's Museum of African American History, to invest the money in a mural for the lobby of the Southwest Detroit Hospital to be painted by Detroit's most renowned muralist, Leroy Foster.

The idea found favor among the Boulevard Hospital staff and Foster was commissioned to paint a 9 x 28 oil, entitled **"Kaleidoscope."** Southwest's administrators were so pleased with this decision that they agreed to share the cost of the mural.

A contract was signed on July 9, 1974, between Dr. Dwight E. Stith, representing the Boulevard General Hospital, and Leroy Foster. Robert Shannon, president of the board of trustees of the Museum of African American History, the patron and sponsor, witnessed the signatures.

During the somewhat extended negotiations, Foster gave considerable thought to the commission. For the title, he chose "Kaleidoscope." Contemplating the blank canvas, with brush in hand, he reminisced:

"The great exhilaration I felt, when I learned that I was to be given the chance to paint a mural in the lobby of Southwest Detroit Hospital, lasted for a few, happy days. Then it began to give way, bit by bit, to a most irritating dilemma. What do you paint on the wall of a hospital? A painter is often hampered by having to illustrate some theme that is complicated, trite, uninteresting, or otherwise not to his liking. But what does he do when given "carte blanche" and no scenario to follow?" (See photo of "Kaleidescope").

Exactly 22 months after the contract was signed, the mural was unveiled on Sunday, May 7, 1976, in the lobby of Southwest Detroit Hospital before a large and appreciative audience. Among them, with words of thanks and praise, were:

1. Augustus Calloway, president of board of trustees, Southwest Detroit Hospital.

2. Delford G. Williams, Sr., M.D. representing the former Boulevard General Hospital Staff.

3. Mrs. Elvin Davenport, member of Arts Commission of the Detroit Institute of Arts.

4. Mrs. Joyce Garrett, executive director, Detroit Bicentennial Commission.

5. Charles H. Wright, M.D., founder and chairman, board of trustees of Detroit's Museum of African American History.

In nearly two decades of the Southwest's stormy course, the mural has dominated the hospital's entire lobby. Most viewers who expressed an opinion of the painting, marvelled at the immensity of the 9 x 28 oil and the skill of the artist who conceived and executed such a masterpiece.

Others, facing the illness and loss of loved ones, praised the artist for the welcomed diversion he provided, during which they were able to replenish their sagging reserves return to the scene of battle and resume their struggles to cope.[12]

In 1993, Southwest Detroit Hospital found itself in a cul-de-sac. In an effort to avoid direct competition with the hospitals in the Medical Center and to profit from their prior hospital experiences, Southwest's developers had chosen a remote section of the city, inhabited for the most part by African and Latino Americans.

Another earlier prediction of the "kiss of death" for Southwest followed the decision to allow the construction of an Osteopathic hospital nearby on Martin Luther King Drive.

Southwest filed for bankruptcy protection in August 1991. In August 1993, a U.S. attorney tried to convince the bankruptcy court to proceed with an immediate sale of the property to a group of investors, Life Choice Quality Health Plan, represented by Robin Barclay and Harley Brown.

After Life Choice's heroic efforts to save the hospital began, the value of the property was reported to have increased "appreciably." They claimed better marketing had increased the enrollment to 26,700 and that health care clinics in Wayne County had increased from 3 to 51. Community Health Care Providers, acknowledging previous mismanagement by prior administrators, tried to convince the bankruptcy court that they had been able to raise the $3 million purchase price and had already accumulated operating funds and sufficient experience to operate the facility successfully.

The bankruptcy court had heard all of this before and was not very responsive to the entreaties of Life Choice's investors. The final epitaph on the burial site of Detroit's long African American hospital effort appeared in the *Detroit Free Press* on November 19, 1993, seventy-five years after Mercy General Hospital opened its doors in 1918: "Hospital unlikely to reopen after auction of its HMO. Its health maintenance organization was sold at bankruptcy court auction, Friday.

"The federal government has begun foreclosure proceedings on the Detroit hospital building and adjacent property and is looking for a buyer," Assistant Attorney Julia Caroff, said Monday.

After the sale, the hospital property reverted to the Department of Housing and Urban Development to be maintained until a new owner is found. For the first time since 1918, Detroit did not have a hospital for which an African American could claim ownership.

The cloudy outlook of Southwest Detroit Hospital's building makes the future prospects of Leroy Foster's mural, **Kaleidoscope,** uncertain. Under the best of circumstances, the building will continue to serve as a public gathering place where those in charge will appreciate and preserve this magnificent painting.

If such is not possible, all is not lost. The mural was painted on a canvas in Foster's studio, transported to the Hospital and hung on the wall on a single canvas. Foster confirmed that the mural's dimensions are as stated above. The matter was discussed with several artists. They seem quite sure that the painting can be removed from the present wall, intact, to another site, if necessary.

Early in March 1995, I learned that Andre Lee had returned to Detroit to reopen Southwest Detroit Hospital. Having met him some years ago, first when he was the administrator of Highland Park (Mich.) General Hospital and aware that he had been the administrator of Meharry's Hubbard Hospital, more recently, I decided to interview him, just before this book went to press, on March 13, 1995. We met in his office at the former Southwest location.

My first question dealt with his background in hospital administration, to try and determine why he had come back to Detroit to take on a responsibility at which others had tried and failed.

"As you know, I have been a hospital CEO four times and four of them, including this one, have been black institutions —Highland Park, Sumby, George Hubbard and this one. I was offered jobs in Houston and Fairfield, Ala., but I didn't take them. I was offered a job at Southwest hospital in Atlanta. It began as a Catholic Hospital but became black.

"A group contacted me who wanted to keep this hospital going, and they wanted someone that could help them to do it. They hired me as a consultant about two years ago. It is about to reopen, and the question is 'how do we go about doing it in light of today's managed care market and increased competition to keep it open?'

"So, I decided to reopen this hospital in light of those conditions. It has to reopen as a hospital of the future, which means that whatever thoughts and plans I have must be realized within the next five years.

"The only way that it can work is that I must be a fortune teller. The hospital must be low-cost in its operation, and we must be creative. It has to be a hospital that is not dependent on patient care, but it has to function as a hospital without walls.

"It also has to be entrepreneurial (a goldmine) that allows for joint ventures and not just medical care, but mainly medical. In this case, it means hospice, home health, billable medical equipment, pharmacy, all those things in the future under medical reform."

Wright: "Isn't this a formidable undertaking?"

"I think so. I'm a businessman. Very few people know this, but I started the first two black hospices in this country: the first in Nashville, Tenn., and the second in New Orleans. I also helped to start the third in Greenville, Miss. I own and operate the only hospice chain in this country—two now, with three more opening this year.

"As an entrepreneur, I have owned and operated a home health agency and other manners of entrepreneurial businesses. I

80

have a business background in hospital administration. Hospices, that I own, make money. I feel that if we structure this thing organizationally, keep costs low, keep it efficient, maintain a flat management structure, place emphasis on direct patient care and a variety of entrepreneurial money with risk-takers willing to invest, I feel that we will make money.

"True, it has been difficult finding blacks to invest, but there are some around. There are a handful but not very many that are willing to come in and do some things. They are going to have to put up some money to start the home health and I will let them make more money up to a certain point. Then the hospital will kick in its shares. I'm affording them the opportunity, and the space for which they pay rent.

"I'm going to open up half of the 156 beds we have here. That means half the space is available for rent and lease to these entrepreneurs. That space has been leased out. That part is done. Then, of the beds we are going to operate, 136 are going to be psychiatric beds. We've gotten indications that we can get a contract for those beds, guaranteeing that they will be filled.

"The gap we have, at this time, is the remaining beds, and an HMO has submitted a tentative commitment for 25% of them. I am trying to get a commitment for 1/2 of the remainder from two HMOs. I'm trying to work a deal, like the Godfather, "that they can't refuse." I will offer these beds at a tremendous discount, if they will guarantee me the income for those patient days. In other words, buy the patient days in advance, and I will discount the beds as close to fixed costs as possible.

"There is a fixed cost, even if you just open the hospital's door. However, it doesn't remain fixed. We have to negotiate contracts very closely. I realize that whatever I do, I will have only six months to a year of lead time before other hospitals with deeper pockets and richer resources start to catch up. At that point, I'd better be able to shift gears and go in another direction."

Wright: "Well, you're in the right spot for that. I discovered that the City's forefathers wanted to get Southwest Hospital, down here, in Spanish town and out of competition with those hospitals that feed into the Medical Center and the Medical School. African and Spanish Americans aren't known for their joint ventures anyway."

"I am going to try, very hard, to employ a balanced mix among African, Latin and Arab Americans, so that the first person seen by a visitor will not always be black. The second thing is that I realize that we were put here for a reason. I will, probably, have well-oiled transportation vehicles at my disposal so that it will be easy for you to come see me."

Wright: "Are there problems between the osteopaths, located close by, and Southwest?"

"There's nothing I can do about that. I take what's there and make do with it. I understand that they're struggling too. As far as I am concerned, they are a part of the competition.

"I am trying to structure this operation so that if I can get some cooperation from HMOs to sell these beds in advance of my opening, it won't matter if AOA is there."

Wright: "Timeline?"

"We anticipate being up and running sometime this summer. That's driven more by Southwest's refurbishing and renovation than anything else. The biggest job is replacing the transformer which contains PCBs. That's an 8-week job. The building is pretty much as it was the day it was closed. They've maintained everything.[13]

"The mural, Kaleidoscope, is one of the most impressive things about this hospital. I thing it is symbolic of what we are all about. And I have no intention of taking it down.

"I had gone back to Meharry to run their hospital. And, I helped with their merger with the City Hospital. My business partners really wanted me to stay, but I had already made a commitment to come here and finish this project. I must stay until I am sure its on solid ground. So, I'll stay as long as I'm useful, then I'll go back to my business.

"As a Mr. Fixit, I must make sure that the project remains open and viable. There's too much money in health care for us to be struggling. People need to realize that this is almost a $100 billion business. From a business perspective, the money shifts around a bit, but, it still flows.

"Cost containment and cost cutting are mandatory in health care. But if you notice, it doesn't change the overall dollar value going through the system. The dollar value steadily climbs upward."

Lee was happy about being chosen to direct the administrative affairs of Southwest Detroit Hospital, as it begins its struggle toward economic solvency and medical responsibility. While our interview dealt almost entirely with the former, Lee's many experiences and contacts must be evaluated objectively to determine his ability to meet, and master, the many challenges of a viably reconstituted Southwest Detroit, now called United Community Hospital.

1. *AMA Journal*, Vol. 252. (Dec. 25, 1984) p. 3391.

2. George B. Catlin, *The Story of Detroit.* (Detroit: The Detroit News, 1926) pp. 481-483.

3. John C. Dancy, *Sands Against the Wind.* (Detroit: Wayne State Univ. Press, 1966) pp. 146-148.

4. Francis H. Warren, *Michigan Manual of Freedmens Progress Commission.* (1915). Republished by John M. Green (1968).

   On page 388 of the same manual, Dr. James Ames wore an inspectors hat for Detroit's Board of Health and offered a sobering look at the health, housing and economic conditions in the congested regions of the city. He reserved his closing remarks for his fellow physicians:

   "A half century of freedom has given to the world several thousand physicians, who are well equipped and ever-ready to do battle anew with death for a long-lived and more efficient people. Negro physicians should lead in urging every community to become actively interested in sanitary methods. It is one thing to be successful in treating sickness and curing disease, but far more profitable to the community-at-large is to prevent sickness and baffle disease."

5. Warren, p. 340.

6. Dancy, pp. 145-147.

7. Roberta H. Wright, *Detroit Memorial Park Cemetery.* (Detroit: Charro Book Co., 1993).

8. Dancy, p.146.

9. Due to overcrowding and congestion, the incidence of pulmonary tuberculosis was always higher in Detroit's African American communities than elsewhere. These conditions worsened in the late twenties, by the city's economic depression and Herman Keifer's Hospital policy of racial segregation that confined African American patients to a portion of one floor of the hospital.

   This wave of TB caused Herman Kiefer officials to face two options: desegregate the hospital or seek accommodations for the overflow of African American patients elsewhere. They chose the latter solution. Dr. Chadwick, of the Herman Kiefer staff, met with a group of African American physicians and convinced some of them to establish several segregated TB hospitals to help control the epidemic. Fairview Hospital at Ferry and Brush, operated by Drs. Greenidge, Markoe, and McClendon, was the community's major responses to the plea.

   Dr. Greenidge had already reclaimed his boyhood training and experience as a photographer by becoming an X-ray specialist. Unable to secure an X-ray residency anywhere, he began the more difficult, prolonged route of periodic, post-graduate X-ray courses at Cook County Hospital in Chicago.

   Although he went on to become a certified roentgenologist in 1941, he was never admitted to the Herman Kiefer staff, nor did he make rounds there. Dr. Rupert Markoe was a pulmonary specialist and Dr. McClendon was a general practitioner. They worked together at Fairview for more than 30 years.

10. According to Stephen Y. Nose, Director of Corporate and Foundation Affairs, "CCS is one of the nation's leading arts education institutions. Located in Detroit's University Cultural Center, its College of Arts and Design offers a Bachelor of Fine Arts. Non-degree programs in music and dance are offered through the institutes of Music and Dance.

11. One of Dr. Daisy Northcross' two sisters was the mother of Dr. Remus Robinson, Detroit's first African American, board-certified surgeon. The other sister was the mother of Dr. William Goins, Detroit's second (to Lewis Boddie) African American, board-certified, obstetrician-gynecologist. All three future physicians, Remus, William and David were cousins. They grew up in and were influenced by the Mercy Hospital environment.

12. The brochure that announced the construction of the Southwest Detroit Hospital, in 1974, disclosed that four smaller hospitals were being merged to realize this goal: Boulevard General, Burton Mercy, Delray General, and Trumbull General Hospitals.

13. "Harley Brown has a pharmacy and other buildings. He has invested perhaps $1.5 million to keep the building up. HUD helps also. The only way that I can see him recovering his investment is for the money to flow into an investment group that agrees to reimburse him over time. Otherwise, he loses his investment. He was committed to the black community to keep it open. He should get an award, and I'll be the first to suggest it."

The Medical Gospel
According to Abraham:
The Flexner Report—1910

Even before the NMA was organized in 1895, members of the AMA had already decided in 1847 that their future members would have to run the gauntlet of approval by other pre-existing members before gaining admission to the AMA.

Since this rule, and others similarly imposed, was made during the period of enslavement, the intent of the measure was quite clear. Nearly every effort by African American physicians to by-pass this strangle-hold on their professional abilities and advancement, since 1847, has been stoutly resisted. The main impediments, as presented above, have been put in place by the members of the medical establishment.

The findings, actions, and the results of the Flexner Committee provide typical examples of how the establishment deals with trespassers who stray into their territory. African Americans who were denied or granted only limited admission to existing medical schools, sought to level the playing field by initiating an institution of their own in 1882. They had established the NMA in 1895 and had also begun to build and staff their own hospitals at the turn of the century.

Such a display of independent entrepreneurship by African American physicians attracted the attention and hostility of the medical establishment. Their response was to create an investigating committee under the sponsorship of the AMA and financed by the Carnegie Foundation, and was chaired by Abraham Flexner.

The Flexner Report

Although he was not a physician, and of doubtful qualification for this enormous responsibility, Abraham Flexner was given the authority, "To investigate and recommend methods for establishing uniform standards of accreditation for operating medical schools."[1]

From 1906-1910, the committee's investigations revealed, according to Flexner: "A proliferation of substandard medical training programs that demanded corrective measures." The findings and recommendations, entitled *The Flexner Report: Medical Education in the United States and Canada,* became the yardstick by which physician preparedness to practice medicine has been measured since that time.[2]

Although the committee indicated that they had investigated many substandard medical schools during their four-year study, those operated by African Americans received the harshest criticism.[3]

These maligned medical schools were created by African American physicians in an heroic effort to survive the pervasive racism tightly woven into the fabric of the AMA, during and following the period of slavocracy.

Reaching for conformity with the prevailing and popular practice of African American enslavement, the newly-established AMA ruled that each of its state's affiliates was sovereign unto itself and would handle its racial matters as it saw fit. This establishment endorsement of a U.S. Supreme Court-approved policy of racial discrimination and segregation rendered the Flexner Committee possible and necessary.

In 1903, AMA President Dr. Frank Billing announced in his inaugural address, "The status of medical college education is very much improved in the last 20 years. The advances in medical knowledge have been greater during that period than in all preceding time."

However, the Flexner Committee found that there was no uniformity in the medical curricula of the uncertified medical schools. A thorough investigation was concentrated on the most prosperous African American medical schools: Howard Univ., Washington, D.C.; Flint Medical College, New Orleans, La.; Leonard Medical School, Raleigh, N.C.; Knoxville College and Memphis Medical Department of the University of Western Tennessee, Nashville, Tenn.; Meharry Medical College and Louisville National Medical College, Louisville, Ky.[4]

Time, space, nor intent will allow an adequate critique of the Flexner Report, so I'll make a few observations, some 85 years later, with regard to the Louisville National Medical College (LNMC) with which I am most acquainted.

When Dr. Henry Fitzbutler, a Canadian, graduated from the Univ. of Mich. Medical School in 1872, there were already two African American doctors in Michigan, and Kentucky had never had any—so Dr. Fitzbutler chose to practice in Louisville. Since internships were unknown, he opened his office soon after graduation.

The University of Kentucky's first medical school was started in Louisville in 1837, twenty-eight years before the Emancipation Celebration and 35 years before Fitzbutler's arrival. The second medical school did not open until 1960. Its freshman class admitted only one African American, Carl Webber Watson of Lexington, nearly a half century after Dr. Fitzbutler's school was closed.

Having never trained an African American physician, and with no immediate prospects for doing so, the grateful Kentucky Reconstructionists assisted Fitzbutler with donations of land, equipment, supplies, and money sufficient enough to allow him to open his school to five medical students in 1888.

Although the endowments from the Kentucky establishment were most helpful in launching LNMC, the personal resources of the founders, alumni and their friends were required to keep the school operational for 24 years. The graduates provided medical care to thousands of victims suffering the legacy of enslavement when no other medical resources were available to them. An increasing number of African American babies were delivered by doctors than by midwives and thereafter until the school was forced to close.

Despite the limitations of these schools and their faculties, the African Americans who were in greatest need for medical care were the patients of those physicians who had graduated under the hammer of the Flexner Committee.

The Flexner Committee issued a blanket charge that these medical school officials were profiteers with "absolutely no regard for the public welfare and without any serious thought of the interests of the public." This statement was a disservice to the African American physicians and patients who were victims of a racist system that neither they, the patients, nor the students had created nor could they control.

Their efforts to survive the system were subjected to ridicule and contempt by the medical establishment. Ultimately, all but two of the schools were closed rather than being assisted toward "acceptability."

Flexner's 1909 report of the status of the LNMC, released a year before the other schools, allowed LNMC unhampered exposure to national criticism for trying to make the best of a bad situation. It had 23 faculty members and 40 students. The facilities were reportedly inadequate and its financial resources were all but exhausted. It was permanently closed in 1912, twenty-four years after it opened. The Flexner Report indicated that only six of the many closed schools were operated by African Americans. The Committee cited them as having few, if any, "redeemable qualifications."

At that time, the U.S. had abandoned all efforts to reconstruct its centuries-old slavocracy. The U.S. Supreme Court had ruled that all of the civil rights laws passed during Reconstruction were unconstitutional. Restored officials of the Secessionist states were busily replacing their slave codes with "black codes." While passage of the 13th Amendment on January 31, 1865, removed the possibility of a return of slavocracy, the implementation of a facsimile was well underway.

The full "gospel according to Abraham," decreed that: "Of the seven medical schools for Negroes in the U.S., only those schools at Howard Univ. in Washington, D.C., and Meharry Medical College in Nashville, were worth saving."

The others "were of varying degrees of proficiency and authority, and were awarding medical degrees to medical students, many of whom were not qualified to practice medicine. ... They are wasting small sums of money, annually, and are sending out undisciplined men (and women) whose lack of training is covered up by the imposing M.D. degree. The upholding of Howard and Meharry will profit the nation much more than the inadequate maintenance of a larger number of schools."

The full report, published under the title: *Medical Education in the United States and Canada; A Report To The Carnegie Foundation For The Advancement of Teaching,* offered a detailed and highly critical study of the status of medical practice at that time in the U.S. and Canada:

1. "The majority of the maligned medical schools were still privately owned and commercially operated for profit at low professional standards. The curricula varied widely from school to school. The M.D. degree was available to charlatans as well as to honest, qualified physicians.

2. "Entrance requirements for some uncertified medical schools were non-existent, and unenforced in others. Anyone who could afford the price of attendance could secure a position in a medical school of choice" [if he or she were not an African American].

3. "There is an enormous over-production of uneducated and ill-trained medical practitioners graduating from these schools."

A reduction in the number of medical graduates (and medical schools) and a radical reform of the methods of teaching were proposed. The goal became "to produce fewer, better-trained graduates who could fill medical positions of high caliber."

A college diploma with credits in chemistry, biology and physics was recommended for admission to a medical school. This premedical preparation was to be followed by a four-year medical curriculum, consisting of fundamental courses taught in laboratories and lecture rooms the first two years, and clinical work in medicine, surgery and obstetrics the last two years. A fifth year of hospital training, the internship—endorsed and advised several years earlier by the AMA—was declared *mandatory* for all medical school graduates.

The Flexner Report was welcomed and adopted by the AMA. Its Council on Medical Education was authorized to prepare and enforce Standards of Accreditation for all medical schools. Within a few years, the discredited medical schools, unable to achieve accreditation under the articles of Abraham, disappeared from the scene.

The implementation of the Flexner Report, with its principal rebuke of those medical schools owned and operated by African Americans, placed impossible burdens of responsibility on Howard and Meharry Medical Schools to supply even the minimum number African American physicians to those communities where they were needed most.

Within a year of the published findings, the Flexner Committee ceased to exist. The Carnegie Foundation and the General Education Board of the Rockefeller Foundation, however, were encouraged to respond to a plea from Meharry's board of trustees; and each organization appropriated a conditional grant of $150,000 to Meharry with one stipulation:

"Upon the retirement of Meharry's president, George W. Hubbard, a man of scientific training in medicine would be chosen to succeed him" and, "Meharry would be reorganized along modern lines."

This $300,000 conditional grant from two of the nation's wealthiest funds was the beginning of the chronic underfunding of one of the two main sources of African American physicians since Flexner.

There is no question that both Meharry's and Howard University's medical schools were improved by the timely intervention of the Flexner Commissioners and the philanthropic infusions that followed. But neither the AMA nor any other agency attempted to eliminate the root cause of the proliferation of substandard medical schools—racism in the medical establishment.

At that time, few American medical schools admitted African American medical students except those being operated by African Americans. None of the medical schools affiliated with the Southern universities did so. The few Northern medical schools that accepted an occasional African American medical student imposed a strict quota policy of one, but not many more than two per year. Those few African Americans who were fortunate enough to be included in the annual quota were not given equal opportunity with their European American classmates. It was not "more," for them, but considerably "less."

In Detroit, for instance, the denial of internships to African American medical graduates is but one of many examples of this inequality of opportunity that the Flexner Committee did not correct.

Against the recommendation of the AMA's own Council on Medical Education in 1906 and its reaffirmation in the Flexner Report that "the internship is an indispensable part of the physician's training," none of the Michigan-trained, African American physicians was accepted as interns in any Detroit hospital until 1926—eleven years after the city-owned, Detroit Receiving Hospital was built in 1915.[5,6]

A casual reading of the Flexner's Report gives the impression that the medical establishment played no role in creating the inadequate medical school and hospital conditions that the Flexner Commissioners criticized and were paid to correct. Such was not the case.

Since the *Plessy v. Ferguson* decision of 1896, and more specifically, since the *Berea v. Kentucky* decision of 1906, the U.S. Supreme Court abdicated its authority to enforce the "separate but equal" provisions of *Plessy v. Ferguson* and allowed the several states, beginning with Kentucky, to do as they pleased.[7]

As seen through the prism of their assumed, white superiority, it was impossible for members of the medical establishment to understand why those "inferior African Americans" were dissatisfied with their "secondariness" and tried so hard to prove that it was not true.

Only when the members of the medical establishment accept their African American colleagues as equal fellow human beings will "gospels according to Flexner" become obsolete, to the benefit of everyone.[8,9]

The net benefit of the investigative work of the Flexner Committee on African American physicians and their patients left much to be desired. Although all of the surviving medical schools emerged stronger, none of those which discriminated against African Americans (which were all of the Southern medical schools excluding Howard and Meharry) was required by the government, the Flexner Committee, nor their funding sources to integrate their classes or their faculties. Those few schools that accepted African American students, interns or residents did so on a quota system that was woefully inadequate to meet even their minimum needs.

During the first half of the 20th century, the few Southern universities that had practiced racial segregation in their medical schools allowed some reimbursement to African American medical students who were accepted elsewhere. These arrangements were both inadequate and condescending.

The Flexner Committee also ignored the accomplishments of the many graduates of these maligned schools who went on to distinguished careers (medical and otherwise.) Among those Leonard alumni elected to the presidency of the NMA were Dr. John Kenney (1913), Dr. John P. Turner (1921), and Dr. John O. Plummer (1924).

Dr. John Kenney, Sr., was the senior member of the only father and son team to serve as presidents of the NMA (1913 and 1963, respectively). The senior Kenney was editor of the *JNMA* for 32 years and was the founder and director of Tuskegee's famous John A. Andrews Clinic until he was forced to flee from the Ku Klux Klan.

It wasn't until the explosions of the civil rights revolution in the mid-20th century, heralded by the School Board (1954) and Bus Boycott (1956) decisions and the passage of the Civil Rights Act (1957) that any significant relief emerged from the racism of the medical establishment.

One of the earliest torchbearers to cast the light of constructive criticism on the Flexner Report was Hubert A. Eaton, M.D., in his informative book *Every Man Should Try.*[10] His father, Dr. Chester Arthur Eaton graduated from Leonard Medical School in 1910 along with four other African Americans.

94

Leonard was established in 1882 and was affiliated with Shaw University in Raleigh, N.C. It is reported to be the first U.S. medical school to adopt a four-year curriculum.

LMC, the oldest of the African American medical schools under seige, was closed as an aftermath of the Flexner Report. On his word, the schools were rated A, B, or C. The C's vanished shortly after his pronouncement.

It is understandable that the Eatons, both Carolinians and physicians with abiding concerns for Freedom and Justice, would question the authority given to Abraham Flexner to shut off an important source of African American physicians when other options were available.

Dr. Hubert Eaton felt that the Flexner Report was "too readily accepted, at face value by the American Public."

When he graduated from the Univ. of Mich. and took the State Board for licensure to practice in North Carolina in 1942, his average passing grade was 89%. Thirty-two years earlier, his father's grade, upon graduating from the Leonard Medical School was 84%. Four of his Leonard classmates also took the medical board examination in 1890 and their average score was 84.4 percent. The remaining examinees were from 12 other "approved" medical schools. Their average score was 85.8, a mere 1.4 percent difference.

When Hubert compared the scores of the Leonard alumni with those of "acceptable schools," he raised some serious questions that suggested a racial motivation fueled Flexner's four-year investigation and ultimate recommendations.[11]

Flexner's poor opinion of African American scholarship was detrimental to the advancement of other such scientists since his "Report." In 1920, friends of Ernest E. Just, the famous African American marine biologist, supported Just's request to Flexner' that he be allowed to continue his experiments in Jamaica, rather than at Howard.

Flexner rejected a favorable opinion advanced by Dr. Frank Rattray Lillie, Just's teacher, who assisted him in earning the Ph.D., but accepted the "cautious and conservative appraisal" requested of Dr. Jacques Loeb, a fellow scientist. Dr. Loeb felt the obligation to express himself with "complete frankness;" was of the opinion that "Just would never be a prominent investigator," but that he could be made into "a better teacher through his research fellowship." The latter opinion prevailed, and Just's proposal for a transfer was denied.

Dr. George A. Johnston gave a timely review of "The Gospel According to Abraham," ten years ago. His closing statement is as timely now as it was then:

"The lesson to be taken from the Flexner Report is that the ultimate answer to the medical manpower problem as well as other health problems in the black community rests, ultimately, on the shoulders of the citizens served by these institutions.

"Were it not for the self-sacrificing faculty, staff and student body as well as the generosity of only a small handful of philanthropic concerns and government subsidy, Meharry and Howard would both be lost in the pages of history, as are the five black institutions that closed as a result of the Flexner Report."[12]

Let us hope that the investigation will be exhumed and given a more objective evaluation.

---

1 Robert L. Green, *The Urban Challenge-Poverty and Race.* (Chicago: Follett Publishing Co., 1977) pp. 250 and 277.

2. Flexner, A., *Bulletin Number Four, Medical Education in the United States and Canada.* (New York: Carnegie Foundation for the Advancement of Teaching, 1910), p. 224.

3. Meharry Medical College, Nashville; Howard University, Washington, D.C.; Flint Medical College, Knoxville, Tenn.; Tennessee Medical College, Memphis, Tenn.; Chattanooga National Medical College, Chattanooga, Tenn.; Shaw Medical College, Raleigh, N.C.; and the Louisville National Medical College, Louisville, Ky.

4. The Flexner Report (1910).

5. Dr. James Ames, a city physician with plenty of professional and political clout, was able to push his son, Chester, through Receiving Hospital's racial barrier in 1926 to become Detroit's first African American intern.

6. It was not until 1943 that Dr. Marjorie Meyers became the second African American to be accepted as an intern at any Detroit hospital.

Prior to Ames and Meyers, nearly all of the African American graduates of Michigan's two medical schools began their Detroit practices without internships or sought and found them elsewhere.

7. Loren Miller, *The Petitioners*. (New York: Pantheon Books, 1966) p. 165, and, especially, after 1906, in *Berea College v. Kentucky* (ibid, p. 197).

8. The Committee's suggestions that these schools were being run by profiteering charlatans who seized the opportunity and took advantage of the U.S. Supreme Court-endorsed policy of racial segregation for their own ends, is an old version of an old game: Blame The Victim!

The criticism ignores the support provided by the various state legislatures, churches and individuals, including the founders, who helped to keep the projects alive. On the other hand, some of the maligned medical schools, The Louisville National Medical College, for example, was established by Dr. Henry Fitzbutler in 1888, with the permission and support of the Kentucky legislature. The need for doctors was so acute that all of their graduates were encouraged to practice within the state.

Dr. Fitzbutler, and his wife, Sarah, a later graduate of the medical school, had six children, one of whom also graduated from the school. LNMC became a life-time preoccupation, at which they practiced for more than 20 years. Many of the staff physicians underwrote much of the operating costs themselves, and rendered other valuable services to an ungrateful society.

The Flexner Committee estimated that the African American physicians who established and operated these schools provided training opportunities for more than a thousand of their graduates. Many of them passed qualifying examinations and provided a wide range of valuable medical and other services to their communities, despite incredible impediments. A review of the listings in several issues of *Negroes in Colored America* and *Negroes in Black America* suggests that many of the these physicians did not fit The Flexner Report's description of "an enormous over-production of uneducated and ill-trained medical practitioners." (Appendix 1, p. 225)

A brief look at some of these graduates should cast doubt on the reliability of the above, sweeping declaration.

Name	Year	School	Comment
John A. Kenney	1901	Leonard	Dir. John A. Andrews Clinic, Tuskeegee, 21 years; founder of Kenney Mem, Hosp, Newark, N.J.; pres. NMA, 1913; Ed. *JNMA,* 32 years
Jon O. Plummer	1904	Leonard	EENT Spec. at Lincoln and St Agnes Hosp. Raleigh; pres. N.C. Med Assoc; pres. NMA,, 1924-25. Had large EENT practice.
John P. Turner	1906	Leonard	Attended Univ. of Penn. for grad work in surg. Appointed by mayor to Sesquicenten. commiss. police dept., surg. pres. NMA,, 1921-1922.

9. The Committee's findings and recommendations led to the donation of over $50 million from John D. Rockefeller to upgrade the nation's better medical schools and persuaded other philanthropies to donate lesser sums. These and other pressures to reform medical education led to a more than 50% reduction in the number of American medical schools from the 148 Flexner studied to 60 or 70 superior institutions in 1930.

10. Hubert A. Eaton, *Every Man Should Try.* (Bonaparte Press, 1984) p. 198-204.

11. I cannot comprehend the logic and fairness of this entire (Flexner) study. I cannot help but wonder: (1) Was Abraham Flexner qualified or competent by virtue of his training and/or experience to conduct a solo study of medical schools, using self-established criteria? (2) Why did he fail to appraise and evaluate the finished products, especially of the schools which he rated as B or C? Could it be that such an evaluation would have discredited his criteria and jeopardized the credibility of his study? Was he aware of the possible impact of his ratings? (3) How did he expect a smaller school to measure up with respect to physical plant, faculty, library and endowment to tax-supported schools such as Johns Hopkins, the University of Michigan, Tulane University?, and (4) Why did North Carolina permit a four-year medical school for Negroes, located in the state's capitol, to close when modest funds would have kept it alive for continuing development? Did public opinion make unacceptable to the dominant race the fact that the first four-year medical college in the state, and, possibly the nation, was for colored students?

With the closing of the Leonard Medical School in 1914, Thirty-seven years elapsed before an African American was admitted to any medical school in North Carolina. Between 1951 and 1969, twelve African Americans were admitted to the Univ. of North Carolina, one African American student every 18 months. Bowman Gray Medical School's first African American enrolled in 1968, well over fifty years after the Leonard Medical School was forced to close.

12. George A. Johnston, Jr., M.D., FICS., "The Flexner Report and Black Medical Schools," *JNMA,* 76 (1984) pp. 223-225.

The National Medical Association Comes to Detroit (1927)

When the NMA's Detroit affiliate was organized in 1917, it was initially called the Allied Medical Society. Then, around 1920, the name was changed to the Detroit Medical Society. The DMS offered professional services to African American physicians in southeastern Michigan.

Whenever a local group grew to such size and influence sufficient to host the national convention, NMA officials would enter into an agreement with chapter officials to make arrangements for such a meeting. In many instances, the NMA conventions provided the members of the sponsoring affiliate with their first, formal opportunity to participate in the learning process of medicine since graduating medical school, sometimes years before.

Although Detroit was considered a major U.S. city, it was not asked to host an NMA convention until 1927, thirty-two years after the NMA was founded. This delay may have been due to the fact that just two years before, in 1925, three of Detroit's African American physicians had experienced tremendous grief, because of their color:

1. Dr. Robert I. Greenidge was ordered out of the Florence Crittenten obstetrical hospital because African American physicians, even Michigan's medical school graduates, were forbidden to practice in that institution.

2. Dr. A.L. Turner, the only African American physician with admission privileges in an approved, general hospital, was forced to flee from his newly-purchased home by an irate, white mob. The mob was enraged because he had dared to move into their restricted neighborhood; they tore the roof tiles off his house, manually.

3. Dr. Ossian Sweet defended his home against invasion by another white mob, one of whom was killed at the scene. The NAACP hired the world-renowned attorney, Clarence Darrow, to defend Dr. Sweet. After the second trial, Attorney Darrow won an acquittal for his client from an all-white, all-male jury. This unprecedented decision brought international attention to the case and to Detroit.

All of these events were highly publicized by the national press. Because of these and other unfortunate events, some of the delegates who had planned to come to Detroit's 1927 convention elected to stay home.

At that time, Detroit had only two hospitals in which African American physicians could practice:

1. Mercy General Hospital—a 20-bed institution owned and operated by the Drs. David and Daisy Northcross. It began operating in 1917 soon after the NMA became affiliated with the Allied Medical Society.

2. Dunbar Hospital—a 30-bed institution, began receiving patients in 1918 when African American physicians were not permitted to practice in Detroit's general hospitals (with one exception).

Despite the scant professional nourishment offered in the clinical sessions in those two bare-boned institutions, the NMA delegates came and enjoyed the camaraderie of seeing and comparing notes with friends and schoolmates of the recent and remote past.[1] Most of the African American physicians were denied internships and they went from the classroom directly to their private offices, such as they were. They had no contact with Detroit's accredited hospitals nor with the members of those hospitals' well-trained staffs.

The convention's clinical sessions were held at Eastern High School on East Grand Boulevard. The major social events attracted many of the delegates to the Belle Isle Casino and the Graystone Ballroom. The more adventurous explorers boarded the Detroit-Windsor Ferry "Britannia" for their first trip abroad to Windsor, Canada.

Unfortunately, Detroit's racial climate did not improve rapidly. Less than a decade after the first NMA convention, a group of

African American physicians representing the Cleveland Medical Association tried to enjoy the customary banquet at Detroit's Book Cadillac Hotel after touring the Parke Davis Pharmaceutical Plant.

The hotel's owners refused to admit the African Americans, so Parke Davis was forced to move the banquet to its plant's cafeteria. Detroit's race riot in 1943 sent another chill through the community.

Downtown merchants were extremely hostile to African Americans and all downtown hotels were off-limits to potential African American patrons. Subsequently, the greatest portion of convention activities were held in the local schools and churches. Members of the Allied Medical Society, the forerunner to the DMS, housed the convention delegates in their own homes and those of their neighbors.

The American Medical Association's Centenary (1947)

These and other similar events were brought into sharp focus during the AMA's Centenary in 1947. Several leaders of the NMA took careful aim and fired a 100th birthday charge of "blatant, shameless, bigotry," at the AMA because of its racist policies.

It was during the NMA's 1947 convention that the delegates learned that Dr. Charles Drew, developer of blood plasma, had sent a 100th-year birthday reminder to the AMA's Committee of Arrangements that the AMA had not changed its racist posture since it rejected the three African American applicants in 1870 and, he added:

"One hundred years of racial bigotry and fatuous pretense, one hundred years of gross distrust in a large section of the American people whose medical voice it purports to regard as the problem of Negroes which it raised in 1870; one hundred years with no program to report, a sorry record."[2, 3]

He challenged the AMA to follow the lead of the American Specialty Boards and the American College of Surgeons and erase its infamous policy of racial discrimination. He hoped that the AMA would not start the second hundred years with

103

unfinished business on its agenda that "makes a mockery of its continuous protestations of leadership in medicine, under the great and free 'American Way of Life.'"

Dr. Morris Fishbein, editor of the *AMA Journal*, responded to Dr. Drew in a letter dated January 22, 1947, that no one could join the AMA except through the county medical societies. "There is no other way in which membership can be secured by anyone."

Dr. Drew reminded Fishbein that it was impossible for a "Negro" to join a county medical society in the South. The position taken by the AMA, with respect to the by-laws, was severely criticized. "Since they (the by-laws) were not made by God," he said, "they are changeable."

Drew recommended that the AMA's board of trustees should "change the by-laws so that black physicians in the South can join the AMA." Their attempt to exercise what should have been their inalienable right to join the AMA was denied for one reason only—color!

Later, the AMA's general manager, George Liel, M.D., advised Dr. Drew that "the troublesome question" that he had raised could only be presented to the House of Delegates by an AMA delegate. Dr. Liel's continuing reply appeared to put an end to any hope for relief from within the AMA:

"I realize that the question is a troublesome one, and I do not have the answer. It is entirely controlled by the county and state associations. As you know, the AMA cannot 'dictate' any policies to such organizations. We are a federally constituent association. Even if a resolution was passed by the House of Delegates, the state and local societies could still refuse to comply with it."

As we shall learn later on, when the AMA's support of the Hungarians, Cubans and South Africa are discussed, Dr. Fishbein's trouble with Dr. Drew's question, and his inability to act on it, occurred only when the applicant was African American.

When the American Bar Association Excluded Blacks

It was at this time that I asked my good friend, Prof. Harold Norris, of the Detroit College of Law (DCL), how the American Bar Association (ABA) handled race issues organizationally. It will come as no surprise to anyone who knows Harold as well as I do, that he had already dealt with the subject, editorially:

"First, the ABA was clearly racist. Despite the purpose stated in the constitution to 'advance the science of Jurisprudence' and 'promote the administration of justice' and the oath of its members to uphold the U.S. Constitution, the ABA barred black lawyers from its membership. An item that appeared in the spring 1977, issue of the ABA publication, *Individual Rights and Responsibilities Newsletter*, read as follows:

"In 1910, when the NAACP absorbed the Niagara Movement and took on organizational form, with W.E.B. Dubois as the full-time staff Director of Publicity and Research, the ABA president elected by acclamation was Morefield Storey. He was to continue in that post until his death, 20 years later, at the age of 84. Hardly had he assumed office when his own profession presented a problem that portrayed well the degraded state of American morality.

"It became known in 1911 that three Negro lawyers had become members of the ABA simply by filling out application blanks and sending them in. Although one of them was an Assistant Attorney General, the reaction of the membership, reflecting the nation's racial animosity, was such that the ABA's Executive Committee "rescinded" the memberships and expelled all three.

"This action by a body of members of the bar pledged by oath to support a constitution guaranteeing 'equal protection of the laws' aroused the wrath of many. One who denounced the action as illegal was the U.S. Attorney General George W. Wickersham. Morefield Storey, as past president of the ABA, took the lead in the protest campaign.

"The battle was won, but the war for the next couple of decades at least, was lost. The three expelled lawyers were reinstated, but the nature of the questionaires changed so that until 1936, only the national lawyers retained the color line."[4]

As mentioned earlier, African American Dentists and Pharmacists were a part of the organizational structure of the

NMA in 1895. Since 1940, they have formed their own associations that continue to serve their professional needs.

What was clearly a response to the NMA's attack against the AMA in 1947 surfaced during the AMA's 1948 meeting of the House of Delegates in Chicago the next year. The New York County Medical Society submitted the following constitutional amendment:

"No association shall exclude from membership any physician for other than professional or ethical reasons."

A resolution was offered which stated: "The exclusion of physicians on the basis of race constitutes an affront to our colleagues, a degradation of this honored profession and a violation of our American democratic ideal."

Instead of acting on the New York resolution, the AMA chairman permitted the Georgia delegation to respond by offering a substitute resolution:

"It is the recommendation of your Reference Committee that the county medical society is the sole judge of whom it shall elect to membership, provided the delegate meets the medical requirement for membership and is so recommended."

Dr. Cobb, then editor of the *NMA Journal*, labelled this action: "a direct slap in the face of the many doctors of both races who had striven for an era of better understanding, good will and unity in medicine."

He described the move as an ill-advised, unnecessary restoration of brutal prejudice, camouflaged as "states' rights." He continued, "so long as the AMA permits its Southern membership to establish policy, racism will continue to reign in the organization."

Dr. Cobb reviewed Dr. Fishbein's new book, *The History of the American Medical Association, 1847-1947*, and demanded that the AMA amend its constitution "so that black physicians in the South can join the AMA." He pointed out the many disadvantages to which the Southern "black" doctor is put by the denial of membership by the AMA.[5] None of these exchanges had any appreciable effect on the course of the AMA.

---

1. *JAMA*, Vol. 39. (1947) pp. 222-224.

2. Kenneth R. Manning, *Blacks in American Medicine*. (Cambridge, Mass.: Institute of Technology Cambridge, Jan. 1989) p. 46.

3. Manning, pp. 51-52.

The following letter was mailed to Dr. Leonidas Berry from Dr. Lynn A. Ferguson of the AMA, advising him not to assume the same position as Dr. Drew.

November 10, 1958

Leonidas H. Berry, M.D.
412 East Forty Seventh Street
Chicago 15, Illinois

Dear Dr. Berry:

I appreciate your sending me a copy of the letter addressed to Dr. Perkel. It has been brought before the Board, and fully discussed. You will recall, of course, that Dr. Nix and I talked to you about the situation while we were in Washington. At the time, I did not realize exactly the full impact of the situation as it is. Now, I believe, I understand it a little better. I am very sorry that you did not choose to attend the meeting, because we had a very excellent and well attended program. There were two-three colored doctors, and a couple of colored interns, who attended all the sessions. The only hitch is this, that the hotel would not serve them food; neither would they give them lodging. I was told that, had you been present, you would have been a house guest of the president of the Dillard University.

This matter of religion, creed, color, and intregation is a little larger than any of us even though, in our small way, we do participate. Obviously, we cannot make the final decisions. Personally, I would not want to boycott New Orleans as a meeting place, because it is an excellent one. These other extra medical problems we each have to work out as best we possibly can. I find that all of the men in the organization in New Orleans are staff members at Turo and the colored hospital and, as you know, Nix, Ochs, and Irving Levin carry on teaching courses for the staff, residents, and interns. I feel sure that, with a patient attitude, these differences of opinion will eventually fade out. It may not be in your generation or mine, but if you will think back a few years, you must realize that your race has come a long ways not only through your own efforts but through those of your white friends, in spite of the fact that their white friends objected. Many years ago, when I was Chairman of the St. Mary's Board for 19 years excepting for two years when I was staff chief, we had a couple of colored doctors on our staff who were fine gentlemen. One was a dermatologist, and the other a general practitioner. The general practitioner never got a chance to do surgery on his own.

Now, we have four or five colored physicians in our city, all fine gentlemen, and all scheduling their own surgery according to their several abilities. I think we have made some gains, and I don't think anything is to be gained by being vindictive, and I don't think the American College of Gastroenterology could accomplish very much by boycotting any of the Southern states. As far as I am concerned, it is the wrong way to go about it. I think that one gains favor by being understanding and cooperative and—above all—humble even though it may take 2-3 generations to accomplish the ultimate end. There are quite a few of use who understand your position thoroughly, and can agree with you on all points excepting the method of solution. Keep in mind that I am not stating the position of the Board of Trustees, by this letter, but only my own thoughts in the matter. We have these problems in Grand Rapids, and you certainly have encountered them in Chicago. In your heart, I am pretty sure, you feel the same way I do, but it is a whole lot harder for you to accept.

I hope you will not let your membership in our organization hinge on that sort of thing, because that attitude is juvenile, and I am pretty sure you are not that kind of fellow. I feel sure that patience and good behaviour will, eventually, win out.

With all good wishes, and best personal regards, I am

Very sincerely yours,

Lynn A. Ferguson, M.D.

4. Harold Norris, *Reflections on Law, Lawyers, and the Bill of Rights*, Vol. 111. (Michigan Law Book Publishing, 1984) pp. 593-610.

5. *JNMA*, Vol. 39, pp. 266-267.

The Hill-Burton Act: (The Hospital Survey and Construction Act of 1946)

The Hill-Burton Act of 1946 could have been one of the most important pieces of legislation of the first half of this century, except for one fatal flaw. Like the U.S. Constitution of 1787, the act failed to acknowledge that African Americans are first-class citizens, too.

As a result of the denial of this irrefutable fact, the act has been the target of expensive litigation, congressional amendments and executive orders to make it a respectable document. During the 18-year lapse from the passage of the Hill-Burton Act in 1946, with the "separate but equal" clause intact until it was finally removed from the Civil Rights Act of 1964, every African American physician and patient was subjected to the degrading influence of Hill-Burton.

A close study of the origin, passage, execution and ultimate amending of the act will reflect, in microcosm, the fate of the African American when left in the hands of his government.

While the passage of this act was not the first time that a self-interest group (organized medicine) has gorged itself at the public trough, few had ever appeared better garbed in the vestments of respectability.

There could be no argument that the state of the nation's health was quite poor in the early 1940s. World War II had underscored many deficiencies in the recruits who showed up for induction. Without a doubt, one of the nation's basic needs was better hospitals and more of them, especially in those areas of greatest deprivation, the African American neighborhoods.

These areas of need were largely determined by the Commission of Hospital Care that was created in 1942 by the

American Hospital Association and the U.S. Public Health Service. Recommendations from the commission formed the basic structure and mechanism of action of the Hill-Burton Hospital Survey and Construction Act of 1946. Organized medicine had a great deal to say for a bill that "expressly forbade governmental interference in the operation of hospitals."

Congressional sponsorship of the enabling legislation was bipartisan to avoid the cross-fires of party opportunism. The two men whose names appeared on the bill seemed to be wise choices indeed. Senator Lister Hill (D-Ala.) was the son of Dr. Luther Hill, a pioneer heart surgeon of Montgomery, Ala.

Hill brought with him a family orientation toward medical matters. In his own right, he was recognized as a sincere and trustworthy, Southern liberal, a rare breed.

The act's co-sponsor, Senator Harold H. Burton, was a former mayor of Cleveland, who had become known in the senate as an "independent liberal." Soon after the act was submitted for legislative action, Senator Burton, a Republican, was appointed to the U.S. Supreme Court by President Truman, a Democrat, in 1945.

The more-favored Hill-Burton Act reached the senate in record time, unlike somewhat similar but more liberal health measures (i.e., the Murray-Wagner-Dingell [M/W/D] and the Jacob Javits bills) that had been awaiting congressional action for two years.

The main stumbling block was Senator Walter F. George (D-Ga.), the outspoken, segregationist chairman of the powerful Senate Finance Committee. It was his option to choose which, among the several bills available, to call up for senate action and funding.

Senator George found the language of Hill-Burton more palatable to his conservative taste than either the M/W/D or the older, even more liberal, Jacob Javits measure, awaiting his action. The senator snatched Hill-Burton right off the top for immediate senate consideration and funding.

The other two acts were allowed to expire quietly, as "crib deaths" in the senate nursery. What had been a two-year bier for

110

M/W/D and Javits, became a launchpad for Hill-Burton. These events occurred in 1945, when the NMA was celebrating its 50th anniversary. The enactment of Hill-Burton, with separate-but-equal still intact, was an anniversary present from the medical establishment of dubious value—16 more years of denial of equal training opportunity for the members of the NMA that would have enabled them to deliver the best of care to their patients.

Close behind, if not alongside, Senator George was Senator Robert Taft (R-Ohio), the North's conservative equivalent of Senator George.

One of the most influential voices heard for the act was that of Dr. R.L. Sensenich, representing the AMA's board of trustees who read the act and reported that "the language of the bill was flexible enough to allow it to be adapted to different regions of the country without the interference of the federal authorities."

After the bill was passed, the surgeon general gave credit to the AMA for the rapidity of its course through the senate, which was brief. Senators Murray and Wagner, whose bill was introduced two years before Hill-Burton, made several attempts to liberalize Hill-Burton by amendments. Senator Taft, true to form, allowed only one minor change.

Only a careful reading of the facts of that period will offer some explanation for the Southern preference for Hill-Burton over the more liberal measures. The appointment of Senator Burton to the U.S. Supreme Court left Senator Hill alone to defend the liberal prerogatives of his act against the well-coordinated assaults by the medical establishment.

This was an 18-year victory for the medical establishment and their conservative cohorts in both houses of congress. The bill was introduced on December 10, 1945, and was passed by a voice vote the following day. There was hardly a word of dissent against the bill during public hearings.

Among the defeats for Murray and Wagner were:

1. To prevent the transfer of public funds to private hands.

2. To insure high standards of operation and maintenance in all hospitals financed.

3. The appropriation of sufficient funds to insure the construction of hospitals in all areas where they were needed most.

The bill (S-191) was passed relatively intact on December 11, 1945. The *NMA Journal* took a dim view of Senator Taft's actions:

"Senator Taft opposed giving the federal government a strong voice in the distribution of public funds, favoring States' Righters."

One of the defeated provisions would have "required the surgeon general to demand that all hospitals receiving federal funds open their staffs to all qualified practitioners." Despite these objections, the President signed the bill "because of the urgent need for a prompt start on the five-year plan, particularly on survey and planning."

Again, the "separate-but-equal" clause escaped even a modest threat of elimination. Despite the fact that passage of the act was hailed by the establishment as a major boost for the nation's health, it continued to be a millstone around the necks of millions of African Americans for 18 more years.

The *New York Times* reported on June 29, 1946, well before the bill became law, that the proposed Hill-Burton legislation had the support of hospital, medical and welfare agencies as well as labor and farm unions.

At that moment, the NMA began a massive campaign to defeat the "separate but equal" holdover from *Plessy v. Ferguson*. Not everyone agreed with the *Times* that the passage of the measure had widespread approval. Midian O. Bousfield, M.D.,[1] a former NMA president, saw the issue from another perspective:

"The Hill-Burton Act was largely Southern sponsored and set a precedent in government help on the basis of need to be calculated through ratio-per-capita income, in relationship to the national average, value of products, and several other factors. This is an important legislation for Southern states."[2]

President Truman's justified alarm over "new ground" that was broken by the Hill-Burton Act only hinted at the real threats that would manifest themselves as soon as the measure was executed. These threats didn't break new ground, they just expanded and increased the institutionalization of the old.

The new measure offered a variable level of financial support for a state, depending on the per-capita income of its inhabitants and other related bases for determining need.

The indices from black communities, in particular, were worse than those from the white communities and favored the Southern applicants. Instead of dealing with the applicants directly, however, the federal government processed the applications for hospital funds through an agency set up by the state's government. If a state-approved application reached the surgeon general, it was almost certain of funding.

The lack of veto power by a federal agency was one of the provisions of the act that disturbed President Truman. Once approved, the project received periodic payments through the state agency as the work progressed. Without question, even if the surgeon general disapproved a request for funds, the applicant could circumvent his rejection through the courts.

The language of the bill underscored the state's complete autonomy in the exercise of its prerogatives in the distribution of public funds—(Section 635, Title VI):

"That except as otherwise specifically provided, nothing in this Title shall be construed as conferring upon any federal officer or employee the right to exercise any supervision or control over the administration, personnel, maintenance or operation of any hospital assisted with federal funds."

Insofar as bed availability was concerned, the Hill-Burton Act (42 U.S.C. 291 {f}) provided:

"That the state plan shall provide for adequate hospital facilities for all persons residing in the state without discrimination on account of race creed or color..." An exception was made as follows:

"But an exception shall be made in cases where separate hospital facilities are provided for separate population groups, if the plan makes equitable provisions on the basis of need for facilities and services of like quality for each group."

Thus, in clear and unmistakable language, the architects of the bill gave congressional license to the guardians of status quo to do business as usual. They were fully aware that in every other such instance (housing, education and employment) where the state was handed "separate-but-equal" mandates, separate-and-unequal mandates were uniformly the result. At that time, Alabama, Arkansas, Georgia, Louisiana, Mississippi, North Carolina, Oklahoma, Tennessee, Texas and West Virginia had laws on their books that required racial segregation in all public facilities. This concession was what AMA trustee, Dr. Sensenich, was referring to when he applauded the "flexibility" of the bill during its senate hearings.

For the first time in the history of this republic, the Southern establishment was able to parlay its mistreatment and deprivation of its African American citizens into a self-interest project, financed by the federal government. This is not to say by any means that the non-South did very much better. In neither area, but especially the south, was there any sincere interest in or effort made to extend equality of medical care to these segments of the population that needed it most—African Americans and Native Americans.

The results were easily predictable. Morbidity and mortality rates, perinatal mortality figures, life expectancy and the incidence of preventable diseases—all favorable to the whites—were published in biostatistical printouts with the regularity of the seasons.

Then, adding insult to injury, these data were repeated in the print and electronic media with an accusing finger pointed at the African American physician as if he were the responsible agent. How could a measure like this emerge in 1946 without a word of challenge from any segment of the liberal community? Where were the watch-dog politicians?

In 1946, President Truman was putting the finishing touches on a new foreign policy that became known as "The Truman Doctrine." Under its influence the people would waste billions of dollars the next quarter of the century before convincing themselves that military defeat of world communism was not possible, a fact recently

114

verified by the confessions, *A Mistake, a Terrible Mistake,* by former U.S. Secretary of Defense Robert McNamara.

Adam Clayton Powell, a freshman congressman in 1946 was, at that time, keeping a low profile and William Dawson, Chicago's African American congressman, was not heard from on the matter.

Taking advantage of this silence, the Truman administration entered into an agreement with South Africa's apartheid government and brokered their political victory in 1948 as well as his own. Those victories, although rarely mentioned in the discussions of American, and especially African American history, deserve more attention than they get.

Racial segregation was so neatly woven into the fabric of American society in the first half of this century, that even the NAACP despaired of a head-on attack. The Supreme Court's 1954 *Brown v. Board of Education* decision was limited to outlawing racial segregation in "public schools" only. There was no way it could have produced all of the results expected and deserved by African Americans.

As late as 1961, the NAACP accused the federal government of pouring millions of dollars into segregated, and otherwise discriminatory, school systems, "seven years after the Supreme Court's Brown Decision."

---

1. Midian O. Bousfield, M.D., graduated from Northwestern in 1909 and was president of the NMA in 1934.

2. Thomas Yenser, *Who's Who in Colored America.* (New York: 1938) pp. 67-68.

Detroit Hosts Her Second NMA Convention (1949)

Due to the racial hostility encountered throughout the city before and during the first NMA meeting that was held in 1927, twenty-two years elapsed before the NMA agreed to schedule another convention in Detroit. By August 1949, some progress was noticeable in the quality of hotel accommodations and the professionalism of some of the clinical sessions.

The Gotham was an attractive and popular hotel owned by African Americans which accommodated most of the guests. Smaller hotels and private homes were used to house others.

At mid-century, however, medical advancement in Detroit's African American community still compared unfavorably with what was available to the European American members of the medical establishment. Only ten, of more than 200, of Detroit's African American physicians were certified as medical specialists; and only about half of them had been accepted for training at a Detroit hospital. Most of the few who had been admitted to staff positions were frozen at the courtesy level.

(No intern or resident was assigned to members of the courtesy staff; thus, he or she was unable to call upon an intern or resident for help, no matter what the emergency. Doctors at the courtesy level assisted each other with operations, deliveries, etc.)

In the 31 years that Receiving Hospital served as Detroit's main city hospital, only three African Americans had been awarded internships in that institution. No private hospitals accepted African American physicians as interns or residents.

Most of the medical lectures for the 1949 NMA convention were held at the Rackham building, an affiliate of the Univ. of

Mich. and at some of the private, small hospitals which served the African American community.

In addition, clinical sessions were held at Providence Hospital on August 9th. Dr. Thomas Billingslea, a Detroit internist, conducted a symposium on diseases of the chest on the 10th of August at the African American-owned West-Haven Hospital. The group went to the Univ. of Mich. in Ann Arbor on the 11th and ended the sessions at Grace and Harper Hospitals on the 12th.

Interspersed among these visits to the medical centers were tours to Wayne Diagnostic, Trinity, and Parkside Hospitals (all except Parkside were relatively recent additions to the hospital scene). The African American owners of these hospitals were the happy hosts and went out of their way to accommodate the visitors.

The highlight on the social calendar was a delegate's party at the newly-purchased, palatial home of Dr. and Mrs. D.T. Burton on Arden Park Blvd. Together they owned Burton Mercy Hospital, one of Detroit's finest, privately-owned African American hospitals.

The delegates and their female companions dressed up in their finest attire and adorned themselves with their most expensive jewelry, to eat, drink and be merry. The beautiful house and its spacious grounds were festooned for the occasion, and a good time was had by all.

Neither the improved clinical sessions nor the more enjoyable social calendar diverted the attention of outgoing NMA President C. Austin Whittier from the real issue. Racism was a constant factor in the lives of the NMA's membership. Although the problem had been referred to on several occasions throughout the sessions, it was the main topic of Dr. Whittier's exaugural address:

"Through a series of rebuffs and disappointments, the realization has been brought to us that if the NMA is to take its place as a viable player in the field of organized medicine, it must come as a result of our own actions. For many years, we have tried to get recognition without the proper expenditure of our energy to a daily program of organization building.

"It is now time that we assert our inward strength. The NMA must become a part of organized medicine. Let us begin with our local units by establishing strong county and state societies. We must let it be known that these affiliates represent our leaders who are to be consulted on matters of policy to which we are expected to subscribe."

Dr. C. Herbert Marshall accepted the president's gavel in 1949 with the following pledge: "For years, the AMA has made the Negro the scapegoat of its own demagoguery. The time has long since passed when the NMA will lean backward to seek and expect accommodations that are due from the AMA.

"It is my firm belief that the one way we are to gain the recognition and respect that is justly ours is for each member of the NMA to conduct his or her activities in the highest ethical plane. We must continue to research and continue to make original contributions in our own fields, knowing well that knowledge knows no racial barriers.

"There is a ray of hope for a change in the attitude of the AMA by virtue of the fact that the key officer, Major General Lane, is the type of man who deep within him, does not appreciate the present attitude of his associates toward the Negro physician. He knows of the competence and the integrity of many of our members. He served in the medical corp in World War II, and I'm sure that experience he received working with members of our group has served us exceedingly well.

"There will be no Liaison Committees between NMA and AMA during my term of office. I shall be prepared to handle any exigency that may arise that would necessitate such a committee and will, impartially, appoint members to function on that committee whose records are clean and whose characters are unblemished."

Unfortunately, such wishful thinking was often heard when a new president was accepting the gavel before his or her inaugural address. After the frustrations of a year in office, we hear a different tune. In upcoming paragraphs, you'll note the contrast in the departing soliloquy of NMA President Leonidas Berry, in 1966, following the disappointment after passage of the 1964 Civil Rights law.

Insofar as the general public was concerned, Detroit's 1949 NMA convention was the last one from which the African

American community drew significant, direct benefit. Being housed in the community and dining in the area's restaurants, the delegates were identified by and with the community.

The presence of several hundred, well-dressed, apparently wealthy, professional men and women with their spouses was very impressive to retired real estate agent, Raymond Caldwell, then, an 18-year old African American student. At the time, he lived near the Gotham Hotel and is still able to recall the beautiful women and confident men driving or being driven in expensive, late model cars—even one with "an alligator-hide interior."

Although the convention delegates were not welcome in the downtown hotels, Hudson's department store clerks and those of other business emporia rolled out the red carpet for any potential customer wearing a convention badge. When the delegates departed Detroit, an appreciable part of their expendable income was left in the hands and pockets of the grateful, local citizenry.

Others recall this "foreign" invasion fondly, and with sudden clarity, as though it had happened last week. The delegates' impact on Detroit's pride-starved, African American public was positive, and profound.

Another event occurred during that August 1949 convention that was not only positive and profound, but altered my life forever. I was offered an ob-gyn residency at Harlem Hospital by Vaughn Mason, M.D., who had succeeded Dr. Murray as chief of gynecology. The doctor who had been chosen to fill the slot fell ill and had to withdraw. Unmarried at that time, I readily accepted the offer and began to close my office, after four years of general practice, and prepared to return to New York.

Louise Lovett and I had been courting for a year and decided to get married in February 1950. It was only during the preparations for the wedding that she became fully aware of my commitment to return to New York. Although this disclosure nearly wrecked the marriage, we reached an understanding and departed for New York the last week in June.

After nearly four years of general practice, my income had grown to nearly $25,000 per year. My starting salary as a resident was reduced to $130 per month. During my three-year residency,

I saw only one private patient for Ethelbert Carrington, M.D., a classmate, who was a family physician in Brooklyn. I received $30 for that consultation.

During my last two years, the National Medical Fellowships, organized in Chicago by Dr. Franklin C. Mclean, supplemented my meager funds with a monthly contribution of $150. Louise and I did not return to Detroit until 1953 and brought along Stephanie Jean, who was born on September 18, 1952.

Fortunately, Dr. Henry Falk, former chief of gynecology at Harlem Hospital, was pleased with my residency and interceded on my behalf with his colleagues in Detroit. A staff appointment at Hutzel Hospital was arranged due to Dr. Falk's timely and thoughtful intervention.

If the Detroit community's active participation in the affairs of the NMA ended after the 1949 convention—and it did—this was the first NMA convention to attract the full attention of the AMA; the general manager of the AMA appeared in Detroit to solicit NMA's support for the AMA's opposition to the King-Anderson (Medicare) Act.

In an all-out, full-press effort to influence the NMA delegates, the AMA rented hospitality suites at the segregated, Book Cadillac Hotel where AMA-sponsored Anti-Medicaid workshops were conducted by Dr. Lorenzo Nelson, the first African American to be elected president of a constituency of the AMA; and Dr. Peter Marshall Murray, former NMA president in 1932 and at that time, the first African American chairman of gynecology at Harlem Hospital. Although Dr. Murray was the first African American to be chosen to serve on the AMA's House of Delegates, Dr. Cobb stated that Murray's appointment was "formally" announced to coincide with his appearance at the NMA convention.

Despite Dr. Cobb's caution about "Greeks bearing gifts," the AMA's resolution to oppose Medicaid was tabled thanks to Cobb's, and other, spirited objections and the measure eventually passed into law with full support of the *NMA Journal* and the Cobb team.

Many politicians remembered how the NMA fought the AMA for the ultimate passage of the Medicare Act, but when implementation became an issue, the establishment sought, and was often given, the advantage.

I could find no further evidence that Dr. Murray ever lobbied his fellow African Americans delegates for the AMA. He continued on as a member of that body, garnering public attention again in the spring of 1951, when final arrangements were being made for the AMA's winter meeting in Houston, Texas.

Dr. Murray insisted on attending the meeting, despite promises to Dr. J.T. Billups, chairman of the AMA's Houston Committee, that he would not. When oil-man, Glen McCarthy, owner of the Shamrock Hotel, learned that Dr. Murray was headed his way, McCarthy objected so strenuously that the AMA's Houston convention was moved to Los Angeles.

Imhotep Conferences

The 1954 *Brown v. Board of Education* decision thrust the nation forward into a long, difficult and, often dangerous retreat from that 1896 racist ruling. While only four years (1892-1896) of deliberation were required to erect this shrine to white supremacy, sixty (1896-1956) years of effort to remove it have not been sufficient.

Efforts to rid "the separate-but-equal" stigmata of *Plessy v. Ferguson* from the new Hill-Burton Hospital Act was encountering great resistance from the same medical establishment that had achieved an extension of the act in 1946. The Imhotep group was determined that the "separate but equal" clause would not survive this encounter.

Sponsors were the NMA, NAACP and the Medico-Chirrurgical Society of the District of Columbia. Dr. Cobb was, or had been, an officer in all three organizations, thus, it is understandable why each sponsor contributed $500 to underwrite the first conference. The remaining conferences were sponsored by the NAACP and the NMA. Only the dogged determination of "Monty" and his dedicated team kept it going for seven, annual sessions.

Dr. Cobb, a man of tradition and letters, chose "Imhotep" (He Who Cometh in Peace) as the theme of the conferences. In retrospect, it may have been Dr. Cobb's first mistake to declare peace before declaring war. He chose this name to honor the memory of Imhotep, an early Egyptian who was the first person to be identified with the medical profession.[1]

The purposes of Imhotep Conferences were:

1. To bring together representatives of all the interests among the public, hospitals, the healing profession and the governmental agencies, which were concerned with this problem.

2. To evolve, in the atmosphere of common understanding and cooperation, some creative recommendations and

programs of remedial action which may be made known to the American people, with the aim of securing widespread public support for their implementation.

3. To provide a complete, comprehensive picture of the situation through first-hand presentations from the various regions, of the country.

4. To make available in the *Journal of the NMA*, form, publications of conference proceedings in a compact, authoritative reference on the subject of hospital integration which may have value both as information and as guidance for continuing efforts in the field and in all parts of the U.S.

Unfortunately, instead of taking the malefactors into court, as the NAACP had done in education and transportation, Dr. Cobb chose to invite all interested parties to meet, look at the facts and everyone would, he assumed, see the logic in following the Supreme Court's lead away from the proscriptions of *Plessy*, into the 20th century.

Yet Dr. Cobb's assumptions were all wrong. He grossly underrated the establishment's commitment to and investment in racial segregation as a profitable way of life. He had also overrated his personal influence among those health-care administrators who could have helped to create a racist-free society, but chose not to.

The AMA sent representatives to the first meeting, but none came thereafter. Although the AHA and other such hospital establishment groups attended the first few meetings as observers, they were too comfortable with "separate but equal" to be identified with its removal from the Hill-Burton Act.

As editor of the *JNMA*, since 1949, Dr. Cobb had brought a level of scholarship and penmanship to the *Journal* which had earned it the respect of the medical community. His signature on an invitation, asking top-level medical leaders to attend a medical conference would, and did, get a good, initial response.

Howard Univ. School of Medicine was listed as the site for the initial conference. However, due to political stress, the site was changed to the 15th Street Presbyterian Church, thanks to the courage and commitment of the pastor, Rev. Robert Pierce Johnson.

The first conference was held on March 8-9, 1957 and was attended by 175 registrants; representing 21 states and 49 separate localities, 16 constituencies of the NMA, 26 branches of the NAACP and four branches of the National Urban League. Among the 32 organizations representing hospital interests were: American Medical Association, American Hospital Association, American Nurses Association, the United States Public Health Service, the Hill-Burton Advisory Committee, National Medical Fellowships, Inc. (NMF), and the National AFL-CIO. All meetings were open to the public.

The conference voted to seek legislation which would amend the Hospital Survey and Construction Act of 1946 and its amendments, so that clauses which provide for separate population groups be deleted, since "such laws, now, seem unconstitutional in the light of recent Supreme Court decisions."

Although many hospital and medical groups, representing a variety hospital interests, were brought together to discuss hospital desegregation, their long-term, comfort factor with racial segregation, as the "American way of life," robbed them of any real desire to change a situation that was, for them, not only socially comfortable but also economically profitable.

Racially segregated health care facilities were often substandard, and located in "out of sight" facilities for African Americans.

Such facilities were usually operated for a fraction of the cost of operating those more accommodating facilities located in nicer sections of hospitals, where African Americans were not allowed.

It was a common consensus among the delegates that the information reported and compiled during the conference provided a solid basis from which to launch an all-out attack against racial discrimination in the nation's hospitals and health care facilities.

Special attention was focused on the Hill-Burton Act, a decree that declared: "Separate but equal facilities would no longer be approved for federal assistance."[2] The various sessions of the first Imhotep Conference dealt, almost exclusively, with the Hill-Burton Hospital Construction Programs in Florida, Kentucky, Virginia and West Virginia, where projects were already underway.

If Imhotep Conferences had proceeded according to Cobb, it would have been his finest hour. The idea, script, selection of actors and sites of performances were all Cobb's. His major failing was as director. His main cast of characters were prima donnas, for the most part, who came to only one or two sessions, but brought their own agendas.

The second Imhotep Conference was held in Chicago in 1958, with the Cook County Physicians Association as co-sponsor. According to Dr. Cobb, "a group of physicians, primarily white, tried to seize control of the organization and departed when the coup failed.

Then, too, the Hungarian uprising of 1956, helped spoil the Imhotep parade. Although described in detail elsewhere, it garnered the attention and support of the AMA and other establishment groups, entirely.

African American physicians, especially those in the Chicago area, took a dim view of this selective generosity by the AMA. Their experience with the AMA, whose headquarters was in Chicago, had been markedly different.

On June 12, 1955, the previous year, Illinois Governor Will B. Stratton had signed into law a measure which decreed that any public business that denied the use of its facilities because of race or color would lose its tax-exempt privileges.

Four state senators had introduced the measure into the Illinois General Assembly with the support of the Committee for Equitable Medical Care, the Committee to End Discrimination in the Chicago Medical Institutions and the Illinois Conference of Branches of the NAACP.

The Cook County medical establishment had tried a wide variety of delaying maneuvers to defeat the measure. One of them was an offer to build a branch of the Cook County Hospital in Chicago's black ghetto. Dr. N.O. Calloway, an officer of Provident Medical Fellowships, led the charge that defeated that ruse.

126

Despite the best efforts of Governor Stratton and the four senators, this 1955 act did not achieve its desired goal.

A year later, when hordes of Hungarian physicians were being welcomed and integrated into the medical establishment throughout the country, African American physicians were forced to abide by the "separate but equal" restraint that was left in the Civil Rights Act of 1946.

In 1959, the third Imhotep Conference was held, again, in Washington, D.C. Due to the intransigence of the members of the medical establishment and the growing fatigue of Imhotep team, so little was accomplished that Imhotep's unfinished business was placed on the agenda of the 1959 NMA Convention in Detroit.

During the first three sessions, reports were heard from many sections of the United States. No matter where the reports originated, the experiences of African Americans were the same. They were the victims of vicious and degrading racist practices by their white colleagues.[3]

As a result of this great wealth of information, collected from a vast and representative number resources, the conference took the following actions by unanimous vote. The matter of hospital integration should be prosecuted continuously and vigorously until racial discrimination has been eliminated from all hospitals in the U.S.

There were seven annual Imhotep Conferences with dwindling attendance and accomplishments each year. Even the most confirmed civil rights workers began to doubt the wisdom of continuing the sessions.

---

1. G. Mokhtar (Editor), *General History of Africa: Ancient Civilizations of Africa II* (California: Univ. of California Press, 1981) pp. 91 and 165.

   Imhotep, one of the most significant personalities in the history of medicine, appeared during the third dynasty (2900-2200) of the old kingdom of Egypt. As vizor and architect, as well as physician, his fame survived throughout Egyptian ancient history through Greek times, centuries before Hippocrates was born.

2. *Commission on Civil Rights*, Special Publication No. 2. (March 1965).

3. *JNMA,* Vol. 4 (May 1957), p. 272-273; Vol. 5 (Sept. 1957), pp. 352-356; (Nov. 1957) pp. 429-433; Vol. 50 (Jan. 1958) pp. 66, 142 and 224.

Detroit Hosts Her Third NMA Convention (1959)

Delegates to the NMA's third Detroit Convention in 1959 were allowed in the downtown hotels and restaurants for the first time. Shop owners were very solicitous to conventioneers who wandered into their shops. One of Detroit's delegates was so moved by the apparent change in attitude of hotel owners and shop keepers that he was quoted in the news media as exclaiming "we have arrived!"

That illusion did not survive the convention's opening session. Detroit Mayor Louis Miriani, preoccupied with more "important" matters, sent a deputy to re-present the "Keys To The City" to NMA President Dr. Edward Mazique and the several hundred physician-delegates.

The delegates' embarrassment was further increased when Supreme Court Justice-to-be, Thurgood Marshall, responding to the widely quoted "we have arrived" statement, issued a timely rebuke from the bench in Washington, D.C. He informed the NMA officials and delegates that they had certainly "not arrived" when a host mayor showed such disrespect for them as to send the "keys" by messenger.

Although Detroit and NMA officials hastily arranged a private meeting for the Mayor to re-present the "keys" to President Mazique, it failed to assuage the rising anger of the delegates. Before they had time to recover from Mayor Miriani's assault on their self-esteem, the program committee chairman announced a follow-up punch to their mid-section.

HEW Secretary Arthur Fleming, scheduled to be the first sitting member of a presidential cabinet to address an NMA convention, sent his regrets and dispatched Assistant Secretary Dr. Aims C. McGuiness to take his place.

These and other developments within the medical establishment forced many African American physicians to realize that what was being offered as integration, was merely a charade. Many Detroit delegates, already deeply involved in the fight for freedom and justice, renewed their efforts to force racial segregation out of the driving seat of their lives.

By the time of Detroit's 1959 NMA convention, the civil rights movement was gathering steam nationwide. The U.S. Supreme Court had admitted *Plessy v. Ferguson* was wrong by partially reversing it in *Brown v. Board of Educ.* in 1954.

Three years later in 1957, the same Court delivered another dismantling blow to the citadel of white supremacy by a favorable ruling in the Montgomery Bus Boycott, ruling:

"Racial Segregation In Public Transportation Is No Longer Legal!"

Also in 1957, two years before Detroit's 1959 NMA convention, President Eisenhower had served as midwife to the birth of the first civil rights law since 1875.

The NMA—AMA Liaison Committee

The NMA-AMA Liaison Committee was the immediate successor to Dr. Montague Cobb's Imhotep effort to democratize the American medical establishment. This drive began in the early 1960s and each phase bore the imprint of the NMA president who happened to be in office at that time.

This mid-20th century NMA bid for a seat "at the master's table" had several things going for it that should have guaranteed a seating, at least in the kitchen.

1. The leaders of the NAACP, the civil rights movement and the Medical Committee for Human Rights were helping to retool the federal judicial and legislative machinery to make it more responsive to their needs. Their goal was to change it into a juggernaught for justice that would undo the physical and psychological damage done by centuries of chattel enslavement and enforced illiteracy.

2. The AMA had selectively violated its own Mission Statement by racing to the rescue and rehabilitation of thousands of immigrant physicians from Hungary (1956) and Cuba, that began in 1960, and continued for many years.

The NMA leaders concentrated, as a team, on what they hoped would be the final battle in what had been a long, bitter, and demeaning struggle for equal access to the medical resources of the community. They felt that, as human beings, citizens and physicians, equality of opportunity was an inalienable right that had been denied them for too long.

What they should have recognized was their notion of having inalienable rights was not shared by the AMA's guardians of white supremacy. These guardians had established their protective position in 1847, and had successfully defended it since that time.

President John Kenney, Jr. occupied the same NMA office that his father, John Kenney, Sr., had held fifty years earlier, in 1913. The senior Kenney, although a graduate of the unapproved Leonard Medical School, not only became president of the NMA, but served in many other high level capacities over the years.

With a family background of a continuous fight for justice and freedom, the younger President Kenney was fully prepared to represent his group before the AMA officials. AMA President-elect Welch was a recognized NMA guest when President Kenney was sworn into office and delivered his inaugural address:

"For seven years, we have invited them (representatives of the AMA, American Hospital Association and other major hospital organizations) to sit down with us and solve the problem. The high professional and economic levels of these bodies and the altruistic religious principles according to which they are supposed to operate seems to have meant nothing. By their refusal to confer, they force action by crisis. And now, events have passed beyond them. The initiative is no longer theirs to accept."

Shortly after being sworn in, President Kenney scheduled the first NMA-AMA Liaison Meeting and led his delegation to the Chicago offices of the AMA. Since the NMA was the instigator of the meeting, Kenney began the discussion by reviewing, at some length, the long struggle that African American physicians had waged to try to achieve equality of opportunity within the medical profession. He referred to several cases, then in litigation, to illustrate the scope and pervasiveness of the problem.

Speaking directly to his AMA hosts, he was emphatic in explaining to them the difficulties encountered, and the shame felt by an African American trying to convince a European American (especially a Southerner) to endorse him for membership in the AMA.

Dr. Kenney demanded a constitutional change in the AMA's by-laws, an adoption in the interim, or an interpretation that comports with the Hill-Burton Act and the Constitution. An added suggestion was that the AMA's central office urge local societies that have the "personal endorsement" as a part of the hospital they control, not to insist on such a stipulation in the case of qualified African American doctors. He felt that the board of trustees could outline the legal liabilities of societies that cling to racially restrictive by-laws.

Toward the end of his prepared statement, Kenney asked for an AMA endorsement of the pending legislative effort to delete the "separate but equal" clause from the Hill-Burton Act. He closed his report with a question that would define their goals of a liaison committee of the two organizations:

"We should like to ask the AMA's board of trustees and the House of Delegates in what way do they feel we can resolve these important questions (of racial discrimination and segregation)? How can the NMA and the AMA work toward resolving these problems?[1]

With many such questions from the petitioners, but no meaningful responses from those who had all the answers, the meeting lasted for two hours and ended, as all others had, inconclusively.

A few weeks later, a second such meeting began with an NMA restatement of the earlier conditions and a plea for change within the AMA. Like the earlier meeting, the AMA officials made few comments and no definite promises to change their policy of racial exclusion. This meeting also ended inconclusively and was, for all practical purposes, a waste of time, money and self-esteem for the NMA delegation.

The four-month interval between the second and third meeting of the Liaison Committee had produced a set of circumstances that offered a small ray of hope for the more optimistic officers of the NMA. They were able to convince themselves that the joint Liaison Committee deserved one more meeting.

AMA President Annis was picketed by members of the Medical Committee for Human Rights (MCHR) after his speech before the 112th Annual Convention in Atlantic City on June 19, 1963.

As soon as he stepped down from the podium, Dr. John Holloman, Co-director of the MCHR and a future president of the NMA, put down his protest poster long enough to enter the auditorium. He walked up to a surprised President Annis and handed him a list of demands for changes within the AMA. President Annis folded the list and stuffed it into his coat pocket, never to be seen or heard from again.

When there was no discernable evidence of movement in the AMA camp, the NAACP joined the fray by ordering a picket line around the AMA's Chicago headquarters. The NAACP picket line was ignored as well.

When AMA President-elect Norman Welch addressed the 68th annual convention of the NMA, he offered what some delegates mistook for an olive branch. He expressed the opinion that progress was being made in the Liaison Committee meetings: "We, of the AMA, are aware that physicians of your race do have problems to overcome in your struggle for equal opportunities in the practice of medicine;" but, he assured the delegates, "the AMA was prepared to do what it could to help them solve these problems."

He "saw" no reason why the AMA would not take a stand on the repeal of the "separate but equal" provisions of the Hill-Burton Act and even went on record as opposed to the racial discrimination in hospital appointments. He said nothing nor did anything to implement his words.

The third meeting of the NMA-AMA Liaison Committee on December 19, 1963, was a final, year-end bid by the NMA to salvage anything from their year-long efforts to force change in the monolithic position of the AMA.

Although Dr. Welch's speech had divested the AMA of any responsibility for the racist repression of NMA members, there remained some lingering hope that another trip to the well might be in order—just to be absolutely sure that it wasn't still dry. They convened, again, at the AMA's Chicago headquarters six days before Christmas.

The AMA, better represented than ever before, brought out its first team: Drs. Edward Annis, president; Norman Welch, president-elect; Percy Hopkins, chairman of the board of trustees; James Appel, vice-chairman, board of trustees; George Fister, past president and trustee; John Blasingame, executive vice-president; Leo Brown, asst. to Dr. Blasingame; Atty. Robert B Thockmorton, general counsel; and Ken David, communications director. Hugh H. Husey, past chairman of the board and director of Scientific Activities attended for a part of the day.

NMA representatives were Drs. John Kenney, immediate past president; Kenneth W. Clement, president; Cobb, president-elect and editor of the *NMA Journal*; and Arthur W. Boddie, veteran chairman of the board of trustees.

Although Dr. Kenney was unhappy because of the meager results for his heroic efforts as president, he still wanted to tangle with the monster "one more time." President Clement, cool and fearless, held himself in high regard and was anxious to match wits with the "best of them." Dr. Cobb was beaten and bitter; almost singlehandedly, he had organized the Imhotep Conferences, which he truly expected would "broaden understanding of the problem and unify action in respect to the elimination of racism, one of the major barriers to making the best in medical facilities available to all the people of the nation."

The Imhotep Conferences, which had met annually from 1957-1963, were kept going by the fierce, dogged, determination and will power of small core of people, primarily Dr. Cobb. Meeting in various cities, their efforts were heroic, but failed to gain the respect or even the attention of the members of the medical establishment. For them, the NMA hardly existed!

Even at the time of this NMA-AMA meeting, five years later, he still felt that Imhotep had failed because of the refusal of such organizations as the AMA, and its powerful influence over the various religious and lay hospital associations, which dared not to be *for* anything that the AMA was *against*.

As president-elect of the NMA, Dr. Cobb felt an obligation to come along with the "brethren," but his optimism for the future and his hope for change in the AMA had already been hemorrhaged out on earlier battlefields.

135

This third joint conference group accepted a four item agenda:

1. A report on the AMA's House of Delegates action in the November meeting.
2. Report on the NMA study regarding county society and staff appointments.
3. Medical Education.
4. King-Anderson (Medicaid) legislation.

It was reported that during the prior AMA annual meeting, the Rhode Island delegation had submitted a resolution that "all qualified physicians should be eligible for membership in the AMA or any constituent association or component society thereof, regardless of race religion or place of natural origin and any discrimination violates Article 2 of the AMA constitution."

The AMA's House of Delegates was then urged to adopt the following resolution:

"That AMA's board of trustees be, and hereby is, instructed to take such action as it deems necessary or appropriate to deny the rights and privileges of membership in the AMA to any member of any constituent association or component society thereof, which denies membership to any qualified physician because of race, creed or color."

The House of Delegates rejected this resolution and adopted the report of membership eligibility from the Reference Committee:

"A copy of this resolution is to be sent to each constituent and component society which urges constituent and component societies having racially restrictive membership provisions to study the question in the light of the prevailing conditions, with a view of taking such steps as they may elect to eliminate such practices."

The Reference Committee reported that some states had black members who had elected not to join the AMA and suggested that they be urged to do so.

Dr. Clement presented several examples of county exclusions of African American physicians from membership, but angrily rejected responsibility for uncovering and reporting all such cases to the AMA. He was "sure that the AMA knew or could learn infinitely more about the manifold ways in which discriminatory practices could be effected than the NMA could ever discover."

Moreover, he recalled that AMA President Welch, in his earlier address before the NMA, had acknowledged the existence of discriminatory practices, in so many places, within the AMA and that "it would be a waste of time to further belabor the issue with a detailed documentation."

After this heated exchange, Dr. Annis was happy to move on to the next issue on the agenda which enabled him to report that the AMA had been the guarantor of 128 loans, totalling $158,000, to Howard Univ.'s medical college and 158 loans totalling $204,000 to Meharry Medical College, since their last, joint meeting.

At that most opportune moment, Dr. Annis went on to call the group's attention that the NMA's support of the Medicare Bill was in direct opposition to the AMA's rejection of the measure.

Dr. Clement's rapid reminder was that the NMA supported Medicare on its merits and that the AMA's position had nothing to do with the NMA. He went on to infer that Dr. Annis' timing of the loan announcements suggested that the self-interest of the AMA was a motivating factor.

Dr. Annis denied that there was any connection between the moral value inherent in working to eliminate racial discrimination and the NMA's position on Medicare. Yet, Dr. Annis could not quite understand "why all the doctors in the country supported the AMA's opposition to Medicare except those in the NMA."

The two issues of much higher priority to the AMA delegation than the elimination of racial discrimination and segregation were the defeat of the Medicare bill and passage of the Hill-Burton Act with the "separate-but-equal" provision from *Plessy v. Ferguson* left intact. It seemed obvious that the large turn-out of AMA attendees and the disclosure of charitable gifts to Howard and Meharry were hardly coincidental.

137

Anyone who knew "Monty" can imagine his almost uncontrollable impatience to join the fray:

"There is no relationship between majority opinion and the truth. In 1492, Columbus was a minority of one, who believed that the world was round. The NMA respects the high caliber and well-trained minds, in the AMA, which had addressed a set of facts and come to a certain conclusion.

"Inasmuch as I am sure that you gentlemen from the AMA would not aver that your minds are any better than ours, I am equally certain that you will respect our judgement in coming to a different set of conclusions after examining the same set of facts."

The silence that followed that sharp exchange seemed eternal and nearly was. As usual, the meeting ended without anything accomplished; albeit, this time, it ended on a sour note. More than two years passed before the NMA asked for another hearing.

---

1. *JNMA,* Vol. 55, pp. 464-447.

Detroit Medical Society

Michigan's African American physicians have been in the forefront of the struggle for justice and equality in medical care for more than a century. Joseph Ferguson, Michigan's first African American physician, was an activist in Detroit's Abolitionist Movement in the middle 1850s. He was one of seven leaders who met secretly with Frederick Douglass and John Brown on March 12, 1859 in downtown Detroit. Although the agenda of that meeting is unknown, it is safe to assume they gathered to assess and extend the fight against enslavement, a viable American institution at that time.

Many disciples have followed in Ferguson's wake and are still involved in this unending fight. Each generation has been forced to adjust its attack in an effort to bag that deeply-entrenched and resourceful beast—racism.

Between the Civil War and World War I, there was a gradual increase in Detroit's population, both African American and European American. When "king cotton" was dethroned by the boll weevil and automobile magnate Henry Ford offered to pay $5 for a full day's work, thousands of African Americans abandoned their cotton sacks and flocked to Detroit, and other northern cities, searching for a better life. Not all of them were destitute and poverty-stricken. As will become apparent, some were professionals and business people who helped to improve the quality of life in the communities wherever they were welcomed or not.

Unfortunately, these immigrants encountered a level of racial hostility in the North that wasn't much different from their Southern experiences. This book will describe, for the most part, the efforts of this group of patients to secure their inalienable right to the best medical care available and their physicians' unending struggles to provide it. These physicians, like their colleagues in other cities, fought segregation and discriminatory practices with whatever weapons that were available.

The Allied Medical Society, Detroit's affiliate of the NMA and the forerunner of the current Detroit Medical Society (DMS), was the first tent under which the society's members launched a group assault against an enemy from whom they had, so far, failed to gain a single, significant victory despite their heroic efforts.

In the "Hospitals" section of this book, reference is made to the establishment of a series of small private, segregated "hospitals" because of the policies of racial exclusion in the hospitals already operating. The abundance of African American physicians attempting to build and manage his own hospital earned Detroit the dubious title "Negro Hospital Capital of the World."

When they applied for staff positions at any of Detroit's general hospitals, the constant refrain of "you're not qualified!" was the admonition heard by the physicians. Qualification meant residency training in approved hospital programs, none of which was made available to them.

This denial of staff appointment on the basis on not being "qualified" and the denial of opportunity to become qualified have produced an American medical establishment controlled by European Americans. As will be shown later, these "guardians of status quo" allowed African American patients and physicians extremely limited access to these hallowed grounds, which they assumed were their private preserves.

Earlier, we saw that the only option for the rejected, untrained African American physician was to seek residencies outside Detroit, wherever they could be found and beg for hospital staff appointments afterwards. Thus, nearly all of Detroit's first African American specialists were trained outside of the city.

Along the way, you will meet some of those intrepid trailblazers who ignored the "no trespassing" signs and established beachheads of medical service on the hostile shores of the American medical establishment and defended them until the NMA, its affiliates and supporters were able to mobilize a proper counterattack.

All of us who helped to blaze a trail through that thicket of bias and denial can cite the penance that we paid to white supremacy for the privileges of training and practicing in public hospitals, an inalienable right that the "guardians of status quo" take for granted.

Mid-Century Developments

Members of the DMS, aided by the NAACP, the Urban League, and other community groups took a hard look at local medical institutions in the early 1950s. By this time, enough African American physicians had been trained outside Detroit and appointed to numerous Detroit hospital staffs for them to begin to appreciate how badly they and their patients were being treated.

These physicians pooled and recorded their personal experiences, along with those of their patients, and sent copies to government officials and the media. Alarmed and embarrassed by these allegations, Mayor Albert Cobo, through his Committee on Community Relations, appointed a group of 35 leading citizens to make a full study of the charges that racial bias was rampant in nearly all of Detroit's medical institutions.

This Hospital Study Committee was chaired by Detroit's perennial peacemaker, Bishop Richard S. Emrich, an Episcopalian prelate; vice-chairwomen were Mrs. Carl B. Grawn and Dr. Marjorie Peebles-Meyers and among the members were: John D. Dancy, exec. secretary of the Urban League; Katherine Faville, dean of the School of Nursing, Wayne Univ.; Dr. Roger DeBusk, medical director (Grace Hospital); Katherine Failing, chairwoman, board of trustees (Woman's—now Hutzel—Hospital); Dr. Luther Leader (president of Wayne County Medical Society and representing Harper Hospital); Dr. Joseph Molner (Detroit's Board of Health); Sister Marie Jean D'Arc, RSM; Alex Fuller (United Automobile Workers of America); Rabbi Leon Fram; and Remus Robinson, M.D.

Investigations began in 1952 and lasted for four years. Areas of study included, medical and nursing education, medical and nursing staff appointments and hospital bed utilization. Eventually, 47 area hospitals, nursing and medical schools were scrutinized. The Report of the Medical and Hospital Study Committee by Bishop Emrich, chairman, Detroit Commission on Community Relations, was filed with the Water Board in April 1956.

The report showed that bed utilization by African American patients in the voluntary hospitals occurred in just about the same proportion as in the general population. About 65% of black babies were reportedly born in the area hospitals. Four hospitals reported no black patients; while thirteen others admitted black patients, rarely. Fourteen church-related hospitals reported racially integrated hospital admission policies.

After their four-year study and evaluation of the findings, the committee concluded that the presence of racial factors in bed assignment not only affected the availability and utilization of hospital beds, but also, was a serious social problem in almost all of the community's hospitals.

In addition to the findings regarding bed utilization, other practices of racial bias were exposed by the Committee's investigations:

1. None of Detroit's private hospitals had ever trained an African American intern or resident.

2. Harper Hospital, one of Detroit' oldest and largest, had never appointed an African American intern, resident or staff doctor since its founding in 1863.

3. Childrens Hospital was being threatened by members of its own medical staff because of its refusal to appoint its first African American to the residency program.

4. Some hospitals, which had appointed African American physicians, limited their staff privileges and treated them as tokens.

5. Both of the state's medical schools, Wayne Univ. and the Univ. of Mich. maintained strict racial quotas in accepting African American students in their freshman medical classes. At that time, Wayne's medical school had a total enrollment of 11 African American medical students; while Univ. of Mich. had a total of 12.

The Mayor's Hospital Study Committee set as its goal the equitable utilization of the area's hospital bed facilities on a non-racial basis for the benefit of the total community. In order to meet this goal, the Committee made the following recommendations:

1. "Individual hospital boards of directors must make an immediate review of their hospital's policy of staff appointments and bed utilization to determine if procedures are followed which guarantee equal accommodation without racial discrimination or segregation."

2. "Race will not be a factor in the selection of the medical and nursing staff in training. All people will be served without segregation or racial bias."

3. "The community's medical, pre-payment plans must ensure equal accommodation to all people without regard to race, as a condition of the contractual arrangements with hospitals which are willing to receive hospitalization payment from white and Negro subscribers' pre-payment funds."

4. "The Hospital Council, Medical Society and Hospital Trustees will promote a common standard of staff member-hospitals, and they must undertake responsibility for an educational campaign to acquaint the general public with non-racial community standards."

5. "That a study be made of patient utilization of government facilities to determine the extent to which bona fide evidence of indigency and emergency, and not race, factor in hospital care or medical practice resulting in the racial utilization of these governmental facilities."

This report was hailed as a breakthrough in the dike of institutional racism through which freedom of choice and fair-play would gush unremittingly. Such optimism was not universally shared by all members of the committee and virtually none of the recommendations was followed, voluntarily.

Dr. Remus Robinson, still smarting from his earlier, personal conflicts with racism at Grace Hospital took a skeptical view of the report. He doubted the sincerity of the hospital's representatives, the accuracy of the committee's findings, and their ability to produce any significant change.

His alternative plan was to secure $4 million for the renovation and certification of Parkside Hospital and bring it to parity with area hospitals for the training of African American physicians. John Dancy, whose brother had been Parkside Hospital's first intern, supported Robinson's proposal.

Although Drs. Meyers and Robinson were personal friends, she led the opposition against his proposal. She was joined by Dean Faville (Wayne Univ. Nursing School) and others in an ultimate defeat of the Parkside option.

Despite his disappointment, Dr. Robinson continued to work fervently to guarantee that the inalienable rights of all Americans would be observed within the operation of the new Medical Center. My subsequent discussions with Dr. Robinson gave me the impression that he was fully persuaded that the Medical Center project would never voluntarily serve the best interest of those physicians who had been denied access to and those citizens who had been uprooted by its development.

On a more personal note, Robinson was unable to cite any reason why, after 30 years of daily contact with them, any African American physician should have confidence that his European American colleagues would be fair and honest.

During the next two-to-three years, DMS members kept the medical scene under close surveillance and filed many reports that justified Robinson's worst misgivings. Several examples cited below show the high price paid for hospital bias by the African American physician in lost income, stunted professional growth and loss of self-esteem. In terms of neglect and physical injury, the African American patients paid an even higher price.

Shortly after the Report of The Mayor's Hospital Committee was accepted, and the committee disbanded, a moonlighting Ob-gyn resident reported what appeared to be a clear violation of the committee's recent recommendations.

An obviously distressed African American couple appeared in the emergency room of a church-operated, Detroit hospital. The wife complained of a missed period, abdominal pain, fainting and sweating. The emergency room doctor (moonlighting as an Ob-gyn resident) made an immediate diagnosis of ruptured, ectopic pregnancy, intra-peritoneal hemorrhage and impending shock. He advised the nurse to admit the patient and called the operating room to arrange for immediate surgery.

Instead, the hospital administrator was called. She countermanded the resident's order, directed the resident to transfer the patient and demanded that the doctor discharge the patient to the city hospital, 12 miles away. The resident refused, explaining the patient was too ill to be moved.

"The administrator called a staff doctor, at home, and ordered him to come in to sign the transfer document. A private ambulance was called and the patient was transferred, despite the fact that she had ample Blue Cross\Blue Shield coverage.

"Upon her arrival at hospital B, some two hours after her arrival at the religiously-oriented hospital A, the patient, now in deep shock, and was taken directly to the operating room for emergency surgery. The diagnosis was confirmed.

"Although the patient survived, her course was eventful. She required 13 units of blood, developed thrombophlebitis, pulmonary emboli and gluteal necrosis at the injection sites of various medications. She had approximately 30 X-rays and at least 100 other tests. After 28 days, the patient was able to return home to her husband and four sons."

Upon hearing about this case from one of my residents, I tracked down the patient's telephone number and called her at home. She corroborated the above story and was hoping for a complete recovery.

My call came too early in her recovery period to determine if Sheean's syndrome was to be a late complication of the misadventure. While it may have been possible to determine the total cost of a month's stay in the hospital and scores of laboratory tests, the most serious losses are immeasurable and may not have been even considered.

Officials of Michigan State Medical Society, the Wayne County Medical Society and Blue Cross\Blue Shield were notified about this case. Neither of the medical organizations responded. Blue Cross informed me that they were not "in the habit of telling a hospital administrator how to operate his or her institution."

The second case occurred in a Detroit Medical Center hospital, and the patient was less fortunate. Within a year of the above case, a patient reentered another hospital two days after discharge, with a diagnosis of post-conization hemorrhage from the uterine cervix.

The patient's doctor, a certified gynecologist, had failed to gain promotion beyond courtesy appointment despite several years of post-certification effort. Thus, he was ineligible for resident assistance and had to provide his own surgical and obstetrical assistance from within the hospital staff no matter what time of the day or the nature of the emergency.

"When the patient arrived, there was an Ob-gyn resident on call for the emergency room. He informed the staff doctor that he was not available, having been instructed to remain at the ready just in case an emergency case came in."

The gynecologist, working alone, had considerable difficulty securing the bleeder. An estimated blood loss of more than 1,000 cc's and a state of mild shock were managed with a transfusion of two units of blood. The patient recovered from the blood loss and the surgery, but died two months later from an acute transfusion reaction.

Dr. Waldo Cain was a board-certified general surgeon and a highly vocal member of those African American doctors who advocated loudly for patients' rights. He, too, was a member of the Grace Hospital's courtesy staff who also had to do his own histories, physicals, and follow-ups on all of his patients.

He provided his own assistance for surgical operations. On some occasions, he brought a colleague in to assist who was not on the Grace Hospital staff. The administration looked the other way, rather than appoint a resident to assist Dr. Cain.

It was about this time that Blue Cross began reimbursing hospitals for surgical resident assistance. If a hospital did not have an approved residency, the doctor's assistant was eligible for an assistant's fee.

When Cain called this inequity to the attention of Grace's officials and threatened to have one of his patients sue the hospital for unequal protection, he was quietly and quickly promoted to the active staff and assigned a resident.

The first case above showed the refusal of three medically-related organizations to accept accountability for gross acts of injustice which caused injury to people whom they represented and should have been willing to protect.

Blue Cross' membership in Detroit's black community approached 40% by that time. Additionally, the hospital involved in the first case had just completed a major expansion project with the assistance of Hill-Burton funds, for which it submitted a resolution not to discriminate. The vindictive practice of freezing activist African American physicians at the courtesy level was fairly universal in the Medical Center.

The event that eventually triggered Dr. Robinson's abrupt departure from Grace Hospital was the arrival of David French, M.D., in Detroit in the late 1950s. French, an African American, had just completed his surgical residency and was immediately given active staff privileges at Grace Hospital. Dr. Robinson, still on the courtesy staff, regarded this as a slap-in-the-face, resigned from Grace and was accepted at Providence Hospital.

Within a year of the release of the Hospital Study Committee's report, the officers and members of DMS were dissatisfied, justifiably, with the lack of real progress in the area hospitals' elimination of discriminatory practices. They decided to seek the support of their WCMS, directly.

Not only did hundreds of DMS members hold joint memberships in the Wayne County Medical Society (WCMS) and the AMA, Dr. Luther Leader, then president of the WCMS, had been appointed by Mayor Cobo to represent organized medicine on his Hospital Committee when it was formed.

147

An appointment was made to address the Society's council meeting. When Dr. Robinson, the chosen spokesman, led his DMS delegation before Dr. Leader in his WCMS headquarters, Leader's first and last, condescending question was, "well, now, what do you boys want?"

Thus, the Hospital Committee's recommendation, with which Dr. Leader concurred, "that the Society undertake to promote a common standard of staff membership and bed assignment among the member hospitals and they undertake the responsibility for an educational campaign to acquaint the public, as well as those who utilize hospitals, with non-racial community standards," was meaningless and had been completely ignored by the WCMS, since the committee had begun its investigations several years prior.

An earlier review of the *Detroit Medical News'* files, the organ of the WCMS for the 1960s, disclosed only one reference to the struggle of the Society's African American members for equality of medical opportunity in Detroit's hospitals. This one exception was an editorial that appeared in the *Detroit Medical News* on May 11, 1959, under the by-line of Horace Bradfield, M.D., associate editor and member of DMS. His editorial caused quite a stir when it was submitted for publication.

Senior editors, Drs. David I. Sugar and William Bromme, strongly urged Bradfield to withdraw the editorial before publication lest it "disturb the power brokers in the area hospitals." Bradfield refused to withdraw it and the article was published in its entirety.

The editorial, entitled "Democracy and Brotherhood," made a plea for the spirit of brotherhood, especially in the black-white relationship. In his support of the Golden Rule as the standard for this human inter-relationship, Dr. Bradfield said:

"Today, the emphasis is on Judeo-Christian duty with emphasis on the positive benefits accruing to Negro and white persons through association."

While Dr. Bradfield congratulated some area hospitals for opening their doors to black interns, residents and staff doctors, he found it "regrettable" that most of Detroit's private, major hospitals had not trained and "do not, now, train Negro interns and residents." He described this as "second-class treatment for the Negro doctor."

Bradfield went on to warn that when private hospitals use government funds, enjoy tax-exempt status and the right of eminent domain to clear land and build their institutions, the beneficiary institutions are no longer private; but blacks, like their white brothers, "have a clear right to the use of such voluntary hospital facilities in keeping with the general rule of the hospital."

Bradfield's final plea must have been embarrassing to his fellow editors; it reminded them of the same entreaty made (and ignored) by the Mayor's Hospital Study Committee more three years before. He continued:

"A positive expression from the WCMS and Detroit area voluntary hospital staffs would have a salutary effect on the center of the power structure of hospital trustees boards and administrators. By increased access to the facilities of these hospitals by patients and qualified doctors, regardless of race, color and creed, an expression of democracy and brotherhood can be achieved."

Dr. Bradfield, now deceased, was congratulated for his foresight and courage. His opposition to the "separate-but-equal" clause of the Hill-Burton Act came more than four years before it was outlawed by the passage of the Civil Rights Act of 1964. His courage was manifested in demanding freedom of speech, despite the attempts of his fellow-editors to gag him.

The temperature of his relationship with other members of the *Detroit Medical News* staff fell precipitously after his editorial was published. Although, the members of the editorial board failed to silence Bradfield the first time he violated their editorial policy, they made sure that he would not be there for the next round. He was not extended the usual courtesy of remaining on the editorial board thereafter.

My research was extended to include a review of approximately ten years of publications of *Michigan Medicine,* the organ of the Michigan State Medical Society. I found only two references to the critical struggle of Michigan Medical Society's African American members for justice and equality. One was a "Letter to the Editor" by Paul Lowinger, M.D., in the early 1960s. Paul was one of only two European American members of the Detroit Medical Society.

Published without editorial comment, the letter asked for support for the Medical Committee for Human Rights (MCHR), a national group of physicians who supported the African American physician's struggle for equality of opportunity. The other, also devoid of comment, merely noted the passage of a resolution in the Michigan State Medical Society's House of Delegates affirming the Society's opposition to racial discrimination.

As DMS girded for its long, overdue battle against its enemies in the medical establishment, a letter came from the Detroit office of the NAACP expressing a desire to launch a more vigorous attack against discrimination in the field of medicine than had ever been mounted. The letter was signed by the president and the executive director of the Detroit Branch of NAACP.

Lionel Swan, president of DMS, sent the following reply:

Dear Messrs. Turner, Johnson:

Your kind and thought-provoking letter, of November 25, 1958, was read before the Detroit Medical Society during its regular meeting on the same date. Its contents, plus your charming representative, served to stimulate and encourage us.

The Detroit Medical Society is aware of the many therapeutic activities being carried on by the NAACP to cure the social ills of our time. To share some of these experiences with you has provided us with a feeling of real accomplishment.

Your desire to undertake a more vigorous anti-discrimination program in the field of medical services coincides with our own activities in this area. As your letter states, this is a multi-faceted problem which does require a variety of solutions.

To this end, the Detroit Medical Society has appointed a liaison committee to work in the field of medical services. We are anxious to meet with you at an early date in order to coordinate our actions. Moreover, we feel that such a meeting should include representatives of other organizations that are already actively girded for the same battle.

We refer to the Urban League and the Cotillion Club, especially. We recognize that each organization has its own approach to the problem but synchronization increases effectiveness. We shall look forward to your suggestions for a meeting, in the not-too-distant future.

Sincerely yours,

Lionel Swan, M.D.,
President, DMS

This letter came at a most opportune time for the DMS' officers and members. Nearly three years had passed since the Mayor's Hospital Committee had submitted its report and disbanded.

Lionel Swan, M.D. (Howard Univ.), had practiced in Birmingham, Ala, until 1951, when he moved to Detroit. He first came to the attention of the members of the DMS with his leadership in helping to establish the NAACP's Freedom Fund Dinner in 1956. He was in the first of his two-year tour of duty as DMS president, when the NAACP's letter was received.

Thus, Dr. Swan was in command of the DMS during the crucial 1950s when the Society launched its all-out attack on hospital discrimination and racial segregation in Detroit's general hospitals. Joint committees were formed with the NAACP, the Cotillion Club, community and church groups to keep up anti-segregation pressure.

It was also during Dr. Swan's regime that Atty. William Patrick, an African American, made his successful bid for a seat on Detroit's Common Council. Dr. Swan helped to deliver the winning financial and political support of an aroused DMS.

Once elected, Councilman Patrick began to take a critical look at the Medical Center, then under construction in Detroit's central corridor. He discovered that the Medical Center's authorities were using federal funds to build a racially segregated Medical Center, a clear violation of the Hill-Burton Hospital Construction Act.

Councilman Patrick notified Dr. Swan that the Medical Center was to be accused of violating the Hill-Burton Act during a council meeting and urged that the DMS be represented. Dr. Swan recruited a team of DMS members to accompany him to the meeting, including Dr. Lawrence

Lackey, DMS vice president. Attorney Patrick formed coalitions with the liberal forces on the Council and a bitter struggle began that attracted national attention.

As a result of the fearless fight to rid the medical establishment of its racism, NMA officials applauded Dr. Swan's fearless courage and elected him to the office of president in 1967 after Lyndon Johnson succeeded President Kennedy in the Oval Office.

Dr. Swan still recalls the great occasion when he, as president, was called upon to introduce President Johnson at the 1967 convention in Houston, Tex. (the first sitting president to address an NMA convention).

It was during that convention that the DMS first presented the medical recruitment film, *You Can Be A Doctor!* It was a joint venture between the DMS and Detroit's Museum of African American History, which I founded in 1965.

Dr. Lawrence Lackey, of Kansas, who had worked closely with Dr. Swan as vice president of the DMS and succeeded him without losing a step.[1]

The liaison committee was formed as proposed by the NAACP and it helped to coordinate the battle plans of the DMS with similar activities within the NAACP and other civil rights groups.

The Cotillion Club, among the other organizations suggested by the NAACP, attracted to their membership some of the city's most active and influential African American leaders. Working together, they have amassed a long and enviable record of successes in the unending struggle for freedom and justice. Its sponsorship of Detroit's annual Debutante Ball is a highlight of the spring season and provides a proper finish to the school year.

The club's successes included, among other things, job integration in banks and department stores and an increasing African American political power through voter registration at the time of election. Their successful drive, which forced Herman Kiefer Hospital to integrate its patients, nurses and staff, provided a good example of how to plan and execute a strategic assault on an implacable foe—the medical establishment.

Prior to 1929, Herman Keifer was a city hospital operating for the treatment of tuberculosis and other infectious diseases. It refused to admit African American patients except on a strictly segregated basis or allow more than one African American physician on its staff; Dr. Rupert Markoe, a fair-skinned Virgin Islander whom the admitting officer at the Univ. of Mich. Medical School had classified as European American.[2]

A TB epidemic, referred to in the chapter on "Hospitals," caused the deaths of many African Americans, in Detroit, in 1929.

Public pressure from the African American community forced the city to relax Herman Kiefer's rigid policy of racial exclusion and a segregated ward of 120 beds was established on the sixth floor. When this number proved to be insufficient, the Board of Health rejected the DMS' recommendation of patient integration.

The hospital administrators elected to extend its policy of racial segregation by sponsoring the growth and development of small, segregated, private TB hospitals to serve Detroit's African American community: Fairview Sanitarium, Good Samaritan, St. Albans General, Bethesda and Dunbar Hospital (which changed its name to Parkside Hospital after it moved to Brush in 1928. See Hospitals).

Swimming upstream against a rising current of blatant racism were Drs. Greenidge, Markoe, McClendon and the Alf Thomases, Sr. and Jr., who managed these institutions.

These institutions were overwhelmed by an epidemic, made worse by malnutrition, overcrowding in the segregated neighborhoods, and limited access to the best health care facilities available. Needless to say, some of these institutions barely offered custodial care. None of them was comparable to Herman Kiefer.

Over the years, the "Herman Kiefer Type Solution" and its implications have enraged the African American community at all levels. Despite discussions with the Mayor's Hospital Study Committee, health commissioner, Dr. Joseph Molner, and other members of the medical establishment, racism remained rampant throughout the region while the death-rate from TB soared to new heights.

Members of the DMS and the Cotillion Club, supported by the NAACP, decided to take on the City of Detroit, Dr. Molner's Board of Health and the medical establishment. A Committee to End Discrimination in Detroit's Hospitals was formed which met with Dr. Molner and his staff on October 22, 1958, at Kiefer hospital.

Representing the Cotillion Club were:

The Hon. Congressman Charles C. Diggs; Thomas Batchelor, M.D.; Leonard Proctor; William T. Matney; Herman Glass; Cassius Pendleton; Atty. (now judge) Damon Keith; and Roland Chapman, M.D. Observers were Richard Marks, Detroit commissioner on Community Relations and Dorothy Quarker, administrative assistant to Congressman Diggs.

In addition to Dr. Molner, the Herman Kiefer officials present were: Dr. Paul Salchow, medical director; Dr. Paul Chapman, TB control officer; Dr. Rupert Markoe, Herman Kiefer's only African American staff member; and Dorothy Schaffer, director of Nursing.

In a heated, two-hour session, Congressman Diggs, speaking on behalf of the Cotillion Club, presented well-documented evidence of the following objectionable practices at the Herman Kiefer Hospital:

1. The admissions clerk demands the racial identity of a patient before admission.

2. Segregation of African American patients on the north and south porch sections of the sixth floor. He demanded that these practices cease, forthwith.

Dr. Molner did not deny the charges but stated that racial identity had nothing to do with the patients' need for treatment and agreed to stop the practice. Hospital officials admitted that patients were segregated racially, but "often" at the (European American) patients' request.

Cotillion Club representatives held that bed assignment should not be left to the patient but should be determined by the patient's need. Evidence was offered to prove that attempts by the nursing staff to integrate the wards had been stopped by the administration. At the end of the conference, Dr. Molner made a commitment to

154

stop the practice of segregation and asked for two months to make the changes effective.

A subsequent meeting was held at the Sheraton Cadillac Hotel on December 17, 1956, seven weeks after the first meeting. Present were Dr. Molner and hospital owner, Dr. D.T. Burton, who had just joined the Cotillion Club's committee. Soon after the meeting got underway, Molner read the following statement and issued a copy to the press:

"All reference to racial identification in Herman Kiefer's admission procedures has been eliminated. It was completely shocking to me that such a practice existed at Herman Kiefer. It was definitely contrary to official policy and will not be tolerated in the future. Patient bed assignment to wards and semi-private rooms are based on patient need, space availability and medical considerations. At present, there are 10 integrated wards and several integrated semi-private rooms."

The commissioner's statement was accepted and signed by William T. Matney and Leonard Proctor, spokesman for the Cotillion Club:

"Dr. Molner's forthright action in correcting inequitable practices at Herman Kiefer represents a milestone of progress in Detroit. Once the charges were substantiated, he moved directly to the crux of the problem.

"The elimination of race as a factor in medical care, treatment and availability of hospital facilities should be the concern of the entire community. It is heartening to know that our city and county health institutions, through the leadership and direction of Dr. Molner, are now setting the pace in extending democratic practices in this vital area."

From Washington, D.C., Congressman Diggs dispatched: "I am elated that Dr. Molner has taken the action necessary to eliminate biased, public hospital practices, which have been a blight on our community for so long.

"I confidently anticipate that Dr. Molner's democratic mandate will be executed faithfully by all city-operated health institutions and hope that his example will be followed by privately-owned hospitals as well.

Congressman Diggs' seeds of "hope" for a more democratic policy in Detroit's health institutions fell on thorny ground. Despite the Cotillion Club's considerable efforts to integrate the hospital, its members were still unhappy with Detroit's Board of Health, in general, and with Dr. Molner, in particular.

They knew he had not negotiated with them in good faith. He had feigned ignorance of the shameful racial situation at Herman Keifer, notwithstanding the fact that he and WCMS president, Dr. Leader, had served on the City's Hospital Study Committee from 1952-1956, when all of the local hospitals were investigated and their findings and recommendations were reported to the Committee.

When the Cotillion delegation challenged Dr. Molner to make on- the-spot ward rounds with them to support their allegations that nothing had changed, he refused. Dr. Markoe was present at the negotiating sessions, but did not say anything in criticism of the segregated conditions under which he worked.

Under Dr. Molner's administration there had never been an African American heading up any department in the Board of Health. He tolerated all kinds of subterfuge among his subordinates to keep the administrative positions lily-white. The entire department assumed a posture of condescension toward African Americans, both employees and the general public.

The physician members of the Cotillion Club provided sufficient personal experience in their dealings with the Dept. of Health to build a strong case for bigotry against Dr. Molner and his department. They decided unanimously that Dr. Molner, an unsalvageable, white supremacist, had to go.

This was an informed decision. The Cotillions knew that Dr. Molner was a prominent and influential member of the medical establishment, a syndicated columnist and, above all else, white. To bring him down would require careful planning, close cooperation and consistent follow through. At that time, the Cotillion Club and the DMS had the will and Detroit's 1961 mayoral election provided the way.

Incumbent mayor, Louis Miriani had run a tight ship at Detroit's City Hall, insofar as the business interests and suburbs were concerned. He was considered a sure winner against the politically unknown upstart, Jerry Cavanagh.

Unfortunately, the law-and-order campaign prosecuted so vigorously against the African American community during Mayor Miriani's first term had alienated many black voters. They were ready to dispose of him.

A group of Cotillion Club and DMS members, including Dr. Thomas Batchelor, met with candidate Cavanagh in Attorney (now congressman) George and Dr. Ethelene Crockett's basement. This was the scene of many major political decisions affecting the African American community during the prior forty years.

They offered to deliver a winning, African American vote to Cavanaugh if he promised not to forget them when he became mayor. This made political sense to Candidate Cavanagh and the pact was sealed with an exchange of handshakes.

The members of the Cotillion Club, the NAACP and civil rights groups launched its most successful voter registration campaign and turned out the winning vote on election day.

Soon after his decisive victory, Mayor Cavanagh was visited by a delegation of Cotillions. They requested that Dr. Batchelor be chosen to fill the vacancy on the Health Commission that controlled the Board of Health.

Batchelor was readily appointed by the grateful mayor. When the newly-appointed commissioner discovered that racial segregation was as prevalent as ever at Herman Kiefer Hospital, he demanded that Mayor Cavanagh fire Dr. Molner. The deed was done by telephone, on a Sunday morning.

According to Batchelor, Dr. Molner spend over an hour pleading, unsuccessfully, to save his job.

The first vacancy to occur at the erstwhile, lily-white departmental level was in health education. The only qualified applicant was Phil Rutledge, an African American. When the chief of personnel, Grover Grimes, hesitated about appointing Rutledge, Batchelor ordered him either to appoint Rutledge or someone else from a lower level; in either case, the position would have to be filled with an African American. Grimes did neither. Instead, he scheduled another exam for the convenience of a white candidate from outside the city.

As soon as Bachelor found out about Grimes' white supremacist ploy, Grimes was demoted to collecting delinquent accounts in the City Hospital. Rutledge subsequently got the job. Eventually, Dr. Batchelor rose to become president of the Board of Health and gained considerable authority over developing plans for relocating the new City Hospital to the Medical Center. It was from this position that Batchelor was able to strike a decisive blow for integration at Grace Hospital, as will be discussed under "DMS Investigates Private Hospitals."

During the next several years, DMS officials kept the Medical Center development under close surveillance. Despite the single, partial success of the Herman Kiefer Solution, in a government hospital, there was no reassuring evidence that the same techniques would succeed in the private sector. As a matter of fact, the medical establishment dug in its heels and treated the Herman Keifer solution as a non-event.

A landmark development in the DMS' fight for our inalienable and equal rights to health care was Atty. Patrick's decision to seek a seat on Detroit's Common (now City) Council in 1958. "Bill" Patrick came to the public's attention as a partner in the highly respected firm of (Hobart) Taylor, (Kermit) Bailer, (Charles S.) Farmer and (James) Lee. The firm's legal menu provided a steady diet of racial discrimination and segregation issues, sufficient to build quite a reputation. This helped Patrick to prepare for the baptism-with-fire that awaited him when he won a seat on the Common Council in 1958, a most opportune time for the arrival of a young lawyer who was as ambitious as he was fearless. It was Patrick's legal skills and his political acumen that helped to direct the inevitable confrontation that became:

"The Detroit Medical Society v. The Detroit Medical Establishment"

Encouraged and informed by the joint venture with the Cotillion Club and happy to follow the courageous leadership of Councilman Patrick, DMS members girded for battle with the real enemy within the medical establishment: racism. By the late 1950s, only a few African American physicians had become qualified specialists through residency training in other cities. Fewer still, had been accepted for residency training in Detroit's private hospitals and admitted to practice there. Almost all of those appointments were to the courtesy staffs, with limited privileges, as described earlier.

Our patients were segregated in the least desirable sections of the hospital, if such spaces were available, or flatly denied admission, outright. I have letters, dated 1960, from Woman's and Grace hospitals that denied staff appointments to Dr. William Bentley, although he was already my partner. No similar denial to a European American physician was found, whether the candidate was a partner or not.

This phase of the showdown had the general support of the entire DMS membership, although the foot-soldiers of DMS' Equal Opportunity Committee were those physicians seeking or who had already acquired staff appointments. They carried the fight for justice directly into the boardrooms of various hospitals.

On-site visits to all of the Medical Center hospitals, except Children's, did include other hospitals in the more distant regions of the city. Different teams were assigned to conduct scheduled interviews with hospital administrators, speak to employees, if possible, and record and report all evidence of integration or the lack thereof. These reports were received and appropriate strategies were mounted by members of a larger committee made up of the NAACP, the Urban League, and several community groups.

One of the most active of these was led by Rev. Louis Johnson, pastor of Friendship Baptist, a Medical Center church located at 3900 Beaubien. Rev. Johnson was an outspoken civil rights activist in the Medical Center community who conducted strategy sessions in his church, issued news bulletins of support and accompanied us on some of our face-to-face sessions with hospital officials.

Over the course of several months, members of the fact-finding missions endured much hostility while carrying out their difficult assignments. A brief description of my personal participation in some of the missions should prove informative.

Three members of the committee: Drs. Waldo Cain, James Robinson and I interviewed a senior medical student, Charles Vincent, on April 4, 1958 at Dr. Cain's home. Vincent reported that he had listed Grace Hospital as his first choice for an internship; but Grace had not selected him, although it had not met its quota. However, all of Vincent's European American medical school classmates, even those with lower grades, were accepted. This was just one of the many misadventures Dr. Vincent encountered while enroute to a medical career. The Committee also confirmed that none of the private hospitals would hire African American externs for clerical duties for which outside, European American help was paid $15 per day.

A few weeks later, another segment of DMS' Equal Opportunity Committee met with officials of Mt. Carmel Hospital to discuss hospital integration. Representing DMS were Drs. Horace Bradfield, Ethelene Crockett, DMS President Lawrence Lackey and myself. Dr. William Carpenter spoke for the hospital, under the watchful eye of the Sister Superior. The meeting was less than cordial and Mount Carmel officials made no commitments to consider integration of their hospital's staff.

In 1959 and again in 1974, Mount Carmel completed multi-million dollar expansion projects with Hill-Burton funds for which non-discrimination pledges were signed.[3] Their obvious disdain for our presence was a clear indication of disinterest in our cause. The Hill-Burton funds had already been allocated and with it went our leverage to force the hospital to be held accountable for its promise to the federal government. This was an expensive lesson.

The Imhotep Conferences, which had begun in 1957 to rid health care institutions of segregation, were still attracting interest and support. The DMS, for instance, sent delegations to nearly every conference to report on the Detroit experience, exchange ideas and learn the legal maneuvers that would make the Detroit fight more effective. Accompanying DMS President Swan to the first (1957) Imhotep Conference was Atty. Damon Keith, representing the Detroit Chapter of the NAACP. Atty. Keith congratulated the members of the DMS for having started the Freedom Fund Dinner the year before. He referred to the recently-released Hospital Study Committee report and pledged the NAACP's assistance in seeing that the committee's recommendations were implemented. Dr. Swan's report described the fruitless meetings between DMS representatives and those of Michigan's state and county medical societies as "much lip service." He cited the fine example of Remus Robinson's 19-year tenure as a trustee of Detroit's Board of Education, many of which were served as president. It was during Robinson's presidency that Wayne Univ., then a city institution under the Board of Education, passed a resolution not to affiliate with any hospital that practiced racial discrimination. Understandably, Dr. Robinson's regular re-elections to the board were supported by members of the DMS. Dr. Swan advised his colleagues to support the NAACP and the Urban League and work for the election of the right men to political office. He made specific reference to the Common Council candidacy of Atty. William Patrick. DMS members mobilized their resources and those of their patients to mount a spirited campaign to help Patrick become Detroit's first African American City Councilman. His strong sensitivity against racial bias was challenged soon after his victory in 1957, which earned him a second term in 1961.

A fair-minded but tough negotiator, Patrick formed a coalition with the liberal wing of the Council and established a close liaison with the DMS, the NAACP, the Urban League and other such groups in the African American community. He was a quick study in catching up on the prior history and pertinent issues of the Medical Center development project and moved quickly to a leadership position from which he defended the rights of his constituency. Councilman Patrick spent the first weeks mobilizing his resources for the fight for medical rights that was ominously looming on the horizon.

In the meantime, two developments in 1959 set the stage for a major confrontation with the medical establishment. First, 1959 was a watershed year for the DMS. Hosting the third NMA Convention provided an opportunity for them to

161

review the past, make a critical assessment of the present and plan a more productive future.

The NAACP's Freedom Fund Dinner, launched with the help of DMS leaders, in 1956, was well on its way to maturity in 1959. The relationship between the two organizations was closer than ever. The dinner was served at the Latin Quarter, on March 22nd. The attendance exceeded 500, thirteen percent of whom were physicians.

Personal greetings were brought to the festive crowd from Honorable Louis Miriani, mayor of Detroit, the Honorable G. Mennen Williams, governor of Michigan, and the Honorable Senator Phillip A. Hart (D-Mich.).

It now seems providential that Michigan's three top politicians would gather at the same time and place to hear the nation's top civil rights advocate, Roy Wilkins, executive director of the NAACP, give his mid-century report. Wilkins was then introduced by Dr. D.T. Burton, owner of Burton Mercy Hospital.

Wilkins had plenty to say to the NAACP's most productive Detroit Branch and about how the NAACP forced th U.S. Supreme Court to reverse itself in a landmark school desegregation decision of 1954 the decision that voided segregation in public transportation in 1956, and the passage of the Civil Rights Act of 1957.

This 1957 act began a series of legislative moves that led to the passage of the Omnibus Civil Rights Act of 1964. Although the passage of C-R-64 did not cause the "sudden death" of the "separate but equal" hangover from the Supreme Court's *Plessy v. Ferguson* decision, it did produce a mortal wound that forced the AMA to vote and accept it.

Since Dr. Cobb was a member and officer of the NAACP's board of trustees, Wilkins knew of the difficulties that Dr. Cobb was having, trying to keep the Imhotep Conferences going. He made a strong plea for their support.

The DMS responded a few weeks later by adding to the agenda of its 1959 NMA Convention the unfinished business of the 1959 Imhotep Conference, held in Washington, D.C. a few weeks before. As we shall soon see, the DMS accepted Mr.

Wilkins' challenge, took on Detroit's medical establishment and things have never been the same since.

Unaccustomed to a defeat of any kind, the guardians of status quo fought back with destructive ferocity. On August 28, 1955, Emmet Till was slaughtered like the sacrificial lamb on the altar of white supremacy by murderers in Money, Miss.

One hundred segregationist U.S. congressmen signed a "manifesto" denouncing the U.S. Supreme Court's rulings against racial segregation.[4] Through articles and editorials in the *JNMA*, Dr. Cobb kept the DMS membership aware of the continuing need to fight racial segregation in the nation's health care facilities. By the time of Detroit's NMA convention in 1959, Cobb's two year-old Imhotep anti-segregation effort was already beginning to lose its forward thrust.

The unfinished business of Cobb's 1959 Imhotep Conference, when added to the agenda of Detroit's 1959 NMA convention, spurred it to a frenzy of post-convention, civil rights activity. The delegates, especially those from Detroit, left the convention with sleeves rolled up, and went to work. Councilman Patrick, who had conversed with many of his colleagues, was now able to distinguish friend from foe and drew up a plan of action.

The second decisive development was the request of Detroit's Hospital Authority officials for permission to acquire a total of 235 acres of land next to the existing corridor hospitals where they would construct a $30 million medical center.[5]

Condemnation procedures precipitated bitter, prolonged discussions between the pro-segregationist members of the medical establishment and the anti-segregationists. The former group wanted to continue observing the "separate but equal" clause; however, the anti-segregationists insisted the clause be eliminated from the Hill-Burton Act.

Their differences semed insoluble—although a small majority of the congress favored eliminating the "separate but equal" clause from Hill-Burton. One hundred members signed a "manifesto" in March 1956 that supported its continuation. Caught in the crossfire, some leaders of the medical establishment decided to sign the anti-segregation clause, get the money, and proceed as usual.

Detroit's four corridor hospitals—Children's, Grace, Harper and Woman's—agreed to move closer together and coordinate their services, creating one of the largest medical complexes in the country.

Now, Councilman Patrick had a place for action. By the end of 1959, plans for the Detroit Medical Center were fairly firm and the hospitals' authorities had signed construction agreements with the Michigan Board of Health (which allocated the Hill-Burton funds to finance the project).

In signing such agreements, the hospitals were expected to acknowledge and implement the integration pledge of the Hill-Burton Act. Moreover, firm schedules had been so tightly drawn that time was a valuable commodity.

The City of Detroit was an active partner in this development and scheduled public hearings before the Common Council so that the private land so desperately needed could be condemned, bought and cleared.

Patrick, ever alert to the welfare of his constituency, notified Dr. Lackey, now president of the DMS, and Dr. Swan, past-president, to attend the hearings. A pre-hearing meeting came first with representatives of the DMS, Urban League, the NAACP and Councilman Patrick in attendance. Still smarting from the contempt and condescension encountered during the hospital survey, the DMS team decided that the hospitals would be forced to abide by the non-segregating rules of the Hill-Burton Act, or they would stop the Medical Center's construction which was already well underway.

The hearings opened on January 15, 1960 before a highly-charged audience of 150 community residents, doctors, businessmen and clergy. Dr. Lackey opened the meeting by reading a prepared statement that charged the corridor hospitals with racial discrimination that concluded: "therefore the project is ineligible for Hill-Burton funds." His findings indicated that the worst offender, Harper Hospital, would profit first and most from the proposed project.

164

Lackey demanded the project be postponed until such time as the accused institutions ended their discriminatory practices. This DMS position was endorsed by Councilman Patrick and supported by the NAACP, the Urban League and other community groups.

Ray Eppert, chairman of the Detroit Medical Center Citizens Committee and president of Burroughs Corporation, took strong exception to Lackey's statement. Skirting the real issue of racial bias, he said, "it will be a sad day for Detroit if these charges of discrimination hinder this tremendous undertaking." His position was supported by housing director, Mark K. Hurley and Atty. Edward M. Welch, assistant corporation counsel. They warned that a delay in approval of the land condemnation would jeopardize the entire project.

Patrick adamantly declared his support for the DMS position and warned that he would ask the Council for a four-week moratorium on the project to allow the hospitals time to act on the charges. He brushed aside the fears from the opposition that such a delay would cause serious harm to the venture.

"The charges of discrimination were highly exaggerated," declared Councilwoman Blanche Parent Wise. She conceded that "black" doctors did not comprise a significant portion of the staffs of the corridor hospitals, but that "this was due to their lack of qualification, not racism."

Patrick's position was supported by a flurry of telegrams, telephone calls, and letters sufficient to win a week's delay in signing a condemnation order to seize and clear the land for Phase 1. During that interval, none of the hospitals' spokesmen said or did anything to suggest they were willing to compromise. As a matter of fact, an event occurred that week to prove they did not intend to make any concessions.

Since Harper Hospital was the most recalcitrant of all the institutions involved, it became the major target of the DMS. As a part of our continuing pressure to break through their haughty walls of hostile complacency, I visited Harper Hospital toward the end of the negotiation period to discuss the matter with Dr. Harry Saltstein, a staff surgeon and true friend. He had agreed to explore the possibilities of integration of the Harper staff.

He listened attentively and sympathetically, but confessed that he could do nothing to change what he agreed was an unfair situation. He reminded me that being Jewish, his staff position was not all that secure, despite his many years of loyal service to the hospital.

Just as I was about to leave, we heard a noise in the adjoining room. Saltstein's mood brightened, and he announced that George Cartmill, Harper Hospital's main gatekeeper, had just arrived next door. He offered to invite Cartmill to come in and talk to me. We congratulated ourselves on our good fortune, as he departed with new-found alacrity in his gait. Seconds later he was back; the enthusiasm was gone, he appeared crestfallen and embarrassed. He hesitated to tell me that Cartmill would not come next door to see me. When I pressed him for a reason, he reluctantly reported, "He said it would be a waste of time' because Harper is not ready to integrate!"

This was an incredible admission in view of the fact that Harper's officials had signed for a multi-million dollar federal grant to replace their 100-year-old institution. The administrators had no intention to comply with the anti-bias stipulations. Not only was the hospital in violation of the terms of the grant, it was defiantly so.

This encounter was reported to DMS officials and the press at the Common Council. When questioned by reporters, Cartmill denied that he'd ever seen or spoken to me in his life, which was true. Despite his denial, the encounter had a salutary effect on hospital negotiations. Having seen Harper's "hold card" of no intent to comply, Patrick and his group of liberals hardened their positions. They demanded an immediate demonstration of compliance or face an indefinite delay in the start of the project. With a May Day emergency in their lap, the mayor once again called on Detroit's most revered arbiter, Bishop Emrich, to try and solve this problem which had grown more acute after festering for many years.

An emergency, closed-door, two-hour session was held in the mayor's office on January 28, 1960. The press was not allowed to attend the arbitration. Across the table from the hospital representatives sat representatives of the Urban League, the NAACP and the DMS. Patrick monitored the discussion from the Council's position.

Dr. Lackey, spoke for his colleagues and made it clear that the DMS did not come to the table seeking favors from the hospitals' administrators: "Since this multi-million dollar project will receive two-thirds of its funding from Hill-Burton appropriations, discrimination in any phase of the project would render the entire project ineligible for federal funds." His list of demands included:

1. "Harper Hospital must admit 12 black doctors to its staff, immediately."

2. "Grace and Woman's hospitals must increase their black doctors to more than token levels."

3. "The city would assign an official to see that these demands are obeyed." Hospital officials objected as much to Lackey's tone as to his allegations of racial bias. Having done his homework, Lackey reported that Hutzel had not appointed a black doctor to its staff since the Hospital Study Committee's report, four years earlier. Harper had never appointed a black doctor to its staff. Moreover, according to the statement attributed to Cartmill, there were no plans to do so in the foreseeable future. Lackey closed his summation with a head count. Woman's Hospital had seven African American doctors; Grace, six and Harper had none. In the entire history of the three institutions, totaling more than 250 years, together they had trained only three interns or residents. Hospital officials declined the offer to rebut or refute Dr. Lackey's figures."

Having exhausted all other options, the hospital representatives reluctantly agreed to sign a pledge to eliminate racial discrimination from their operations. This agreement was greeted exuberantly by Mayor Miriani, a dreamer who said, "There will be no further discrimination." Bishop Emrich, glad

167

to be over with the matter for the second time, exclaimed "there are no blocks (to passage), at all, as far as I can see." Dr. Lackey, being fully aware of the resourceful intransigence of the medical establishment was cautious: "I feel that progress has been made—not so much as we wanted but, still, progress."

After this presentation and with the clock ticking away, Harper officials agreed to appoint a token count of four African American physicians to the hospital staff (instead of the 12 demanded by Dr. Lackey) if the DMS would agree to lift the moratorium. The compromise was accepted. Lackey's demand for immediate staff appointments created a problem for Cartmill. Although several African American physicians had applied to Harper over the years, Cartmill had treated them as he treated me, with blatant disregard. Since an interview was a pre-requisite for receiving an application, all four of the applicants had to endure the entire process. The experience of Thomas Flake, Sr., M.D. (Wayne Univ., 1951, surgeon) is illustrative and fairly typical of how Harper Hospital's officials met this crisis and beat the deadline of the Medical Center's moratorium.

Dr. Flake was the first African American surgeon to be fully trained in Detroit through an approved surgical residency. Foremost among Dr. Flake's teachers, both as student and resident, was Dr. Eugene Osius, chairman of the dept. of surgery at Wayne State Univ. Medical School and chief of surgery at Harper. Dr. Flake had tried unsuccessfully to accompany his European American fellow classmates, who were readily accepted to Harper's staff following their residencies.

Left alone, Dr. Flake sought the advice of Dr. Osius, his mentor and former teacher. Dr. Osius informed Dr. Flake that before he could be given an application, he would have to meet for an interview with Cartmill. Since Cartmill was "too busy" to give him an appointment anytime in the foreseeable future, Dr. Osius advised Flake to "sit tight until you are called." He assured Flake that he would personally let Flake know, "When we are ready for you."

After many weeks of no calls, Dr. Flake applied to and was accepted on the active, teaching staff of Memorial Hospital. He also began teaching at Wayne State Univ. Medical School. After several months, his interest in an affiliation with Harper Hospital dimmed considerably.

Early in 1960, Dr. Flake received an urgent call from Dr. Osius inviting him to join Harper's staff that day. Unaccustomed to such urgency and generosity, Flake hesitated; "Even if I didn't have anything else to do, I couldn't join today. You see, I haven't had my interview with Mr. Cartmill."

Impatiently, Dr. Osius swept that excuse aside with the assurance, "This time you don't need to wait for an interview." After a brief pause, he added, magnanimously, "Do you remember that I promised to call you when we were ready for you. Well, now we are ready for you!"

"But Dr. Osius, that was well over a year ago," Dr. Flake countered.

"Well, these things do take time," Dr. Osius said. "So let's not waste anymore of it in discussion. Come on by here now and let's get it over with." Dr. Flake was finally admitted to the Harper staff, along with three other African American physicians, each from a different specialty: Addison Prince (ob-gyn), William Gibson (internal medicine) and James Collins (pediatrics). They met for a privately-conducted tour of the hospital by Cartmill, who had suddenly become available. Gracious and condescending, he informed them that admitting privileges were already in effect. Each was encouraged to admit patients as soon as possible to certify their affiliations.

Once Harper's gesture toward justice got the Medical Center project going again, the steam seemed to dissipate from the integration drive insofar as the other Medical Center hospitals were concerned. Woman's Hospital had appointed an African American intern by mistake in 1959. It took them four years of recovery and adjustment before they appointed another one. Harper had one African American intern and would wait even longer for the second. Visiting staff appointments were sporadic and unpredictable.

With hospital staff integration moving at a snail's pace, there was no improvement whatsoever in patient segregation, hiring of African American externs, job assignments, etc.

Hospital officials were still protected by the "separate-but-equal" clause of the Hill-Burton Act and took full advantage of it.

In the late 1950s and early 1960s, even the NAACP felt that the clause offered extremely difficult problems as the basis for a suit. Many administrators of formerly segregated hospitals felt secure with their segregationist practices and made no bones about their percentages of allowable African American patients.

At Woman's Hospital, for example, the gatekeeper was perennial Superintendent Catherine Malloy. Her allowable number of African American patients was less than 20%. She checked the figures regularly. If the African American count approached 15%, she would institute "Code Black," calling those European American doctors with large African American patient practices and warning them that they could not admit more black patients until there were some discharges. She even encouraged some of those doctors to become affiliated with other local, segregated hospitals for their African American patients. "Code Black" also included the suspension of admissions of all African American patients, if other measures failed to reduce the undesirable "black" percentage.

Supt. Malloy never discussed her strategy with me. Dr. James McClendon, another African American, reported that she confided her fears to him that the hospital would become "too black" and felt that it was her responsibility to avoid such a calamity. She even sought his concurrence and support, which she never got. Some of the unfortunate by-products of such segregation practices were presented to Mayor-elect Jerome P. Cavanagh in 1961, soon after his upset victory over Mayor Miriani. Since his victorious balance of power had come from the African American community, DMS officials felt that he would be responsive to their problems. To that end, the officers sent the following letter to the mayor:

November 28, 1961

The Honorable Jerome P. Cavanagh, Mayor-Elect
2312 Guardian Building
Detroit 26, Michigan

Sir:

Your announcements and actions since your political victory on November 7, 1961 indicate a genuine and informed concern for the future growth and development of our fair city. You may be sure that thousands of your supporters stand ready to do anything to make your term of office a monumental milestone in the history of Detroit.

There is one area of particular concern to us and many of our colleagues that has not received notice in the local press that it deserves. This is the area of Public Health. A close and objective inspection of this department will reveal that many opportunities exist for its improvement. One specific example will point out one such opportunity.

It is impossible for Receiving Hospital to admit every patient who seeks hospitalization. Hospital officials, there, generally accept the most desirable cases—those that offer interesting diagnostic and therapeutic challenges and those that provide a surgical opportunity for the residents. The other cases may be farmed out to other hospitals in the city.

Unfortunately, many of these cases are critically ill, requiring emergency operations or acute medical management. The hospitals, where most of the less desirable patients are sent, are not always prepared to give them the care they need most. As a result, patients are dying who shouldn't; and many who survive suffer unnecessarily.

We have discussed this matter with the Health Commissioner, and the encounter generated much heat, very little light but not much hope for improving this poor medical care. Our talk did reveal that the Commissioner had little concern about or control over the facilities of the hospitals to which these patients are referred. The smaller hospitals, on the other hand, try to make a profit. So the poor patient is caught between these two imperatives, often at his or her peril.

The Commissioner denied that the patients are referred on a racial basis, but it is a well-documented fact that a white patient is almost never referred to those several hospitals where the most flagrant violations occur. A review of the maternal morality records of Wayne County will reveal that the above statements are not only true but are recurrent.

The matter of economy comes into the picture when a patient is sent to hospitals where unnecessary time is spent while the hospital moves, leisurely, to care for the patient. This same lack of dispatch can, and does, contribute to prolonged hospitalization and a waste of the tax-payer's money.

If the present Commissioner is unable to manage his department efficiently and fairly for all the citizens, there are many physicians in the city who are willing and able to do so.

Yours very truly,

The Detroit Medical Society

The struggle to end patient segregation at Detroit general hospitals was one of the most difficult facing the members of the DMS in this pursuit of justice for themselves and their patients. Each hospital had its own peculiar set of circumstances requiring a unique solution. While Harper and Sinai Hospitals suddenly ended their practice of patient segregation by administrative edict, Grace and Woman's remained stubborn and vindictive.

Grace Hospital was divided into the downtown (old) and the Northwest (new) sections. Few, if any, African American physicians were permitted to admit patients to the Northwest branch. In both hospitals, the room clerk decided who was allowed in and who was not, with the full authority from the administration.

She queried each of us, and those European American doctors who had a significant number of black patients, as to the color of the patient before deciding if a bed was available. When an African American patient was allowed admission, the room clerk managed to convey to the doctor that she was doing him a favor, that time, but that such generosity must never be assumed. The patient was sent to a segregated, multi-bed ward or a semi-private room in the "19th century" part of the hospital, and only if both beds were empty or if one bed was occupied by another African American patient.

In an effort to put an end to this degrading charade, Grace's African American doctors held a series of discussions with the executive committee and various members of the trustee board, over several years. One such encounter occurred in the late 1950s, with the DMS represented by Drs. Waldo Cain, Alegro Godley, A.D. Harris and Ethelene Crockett. Grace was represented by the vice president of the board of trustees; Drs. Roger DeBusk, medical director; Dan Meyers, chief of medicine; Don McLean, chief of surgery and the chief of staff.

Dr. Cain presented, "chapter and verse," an exhaustive study of the hospital's segregation practices. Hospital officials feigned

172

surprise but would not promise any definite changes. During the discussion, Cain criticized the practice of denying bed space to black patients when there was an empty bed available in a room with a white patient. Suddenly, Dr. McLean turned on Cain, eyeball to eyeball, and demanded to know if Cain thought his black patient should be in the room with his (McLean's) white patient. Cain, staring back, allowed that he could not see anything wrong with that arrangement. McLean disagreed arduously. The remainder of the meeting was a disaster and ended discordantly.

It was after that meeting that the DMS, aided by the NAACP and Councilman Patrick, threatened a work stoppage on the Medical Center Project. As a result of the general agreement between the DMS and Harper, Grace and Woman Hospitals, there was token, transient improvement in the segregation practices at Grace; but, as soon as construction resumed, so did the discriminatory actions.

What was perhaps the last face-off between Grace administrators and members of its African American staff occurred on January 9, 1963. Representing the DMS were Drs. Thomas Batchelor, Ethelene Crockett, Melvin Fowler and Charles Wright. Speaking for Grace were Drs. E.S. Gurdjian, chief of staff; Dan Meyers, chief of medicine; Roger Debusk, medical director; "Pinkie" Miller; Floyd Levagood and George Fisher.

Crockett and Wright opened the meeting by presenting documented acts of racial discrimination by Grace Hospital's room clerk. The tone of the meeting was set by Dr. Levagood's customary, snide challenge of Wright's report. He complained that it confused him. Dr. Batchelor immediately retorted, "The fault was not in the report, but in your hearing." Both Miller and Fisher supported the allegations of the DMS group. They recalled that the room clerk always inquired if the patient was white or black, supposedly because of their hospital's large African American clientele. They remembered that African American patients were always sent to the older, more congested section of the hospital. Until the pattern of discrimination was called to their attention by Crockett; Miller and Fisher had accepted the racial discrimination for what it was, "the American way." Now aware of the inherent racism that we were opposing, they found our charges valid and supported them.

Dr. DeBusk did not deny the charges—as a matter of fact, he admitted that "there is a problem," but he was under the impression that conditions were improving. He referred to related directives that had come from the board of trustees, which he tried to implement with variable results. He refused to commit himself to a firmer policy of implementation. Encouraged by Dr. DeBusk's ambivalence, Levagood went on the offensive although he was still smarting from Batchelor's sharp rejoinder. He stated that we were demanding too much and that as members of the DMS, we were seeking special privileges to which we were not entitled. He sneered, "I might be better off joining the DMS myself."

I suggested that he submit a list of his Grace Hospital admissions to DMS. "If we find that 90% of your patients go to Grace's large, congested, segregated Wards B and C, where the services of the short-handed, over-worked nursing staff leave a lot to be desired, you may pass the first test for membership in the DMS."

The meeting lasted more than an hour and ended, as did all the others, inconclusively. It was now abundantly clear to the DMS delegation that unless some outside force could be brought against Grace, nothing was likely to change.

It was at this time that Dr. Batchelor made a decisive move. As president of the Board of Health, Batchelor was an integral part of Detroit's decision makers on health matters. At that time, plans were developing to transfer the city hospital, Detroit General, to the Medical Center. Several sites around Grace Hospital were being considered. Suddenly, Batchelor began to give strong support to a site just north of Grace Hospital where he knew Grace officials had petitioned to build a parking facility.

The distressed officials dispatched a delegation to the Health Commission to plead their case, only to discover that the purchase price of the land included patient integration at Grace Hospital. Activation of an integration agreement by an unhappy Grace Hospital administration left Hutzel (formerly Woman's)

Hospital as the last bastion of officially sanctioned bigotry in the medical center area.

Despite their promises to end the racism as promulgated in the Hospital Study Committee report of 1956, and notwithstanding the 1960 agreement signed with the City of Detroit to end it in order to resume Medical Center construction development, Hutzel Hospital's discrimination continued.

Job categories were sharply divided. African American employees were confined, for the most part, to the food services and housekeeping departments. Patients were separated racially even to the point of denying an African American patient admission or placing the patient in the hallway if a private room or a bed in a segregated ward was not available. In some instances, the African American patients would lie in the hallway outside a semiprivate room that was occupied by only one European American patient—with the responsibility for this practice often placed on the preference of the European American patient. Miss Malloy, who had been appointed to Hutzel's staff in 1953, and I had completed a decade of internecine warfare by 1963. She was a worthy adversary—honest and above-board in her belief that African Americans are inferior and do not deserve equal treatment.

One of my most unpopular ploys was to conduct a personal, well-publicized bed count after the admitting clerk denied a bed for one of my patients. I would ask the nurse to accompany me on an impromptu investigation of the wards. The nurse was asked to verify that each empty bed was, indeed, empty. Some of the nurses didn't approve of the hospital's segregation policies, and were even less happy with my strategy. Some would go off on an impromptu coffee break or secrete themselves in their offices upon hearing that the "bed count" was in progress. Still others would call ahead to their colleagues to announce that I was headed their way.

My fourth, yet far from final, encounter with the intransigence of the medical establishment began on July 19, 1963, thirteen years after closing my general practice office in Detroit. I had returned New York to serve a residency in obg. at the Harlem Hospital, ten years after my appointment to the active staff of Detroit's Woman's (Hutzel) Hospital in 1953. This was also eight years after I had become a certified obstetrician-gynecologist in 1955.

The news media quoted Senator Philip Hart (D-Mich.) as having said the federal government had approved a grant of several hundred thousand dollars, under the Hill-Burton Act, to allow Woman's Hospital to renovate its Hancock Street facility in connection with the Medical Center development.

That very same day, I wrote to Senator Hart requesting a delay in the Woman's Hospital's appropriation until my charge that the hospital was ineligible for the funds was thoroughly investigated. I sent along supporting documents and advised him to drop by *any day* to see for himself. The senator responded in several ways.

He sent copies of my letter, supporting documents and a request for an explanation to Mrs. Katherine Failing, chairwoman of Hutzel Hospital's board of trustees. Mrs. Failing's reply side-stepped the main issue of patient segregation and physician discrimination and created her own agenda:

...The appointment of physicians to the ob-gyn. Each applicant is judged on his own merit—not his color. We are a very specialized hospital, a university affiliate, and a major part of the Medical Center. Our standards are necessarily high and we have had to reject many applicants (including Dr. Wright's associate).

Senator Hart sent me copies of this and the following correspondence related to this matter. I conducted an obg. staff count and had kept the names of nearly a dozen physicians who were appointed during that period—some as partners, others as solo practitioners. All were European Americans.

No one else mentioned "high standards, morality and ethics." Albert E. Huestis, M.D., Michigan's state health commissioner, was reminded of the anti-discriminatory provisions of Section 635 of Title VI of the Public Health Service Act, better known as the Hill-Burton Act. Commissioner Heustis, through whose office such funds were distributed to health-related organizations, in Michigan, promised the senator, on August 28, 1963:

We are doing everything possible, within our ability, to see that hospitals constructed with federal funds render a community service and provide service to all patients within the area served. We will continue to work in that direction.

A reply from Dean Gordon Scott said that neither the university, nor its College of Medicine, practiced racial or religious discrimination. As further evidence that he was not aware of the struggles for justice that we were waging in Wayne's Medical School, Dr. Scott informed the senator:

The residents and interns within the obstetric and gynecologic programs of the university have rotated through the Detroit Receiving, Woman's and Harper Hospitals without regard to color or religion. There have been negroes (sic) in the intern and resident groups in considerable numbers. We have never had an incident which would indicate that they might have been embarrassed.

After considerable defense on behalf of the university, Dean Scott concluded: "We are proud to state our university has no reason to be embarrassed because of its past or present human relations record."

A copy of the dean's letter was also sent to Congressman Charles C. Diggs, who had read my letter to Senator Hart in the *Michigan Chronicle*, on August 17, 1963, and he wrote to Dean Scott.

I am not sure that Senator Hart ever paid a personal visit to Woman's Hospital but his letters to key people and copied to me, drew responses from a congressman, the state health commissioner, the dean of a medical school, the chairman of a hospital's board of trustees and the animosity of some of my erstwhile friends at the hospital. Whether he came or not, the ever-present threat that he might "drop by anytime" may have been partially responsible for the overnight disappearance of overt racial segregation from Woman's hospital.

After some years, Dr. Bentley was admitted to both Woman's and Grace Hospital staffs. For the first time, our partnership was able to function properly and our patients enjoyed better care. But our relief was short-lived. Less than ten years after the Bentley by-pass for staff appointments, he and I added another partner, Dr. N.S. Rangarajan following his obg. residency at Wayne State Univ. By this time, Dr. "Rajan's" extraordinary teaching skills had become legendary throughout the obg. department; and, he had been appointed an instructor in the medical school with a special responsibility for medical students, interns, and residents.

Upon discovering that he was being paid a fraction of what his junior fellow European American instructors were being paid, Dr. Rajan confronted Dr. Tommy Evans, Wayne State Univ.'s chief of obg. with his findings. Dr. Evans seemed neither surprised nor embarrassed. Rather, he informed Dr. Rajan that because of his Indian ancestry he was not worth as much as a European American; hence the difference in salary. Dr. Rajan, who had memorized his classmate's *Gray's Anatomy* text book during his freshman year at India's Madras Medical School, did not take kindly to this malicious comparison. There was a brief exchange of unpleasantries between the two that was so bitter, Chief Evans fired instructor Rajan from the faculty and forbade any obg. student, intern or resident to call on him for any reason whatsoever.

Dr. Bentley and I offered the unemployed doctor a partnership which he accepted. As soon as he learned of our, "stab in my back," Dr. Evans informed me, in no uncertain terms, that we, Dr. Bentley and I, could not accept Dr. Rajan into our partnership because he would soon be dismissed from the hospital. We disagreed, rather loudly, on whether his dismissing privileges were limited to the medical school faculty or extended, also, to the private staff at Woman's Hospital. When he discovered that his authority was limited, he cancelled my clinical professorship at the Medical School, too. That was the last time I was on the teaching faculty of the medical school. Dr. Evans let it be known that if I chose to reapply, my transcript would have to include my high school grades.

Dr. Evans and I had been on a collision course ever since we first met many years before. He was an unreconstructed Southerner who had graduated from Vanderbilt Univ.'s Medical School and completed his obg. training at Univ. of Mich. He had risen to the peak of his profession and was considered untouchable early in his career.

Unfortunately, he brought with him the kind of baggage that made the civil rights movement necessary. On several occasions, I complained of off-color jokes, snide comparisons, and biased behavior to Wayne's medical school, as well as to Hutzel's administrative faculty and trustees. But, he remained untouchable. Evans' loss of untouchability, although slow and painful, may have begun with his failure to prevent Dr. Rajan from joining our partnership. Gradually, others found his jokes less funny, his snide comparisons fell on deaf ears, and his biases became more obvious. Finally, he was asked—even paid—to depart Detroit. My final, indelible memory of Dr. Evans was the day of his smiling departure, waving good-bye with a severance check in hand, which he had rumored, ran into six figures.

The Detroit Common Council did hold the hearings referred to by Dr. Heustis in his reply to Senator Hart in 1963. As a result, the following ordinance was adopted:

Article XI

Discrimination in Hospitals

Section 28-12:2

"No hospital, nor any person acting as superintendent or manager or who is otherwise in charge or control of such hospital, nor any person connected with or rendering service in any hospital in any capacity whatsoever, nor any agent or employee thereof, shall, directly or indirectly refuse, withhold from, restrict or deny to any person admission for care or treatment, equality of care or services relating to care in treatment of such persons on account of race, color, creed, national origin ancestry, age or sex, except that the hospital management may adopt a policy restricting placement in hospital rooms on the basis of age or sex, provided that a member of the medical staff of a hospital or an authorized physician designated to act for him may examine such persons and determine the need of such persons for medical care or treatment. (Ord. No. 813-F #1 -Ord. No. 859-G#1)"

Section 28-12:3

Prohibits Discrimination in Employment of Personnel.

Section 28-12:4

"The City Commission on Community Relations shall collect, analyze and study results of investigations and report to Common Council for enforcement. Results may be made available to duly authorized agencies and departments of the state engaged in the work of preventing discrimination against and protecting the health of its people."

Section 28-12:5

"In the event that the City Commission of Community Relations is unable through conciliation to gain compliance with the article, the Commission is hereby authorized, through the agency of the Corporation Counsel, to seek injunctive relief or other appropriate civil remedy on behalf of any aggrieved person.

Section 28-12:6

"Enforcement—The City Commission on Community Relations shall have the power to enforce the provisions of this article and to investigate all complaints or initiate investigations under this article. It may sign complaints against any person in the city for trial before the traffic and ordinance court of the city for the violation of the terms of this article."

Public pressure was necessary to force the passage of this ordinance in the middle 1960s, testimony to the fact that racism was and is still very much alive. While the foregoing events describe some of the major battles for freedom of choice and justice in Detroit's medical community, when the NMA celebrated its Diamond Jubilee in 1970, the struggle did not end there. Some of the more vigilant freedom fighters have had to carry on continuous mopping-up operations since that time.

As we approached the 1970s, the doors of medical opportunity for the young, black doctor were open wider than they'd ever been. Unfortunately, many have approached these portals in wheel chairs and on crutches, claiming a wide variety of excusable infirmities suffered enroute. An objective appraisal of these claims suggests that "shucking and jiving" and inattention to essential business are significant factors in their lameness. Dr. Cobb, a long-time observer of the social scene and one not often at a loss for words, expressed his appraisal succinctly and with understandable exasperation:

"The Brother won't read!"

Let us hope the facts are no worse that Monty's conclusion suggests. However, there are those who claim, with equal vehemence, "the brother can't read!"

1. Dr. Lawrence Lackey served as president of the DMS in 1958-59.

2. Rupert Markoe, a fair-skinned, accented, Virgin Islander did his premedical work at the University of Puerto Rico. His fluent Spanish attracted Ann Arbor's red carpet, including housing with an European American family and an appointment at Herman Kiefer after graduation. During his four-year course, Markoe's hosts moved and the University found him housing with another, similar family. At that time. Markoe divulged his true identity. He was advised to let sleeping dogs lie. He felt that had he not done so, the Herman Kiefer appointment may not have occurred.

3. All representatives accepting federal funds via the Hill-Burton Act of 1946 were required to sign a resolution pledging "not to discriminate" before the funds were dispersed.

4. *The Ebony Handbook.* (Chicago: Johnson Publishing Co., 1974) p. 88.

5. *Medical Center News.* (Jan. 25, 1960).

The Beginning of the Move Toward Title VI of the Civil Rights Act of 1964

Historians have placed so much emphasis on racism in education and transportation that we tended to be distracted from even worse actions being perpetrated against even more vulnerable citizens in our society; those who are ill.

Such a case, *Dr. Hubert Eaton et al. v. The James Walker Memorial Hospital*, was litigated all the way to a favorable, congressional decision and played a significant role in the formulation of the omnibus Civil Rights Act of 1964. This legislation jettisoned, finally, "the separate-but-equal clause" out of the Hill-Burton Act and Dr. Eaton and his patients were among the earliest beneficiaries.

Despite their bleak prospects, a group of African American doctors from North Carolina made the first effort through the courts to break society's strangle hold on justice in health care institutions. The case was initially filed in Wilmington, N.C., in 1956, the same year that Dr. Cobb prepared his Imhotep Conferences.

After three years of expensive, irritating litigation, a federal judge dismissed the case in 1959. The plaintiffs made plans to reintroduce the case, but at the same time, sought other ways to bring pressure on the medical establishment of North Carolina. To this end, a group of African American physicians left North Carolina for Washington, D.C., on November 11, 1961, to hold a series of conferences with federal officers.

The group, consisting of Drs. Hubert Eaton, of Wilmington, N.C.; Charles Watts, of Durham; and Wiley Armstrong, of

Rocky Mount, comprised a committee of the Old North State Medical Society which sought:

1. "To discuss, in general, segregation and discrimination in hospitals built and to be built in North Carolina with the aid of Hill-Burton funds."

2. "To officially protest such practices of segregation and discrimination to the Department of Health, Education and Welfare (HEW), on behalf of the Old North State Medical Society."

3 "To seek ways and means, as well as assistance, towards the best possible approach to this problem, the solution to which should be the repudiation of the 'separate-but-equal' policy in Hill-Burton-built hospitals in North Carolina and its elimination in these institutions with respect to doctors, patients and personnel."

The delegation held disappointing interviews with representatives in the U.S. Senate, the Department of Justice and, especially with HEW. They found that:

1. The anti-discrimination clause of the Hill-Burton Act was so weak that "assurances as to compliance by applicants had never been questioned, and there was no procedure for checking on the validity of their assurances.

2. There was no authorized course of action in the case of violations. The department stated that "they had never had a case of violation to consider." The group got the distinct impression that the Department of HEW did not consider it its responsibility to know what went on in hospitals after grants had been made and also was not anxious to become involved in the matter of enforcement.[1]

Despite such indifference in high places, the intrepid group of North Carolinians prosecuted their second case vigorously when it was reintroduced in 1961. Taking advantage of favorable rulings since filing their first brief, lawyers from the NAACP Legal Defense pool were able to present pleadings of sufficient scope to yield a landmark decision three years later.

Initially, the defendant hospital officials hoped to repeat their success in *Simpkins*, the first case, and thus move for dismissal.

The judge's prompt denial of their motion was an early warning that things were different this time.

A comparative review of the briefs in the first and second Eaton cases produced the opinion that: "...the present complaint is far more specific in its allegations of state involvement than the first Eaton case.

"Also, it sets forth, in detail, the construction subsidies which have, it is asserted, perpetuated and enhanced the state's involvement in the hospital.

"As we said in *Simpkins*, the opinion of the Court (in the first Eaton case) does not deal with governmental construction subsidies and indeed, shows no awareness of it, nor was this argued in the court. Certainly the decision can scarcely be relied on as authority for a proposition not considered.

"Finally, and most importantly, the first Eaton case did not consider the argument being made (this time) that the hospital was fulfilling the function of the state. The plaintiffs held that the reverter clause (providing that the hospital would revert to the government in case of disuse or abandonment) in the hospital's deed offered irrefutable evidence of the state's involvement in the affairs of the hospital."

Additionally, it was revealed that the state agency for Hill-Burton controlled the operation of all hospitals in North Carolina, whether the hospital received Hill-Burton funds or not. Further evidence showed that the hospital had been granted tax-exemptions in excess of $50,000 per year.

When all of the facts were placed before the Court, it found that "the record in its entirety leads to the conclusion that the hospital is performing the state's function and is the chosen instrument of the state. Under our Constitutional commitment, the James Walker Memorial Hospital is, therefore, bound by the provisions of the 14th Amendment to refrain from the discrimination alleged in the complaint.

This majority opinion of the Fourth Circuit Court of Appeals on April 1, 1964, reversed the lower court's decision. The defendant medical establishment, realizing that 66-year *Plessy v. Ferguson* segregationist reign was coming to an end, mounted a massive appeal to the Supreme Court. Fortunately, the Warren Court was still intact and the appeal fell on deaf ears.

On July 2, the Civil Rights Act of 1964, the most comprehensive piece of civil rights legislation ever proposed, was enacted by the U.S. Congress.[2]

Unlike *Simpkins v. Moses Cone Hospital*, favorably decided earlier, the James Walker Hospital did not receive Hill-Burton funds. Thus, a decision for Eaton was much broader in its concept and ultimate effects.

The NAACP attorneys, Jack Greenberg, Constance Baker Mottley, Michael Meltsner, Robert R. Bond and Conrad O. Pearson, had entered the suit as a class action. They interpreted the finding as a landmark decision that was more far reaching than *Simpkins*.

Secretary Anthony Celebrezze, under the authority of these two decisions, issued a national call for a Conference on Elimination of Hospital Discrimination for July 27, 1964, in Washington, D.C. Representatives came from the White House, the Dept. of HEW, the AHA, the AMA, the American Dental Association, the NMA, the National Dental Association and the American Nurses Association. Secretary Celebrezze asked for the active and vigorous help of the delegates and the organizations they represented, in assuring equal opportunity for health care to all Americans regardless of race, creed or color. He cautioned the group to realize that the federal government had certain well-defined responsibilities to carry out Supreme Court decisions relating to the elimination of racial discrimination in hospitals.

He warned that his department would carry out its responsibilities under the law. He was aware, he continued, that his task would be more successful if he had the help, advice and guidance of all the organizations in attendance. He closed his remarks with a final plea:

"I appreciate, most sincerely, all of you coming here today to discuss ways of assuring the elimination of racial discrimination in hospitals. This is a job that must be done, a job that we in the government cannot do alone, and a job on which I hope you will let us have your help.

186

"I hope that before this day is out, you who represent the major health professions of the nation, in cooperation with persons representing this department and its Public Health Service, will have had a fruitful exploration of ways for moving affirmatively toward that end. You are engaged in an important task. I wish you well."

The two most powerful organizations represented at the Conference, inasmuch as implementing the Federal Court's ruling was concerned, were the American Hospital Association and the AMA.

On August 28, 1963, the AMA had already voted to recommend the deletion of "separate-but-equal" language from the Hill-Burton Survey and Construction Act.[3] On the other hand, despite a strong plea from the NMA, the AMA never issued a clear resolution against the discriminatory provisions of the act. On the contrary, the AMA requested a change in the language of the new ruling that NMA President Kenneth Clement said would have weakened the law. Those differences remained unresolved.

President Johnson's signature on this bill in July made it the Civil Rights Act of 1964.[4] On August 18, 1964, he signed into law H.R. 1004, extending the Hill-Burton Act for five years. But, for the first time since 1896, the "separate-but-equal" clause was eliminated.

Despite all the hoopla, the 1964 Civil Rights Act still made a significant concession to the segregationists. Federally financed medical establishments, existing at the time of the passage of the amended Hill-Burton Act, were not required to integrate unless they did so voluntarily "by city or state ordinance or by court action."

Title VI of the Civil Rights Act of 1964 prohibited racial discrimination in federally-assisted programs and provided that:

"No person in the United States shall, on the grounds of race, creed, color or national origin, be excluded from participating in, be denied the benefits of, nor be subjected to discrimination under any program or activity receiving federal assistance."

Just as he had done in the case of the amended Hill-Burton Act, Secretary Celebrezze called together representatives of the nation's top health agencies for a briefing on the new Civil Rights Act, on January 28, 1965. He reminded the delegates that congress had recently passed a historic piece of legislation that established public policy "to secure the inalienable rights that are assumed for all Americans under the Constitution."

He described Title VI of the Civil Rights Act of 1964 as the vehicle by which to implement the policy of using tax dollars collected from all Americans for the benefit of all Americans on the same non-discriminatory basis.

Secretary Celebrezze showed empathy with some of the delegates by assuring them he was aware they would have difficulty carrying out the mandates of Title VI in some areas of the country. But he left no doubt of his intentions with respect to the law:

"We intend to exercise this new, clear authority with firmness but understanding...The regulations which went into effect early this month call for formal assurances of compliance from every agency, every individual, every institution receiving HEW funds...We extend to you, now, our good will and good faith and our willingness to reason... (but) let no one see, however, in our exercise of reason an absence of resolve to obtain the absolute justice that the law and our own principles require."

Celebrezze was followed by Luther Terry, M.D., surgeon general of the U.S. Public Health Service. Admitting that the job of implementing the responsibilities of Title VI would be difficult, he gave three principles that would guide the drive toward compliance:

1. "Speed is essential to early attainment of the act's objectives."

2. "The objectives should be pursued with a minimum of disruption to important health programs which merit federal assistance."

3. "Voluntary compliance with the law is always preferable to punitive action."

Dr. Terry went on to explain that to comply with Title VI, every institution which received Public Health Service grants must give assurances that there would be no discrimination on the grounds of race, creed or color or national origin in all aspects of its program.

These requirements, he announced, called for a single statement of assurance to cover all the financial assistance programs administered by the Public Health Service. The Statement of Compliance either affirmed that the grantee agency was conducting its program without discrimination or that the agency pledged its intent to do so in the future.

The surgeon general ended his plea for voluntary compliance on a hopeful note that was clearly out of tune with the times:

"We sincerely believe that the day is fast approaching when discrimination in health programs and services is a thing of the past." The court's decisions, affecting the Hill-Burton Act and amended by the Civil Rights Act of 1964, were a considerable improvement over the act of 1946.

Both, however, fell short of the intended goal. The ambivalence of the congress, exempting those institutions built or supported with federal funds before 1946 reflected the pivotal political power of the Southern dixicrats and conservative republicans. Together, they were able to scuttle many serious efforts at enforcement of civil rights statutes, even after the passage of the Civil Rights Act of 1964.

Even worse was that the two men who had the authority to enforce compliance, Celebrezze and Terry, took the unrealistic position that voluntary obedience of the law would be forthcoming from confirmed segregationists. Thus, it was not surprising that an NAACP survey, conducted several months after this conference, found widespread non-compliance among agencies funded with federal money.

Also, there was an equally widespread indifference among H.E.W. officials and staff toward enforcement of the provisions of the new regulations. The lack of sincere commitment to the civil rights legislation in general, and that related to health institutions in particular, spurred the NAACP to expand its investigation of non-compliance. Reports were given at sectional and annual meetings of the associations.

Other, less durable, pressure groups entered the field to protest non-compliance. One of the most visible of these was the Medical Committee for Human Rights. Spawned in 1963, the MCHR took to the streets in many cities to try to embarrass the AMA and related medical institutions into a more responsive posture toward the plight of their African American colleagues. They failed, for the most part, but the efforts made international news in the middle 1960s.

Another development that was not well publicized was a movement by a group of young turks to take over the NMA. They held caucuses during the 1967 and 1968 annual conventions to plan the seizure of power from the "old order." The coup was never staged, but it was a reflection of the explosive period that saw the torch put to Watts, Detroit, Newark and many other cities after the death of Dr. Martin Luther King.

While these pressure groups had little effect on the monolithic AMA, federal officials became a bit more forceful in seeking compliance with civil rights provisions toward the end of the decade. In a few instances, funds were withheld or the threat to do so was voiced to force compliance.

As the 1970s approached, the position of the Executive Branch of the federal government, under President Richard Nixon, became increasingly clear. His appointments to positions of power in his government and on the Supreme Court bench were causes for justified alarm.

In retrospect, the 1946 Hill-Burton Act prolonged the shame and degradation of the "separate-but-equal" clause for another 18 years. Yet, it was greeted with shouts of pleasure from millions of white supremacists.

They were unmindful of the fact that those practices that bring them pleasure and fullfillment cause suffering, pain, and death to millions of other Americans. The cause of this waste and grief was the act's central core of racism, covered by altruistic promises that permitted its passage with little notice. Perhaps the segregationists and their sympathetic fellow law makers profited from that corrupt measure, but the nation, as a whole, suffered irreparable harm.

The first attempt by the federal government to translate a generalized health planning concept into action came in 1946, with the passage of the first Hill-Burton program. The stated intent of the act was to improve the hospital bed-to-population ratio in rural areas and to upgrade facilities and standards of the hospital's operation.

Federal grant assistance was authorized to the states for surveying their needs and developing state plans for hospital facilities based upon those surveys. With plans in existence and minimum standards for hospitals incorporated in state licensing laws, federal funds were to be made available on a matching basis (up to one-third federal) to construct and equip public and voluntary, nonprofit general, mental, tuberculosis and chronic disease hospitals, and public health centers.[5]

For the first time, a determination of need was to form the basis for action; and such priorities were to be explicitly stated. Centering the responsibility for such action in a single authority was also new. However, the law's emphasis on construction and coordination of facilities supports the interpretation that the single agency requirement was adopted primarily for the orderly management of funds.

Between 1949 and 1970, the Hill-Burton program was amended to provide additional grants, loans, and loan guarantees to improve geographic bed distribution. Moreover, from 1956, the U.S. Public Health Service received appropriations under the law for research and demonstrations relating to the development, utilization, and coordination of hospital services, facilities, and resources.

From the planning standpoint, however, the most significant additions to the Hill-Burton program came in 1964 with the Hospital and Medical Facilities Amendments. Along with $1.34 billion for the construction, modernization, and replacement of health care facilities, project grants were made available to develop comprehensive plans for health and health-related facilities on a regional, metropolitan, or other basis.

Furthermore, the arbitrary bed-to-population ratio utilized in determining priorities for grant and loan requests was abandoned. A new formula, incorporating known hospital utilization data, projected population estimates, and a desirable standard of occupancy (80%) was instituted as a more sensitive measure of area hospital needs.

1. Loren Miller, *The Petitioners.* (New York: Pantheon Books, 1966) p. 418.

2. Albert P. Blaustin and Robert L. Zangrando, *Civil Rights and the American Negro.* (New York: Washington Square Press, Inc., 1968) p. 524.

3. Miller, p. 418.

4. Blaustin and Zangrando, p. 524.

5. Public Law: 79-725.

A History of the Auxiliary to the National Medical Association

On August 20, 1936, the dream of many NMA members and wives became a reality. A group of approximately 44 wives of members of the NMA met at a convention in Philadelphia, Pa., and formed a temporary auxiliary.

The wife of John T. Givens, Alma Wells, of Norfolk, Va., served as temporary chairperson and Mrs. J.J. Thomas, of St. Louis, Mo., served as secretary. Drs. D.W. Byrd and John Hale were chosen as their advisors. A committee was appointed and charged to draft a constitution. The group decided to meet the following year to form a permanent organization.

In 1937, the group met in St. Louis, and Mrs. Givens, elected as president, was proclaimed to be the founder of the Women's Auxiliary to the NMA. The Auxiliary's primary aim, prior to the NMA disaffiliation from dentists and pharmacists, was to encourage a better relationship among families and render a service to their communities. The membership was drawn from more than 16,000 African American physicians, dentists, and pharmacists in the U.S., Puerto Rico, and the Virgin Islands.

Many local and state auxiliaries were organized individually, each year, but were later grouped into six geographic regions, each headed by a president. In 1938, the publication of the *Mouthpiece* became the Auxiliary's annual newsletter.

Four years later, in 1942, Dr. Bessie B. Small established the Alma Wells Givens Scholarship Fund in "honor of our founder." Subsequently, scholarships have been presented each year to medical students at Howard Univ. and Meharry Medical College. More recently, scholarships have been awarded to qualified students studying medicine at Atlanta's

Morehouse School of Medicine and the Charles R. Drew Univ. of Medicine and Science at Los Angeles.

The Omega Mason scholarship, presented to a nursing student, annually, during the Auxiliary's convention, was established through the Auxiliary by Mrs. Omega Mason's two sons. In 1950, the Five-Point Program was launched during Mrs. I. Matthews' administration, and green and gold were chosen as the official colors, three years later. An official pledge, motto and song were also adopted.

In 1975, the Auxiliary adopted a "Two-Point Program" on health and education, with subcategories on legislation, community needs and human relations. The programs are implemented by one of the local affiliates. After 1960, membership was restricted to spouses of physicians and the organization's name was changed to the Auxiliary to the National Medical Association (ANMA), so as not to restrict male members, several of whom were already active members.

During the 1979 national convention, hosted by the DMS, the membership voted to initiate a new structure, the House of Delegates, which serves as the legislative body of the ANMA. Also, in 1979, the Advisory Board, consisting of past national presidents, officially became the President's Council. In 1980, the Council became a separate body from the board of directors, with the rotating chairman serving as the official representative for the Council on the board. At the Dallas meeting in 1980, the House of Delegates voted to include new categories of membership classifications: Resident's Spouse, Life and Honorary. The Council continues to serve in an advisory capacity.

President Leonidas Berry Resumes the NMA-AMA Liaison Committee

In August, 1965, the renowned Chicago internist, Dr. Leonidas Berry, assumed the presidency of the NMA. His opening salvo, against the AMA's hostility toward Medicare, was designed to serve notice that he was his own man:

"I have every confidence that members of the NMA will not boycott the implementation of Medicare and other progressive legislation for extension of medical care." He invited all fair-minded European American physicians to join the NMA.

Soon after taking office, Dr. Berry reactivated the NMA-AMA Liaison Committee meetings which had been suspended by an impasse between the two organizations in 1963. It was hoped that passage of the 1964 Civil Rights Act would render such meetings unnecessary. Such was not the case in health care, nor in other areas of voluntary compliance with Title VI of the act. Thus, Dr. Berry, also a Chicagoan, apparently hoped that he could do what no other NMA president had ever done, influence change for the better in the medical establishment.

The first meeting was held on September 25, 1965, at the AMA headquarters. On April 1, 1966, the NMA Liaison Committee was the guest of the entire board of the AMA. On Sunday, August 7, 1966, both liaison groups assembled during the NMA convention as luncheon guests of the NMA's Trustee Board.

The Liaison Committee of AMA-NMA met again on September 27, 1966 at the AMA headquarters. Representing the NMA were Drs. Wiley Armstrong, NMA board of trustees; Leonidas Berry, president; Rann, speaker of House of Delegates; John Holloman, pres.-elect; John Kenney, past president; and Attorney John P. Morris.

Dr. Berry's opening remarks took note of the fact that this was the first Liaison Meeting since December of 1963. He observed, somewhat impatiently, that since the turn of the century, there have been many efforts on the part of the officers of the NMA to remove the principle cause or reason for the origin of the NMA; discriminatory practices against qualified physicians because of race. For at least 25 years, he recalled, there had been utilized, off and on, the concept of Liaison Meetings between the two organizations.

As to what the AMA may or should do toward eliminating the barrier of basic membership in the AMA, and its component and constituent societies; this practice has been carried out by constitutional requirement in the South and some border states and by tactful permissibility on the part of the AMA.

Dr. Berry threw down a challenge to the AMA by demanding help to steer the course of implementation of new health laws and, hopefully, to help in the direction of pending legislation of organized medicine. They must effectively close ranks by bringing into the fold thousands of physicians, black and white, who have been rejected or alienated by entrenched racial and socio-economic discriminatory practices of our modern culture, inherited from the beliefs and practices of our forebearers.

The fifth meeting between the factions, held on April 1, 1966 at the AMA headquarters, lasted four hours. The AMA delegates were: Bernard L. Hirsch, LLB, director AMA Law dept.; Drs. Raymond M. McKlown, secretary-treasurer; W. Andrew Bounten, vice pres.; Trustees L.O. Simenstad, Alvin J. Ingram, Homer L. Pearson, Gerald D. Dorman, Lester D. Bibler, Robert Long, J. B. Copeland; F. J. L. Blasingame, exec. vice pres.; Milford O. Rouse, speaker of the AMA House of Delegates; Wesley W. Long, vice chairman of the board of trustees; Donovan F. Ward, past president; and Ernest B. Howard, asst. executive vice president.

NMA delegates were: Drs. John L. Holloman, president; William H. Grant, trustee; John A. Kenney, past president; Leonidas Berry, president; and Lionel Swan, president-elect. The group agreed on the following cooperative programs:

1. African Americans should appear more frequently in AMA publicity releases.
2. The Liaison Committee will deal more often with issues of common interest.
3. The AMA's House of Delegates will appoint NMA members to top-level committees and councils of the AMA.
4. Appoint a special committee of the AMA's board of trustees to contact local societies and urge their compliance with anti-discriminatory resolutions previously passed by the AMA.

This list of actions was approved at the AMA's Chicago convention on July 1, 1966. With hardly a murmur of dissent, the House of Delegates voted to set up an appeal procedure for physicians who allege racial discrimination at the state and county levels of membership. The news media took note of the fact that this was the first action that the AMA had ever taken to establish an appeal mechanism.

While the AMA still did not agree to alter its by-laws (as the specialty college associations had done) or take punitive actions against the accused, it was hoped that this move would yield more relief for the aggrieved African American doctors than the meaningless repetitive pronouncements released by the AMA since 1950.

The action of the Chicago convention was not a mandate for immediate implementation. The language of the motion was that the request for an appeal procedure would be presented to the next meeting of the clinical session in Las Vegas, in December.

While this step fell far short of the request for disaffiliation of racist component societies, as requested by AMA delegations from Connecticut, California and New York, it did finally recognize that all prior pronouncements were meaningless without an appeal mechanism.

The NMA delegations to the NMA-AMA Liaison Committee can take some credit for this acknowledgement on the part of the AMA. Pressure from 400-500 MCHR pickets outside the convention headquarters was, also, a spur to action by the AMA.

Pres. Hudson's next address to the AMA's Las Vegas convention did not mention the NMA:

"I propose that the AMA, state, and county societies launch a continuing program, under predominantly private auspices, to improve existing health care services and establish new services where they do not exist for all persons of whatever age, race, creed or color."

No mention was made of the NMA nor the activity of the Liaison Committee in 1966 or 1967. Since there were no further NMA-AMA contacts through this Liaison Committee, there was no follow up to ascertain if the appeal procedure was ever approved, passed and made operative. Efforts to find cases that came to appeal were fruitless.

On October 24, 1966, the AMA's Council of Constitution and By-laws reported that it was considering possible by-law changes that would authorize appeal to the Judicial Council by physicians who allege that they were unfairly denied membership in local or state medical societies.

The committee reviewed the actions of prior meetings and discussed ways of implementing the articles approved by their respective Boards of Trustees. A decision was rendered to announce their decisions at the AMA's annual convention held in Chicago, in July, three months later. It was hoped that the timing of the announcement would help to defuse the expected public demonstrations against the AMA that had been an embarrassment at the 1963 and 1965 conventions. This was not to be.

An important question was raised by Dr. Berry, at the end of his term. What was accomplished by these meetings? His answer seemed to be a fair assessment:

1. "We agreed on a program of joint recruitment in medical careers, and AMA officials agreed to increased usage of Negro faces in physician recruitment literature and stories about medical careers.

Author's note—With no knowledge of Dr. Berry's request to the AMA officials, we, of Detroit's Museum of African American

History, produced a 15-minute recruitment film, *You Can Be A Doctor*, in conjunction with the Detroit Medical Society about that same time. Our target audience was African American students.

The film was shot in Detroit's African American-owned Kirwood Hospital and featured African American doctors, nurses, technicians, patients and students. Although the film was shown at the 1967 NMA convention, it attracted very little interest. However, it was distributed nationally by the McGraw-Hill Book Co. for the benefit of the Detroit Museum.

2. The Liaison Committee should meet more often.

Author's note—Insofar as I was able to determine, this was the last, direct, in-house appeal by NMA officials for justice and fair-play from their AMA colleagues.

3. The AMA House of Delegates would appoint Negro members of NMA and AMA to top level committees and councils of AMA. (The names and curricula vitae of 25 candidates were submitted.)

Author's note—If any such appointments were ever made and activated, they, and their accomplishments, should be publicized.

4. AMA President James Z. Appel and board chairman, Dr. Percy Hopkins, extended special invitations to NMA officials to attend AMA convention and other ceremonies as special guests of the AMA.

Author's note—meaningless.

5. A special committee of the AMA board of trustees was appointed to contact local societies and urge their compliance with anti-discriminatory resolutions previously passed by the AMA. This committee would also be charged with devising ways of achieving voluntary improvement in racial discriminatory practices in societies, in hospitals and in patient care.

Author's Note—What did the "special committee" find and do?

6. Of considerable significance is the action of the AMA House of Delegates. During their June 1966 convention, they

199

passed a resolution to amend their constitution, which would have allowed their Judicial Council to hear and consider the charges of any doctor alleging racial discrimination in any area of the United States.

Author's Note—The words, "hear," "consider" and "alleging" all suggest inaction. What was done?

Dr. Berry concluded his appraisal of this third NMA effort to cut off the AMA's prior support for racial segregation with the following observation:

"Considering the AMA's stand, for more than a hundred years, that their organization could have no responsibility for the practices of racial segregation in their component societies, this could be a crack in the iceberg." (Appendix G, p. 221 Marias)

Author's Note—"Fissure" would have been more accurate.

President Berry's Liaison Committee, like President Cobb's Imhotep effort, was undermined by the cold war. The Hungarians rained on Cobb's parade. For Berry, it was the Cubans. The AMA pretended to be interested in establishing an appeal mechanism for those physicians who "charge" that they have been discriminated against, but, they refused to alter their by-laws which made such action legal. Nor did they authorize punitive measures against those who violated the 1964 Civil Rights Act.

Since 1960, well before the first NMA-AMA Liaison Committee was convened, the AMA was heavily involved in a major resettlement operation of anti-Castro Cuban physicians which dwarfed the Hungarian episode by a wide margin. (See The Hungarian Uprising and the Cuban Physician Invasion).

Exaugural Report by NMA Past-President Leonidas Berry on AMA-NMA Liaison Activities, 1966

Since Dr. Berry lived and worked in the same city which the AMA calls home, he approached his presidential term in office with high hopes that he would be able to work through the racist barriers against African American membership in the AMA. He included a report of his efforts during his exaugural address to the NMA on August 9, 1966:

"After one or two years of a moratorium on conferences forced by an impasse, our administration reactivated the liaison conferences between the AMA and the NMA. Once again, these forums were seeking to remove a senseless social embargo which still exists against licensed and practicing physicians based upon a criterion of race in some societies and tokenism in others. I am happy to report to you that three such meetings were held during our tenure (August 1965-August 1966), breaking all previous records for the number of meetings in one year. The first meeting was held at the AMA headquarters on September 25, 1965. On April 1, 1966, the NMA Liaison Committee was the luncheon guest of the entire AMA Trustee Board, at which time problems of discrimination were further discussed.

"On Sunday, August 7, 1966, the liaison groups assembled for a conference with the NMA Liaison Committee and Trustee Board, serving as hosts during our convention at the Pick-Congress Hotel in Chicago.

"What has been accomplished by these conferences, other than frequent meetings? Some will say 'very little.' I would say probably more than ever before in the same length of time; and enough, so that I strongly recommend continuation of this type of communication.

"First, we agreed on a program of joint recruitment in medical careers and AMA officials agreed to increase usage of Negro faces in doctor-recruitment literature and stories about medical careers. Second, frequent meetings of liaison groups were agreed upon, as mutually desirable. Third, there was an agreement that AMA's Trustee Board and House of Delegates would appoint Negro members of AMA and NMA to top-level national committees and councils of the AMA. At least 25 or more names and curricula vitae of volunteer candidates were submitted. Fourth, President James Z. Appel, who, along with AMA Board Chairman Dr. Percy Hopkins, were the AMA leaders in our deliberations, extended a special invitation for your president to attend AMA convention ceremonies and other affairs as a special guest of the AMA.

"Fifth, a special committee of the AMA board of trustees to contact local societies to urge compliance with resolutions, previously passed by their House of Delegates, and to devise some means of achieving voluntary improvement in racially discriminatory practices in societies, hospitals and patient care.

"Sixth, and finally of considerable significance, is the action of the AMA house of delegates at their June '66 convention to amend their constitution permitting their Judicial Council to hear and consider the charges of any doctor alleging racial discrimination in any area of the U.S. Considering the AMA's stand for nearly 100 years that their organization could have no responsibility on the matter of racial discrimination in their local component societies, this would seem to be a crack in the iceberg.

"To be sure, our liaison conferences could only have a small share of credit for this resolution. Of equal importance were the AMA delegates who presented resolutions calling for the expulsion of racially discriminating societies and the 250 interracial picketers outside the June 1966 meeting."

During his departing address for his 1965 term, Dr. Berry revealed a very significant fact. Since its founding in 1842, the AMA has adhered to a promise made to its affiliates at the beginning—that the AMA would have no responsibility in the implementation of racial discrimination in the local component societies. A promise that was made 25 years before slavery ended was still being strictly adhered to 130 years later.

Access, or the lack thereof, to the AMA has been on the NMA agenda constantly for the last 70 years, and it is reputed to represent all of the physicians who practice medicine in the U.S. Since 1895, every president of the AMA has had to address this violation of medical rights in one fashion or another. It was in the early sixties that the issue gained special significance, especially during the presidency of Dr. Kenneth Clements.

In his inaugural address to the August 1963, NMA convention in Los Angeles, Dr. Clement said, "In this hour of the Negro's greatest struggle for his civil rights and his civil freedom, it will be well to remember that the overriding cause is bigotry within the institutions of this republic."

Again, our government is postponing its moment of truth. The first opportunity to shed the shackles of the wicked past occurred during the Reconstruction. The Hayes-Tilden Compromise of 1876, on the withdrawal of Northern troops from the South was paid for with the rights of African Americans.

The Southern strategy of today is exacting the same ransom from them—for those who seek only political advantage for themselves. What right has anyone to traffic with the rights of others?

Every time this inevitable confrontation is postponed, the ultimate cost escalates. Already, the malignancy of racism is gnawing at the very vitals of this establishment. Only radical surgery offers any real hope for survival.

Perhaps, we, too, may have a 21st century Gibbons to record the rise and fall of the American Empire. Like the Romans, our rulers have sent their gladiators forth into the four corners of the world to astound others with the magnitude and invincibility of their strength and vitality. Moreover, they, also, have sacrificed the rights of others to pay homage to the false god of white supremacy. The prediction of a "fall" is a foregone conclusion.

The American Medical Association and the Hungarian Uprising

One of the first instances during which the U.S. cold war foreign policy profited from the AMA's timely intervention began in Poland, in June of 1956 and underwent a more serious resurgence in Hungary the following October. Hungary's anti-communist rebels toppled Stalin's statue in Budapest, took over the radio stations and demanded the withdrawal of Soviet troops from their country.

Just as the surprised Russians were withdrawing, the Hungarians quickly restored their Russian-deposed Prime Minister, Imy Nagy, to office; promised their people free elections; withdrew Hungary from the Warsaw Pact, which prohibited direct U.S. intervention against the Soviet Union during the early 1950s; and asked the United Nations for help. The Hungarians grossly underestimated the effect of their unilateral cancellation of the Warsaw Pact, believing the U.S. would be free to come to their aid against the Russians.

Charging that Nagy had gone too far, too fast, the Russians re-invaded Hungary and replaced Nagy with their own Janus Kadar. He put down the rebellion, killing and wounding thousands of Hungarians. Subsequently, several hundred thousand Hungarian refugees fled to neighboring countries, mostly Austria.[1]

The Hungarian appeal for aid went unanswered by the U.S. government because the "nuclear stalemate" between the U.S. and Russia, maintained under the protocols of the Warsaw Pact.[2]

The members of the AMA did heed an appeal from Dr. M. Arthur Kline, secretary of the American Medical Society of Vienna, Austria. His plea for assistance was read during a fall meeting of the AMA's board of trustees in Seattle, Wash. An AMA editorial of support appeared in the *JAMA*:[3] "The courage of these unfortunate people is known throughout the world; and to those who live in more fortunate countries, it becomes a symbol for the men and women who believe enough in freedom to fight for it."

The report described the plight of and care being administered to hundreds of destitute Hungarian physicians who had fled to Austria to escape the wrath of the returning Russians. They were charged with treating the injuries of thousands of their fellow citizens.

The AMA trustees immediately appropriated $5,000 through the American Medical Society of Vienna for emergency relief. Mobilization of vast U.S. resources for long term support included a Presidential (Eisenhower) Committee for Hungarian relief; landing privileges at McGuire Air force Base for the rapid deployment of thousands of Hungarian refugees; and the sequestration of the facilities at Camp Kilmer, N.J. as a staging area for their rehabilitation.

Hundreds of these physician refugees became the special wards of the medical establishment and were provided a wide range of services which led to jobs, AMA membership, citizenship and full rehabilitation of their normal lives.

Some of the refugees arrived as "parolees"—without passports. Community leaders were encouraged to assist in all aspects of the welcoming process. Language training and refresher medical courses were established. The Health Resources Advisory Committee of the Office of Defense Mobilization called upon all health organizations and educational institutions "to cooperate with voluntary organizations in the professional integration of hundreds of Hungarian physicians—dentists, medical and dental students—and other health personnel being flown into the United States."

The enabling resolution, which provided this directive with a mandate of urgency, said: "With our national shortage of health personnel of all types, these new 'Americans' can make a distinct contribution to our health resources. To the dignity of political and personal freedom, let us help give them the dignity of professional status." The directive ended with a list of 10 health organizations and agencies which had formed a network of support for the Hungarian refugees. Members of the AMA were "urged" to contact them.[4]

Hungarian physicians were dispersed to many U.S. cities and were given every opportunity to become productive members of the American medical establishment. The transition from immigrant to citizen was incredibly smooth, thanks to the all-out, voluntary support of the AMA.

Many of the grateful beneficiaries were happy to be on the right side of the cold war and wrote extravagant letters of praise and gratitude to their European American benefactors.

1. Marvin Perry, *A History of the World*. (Boston: Houghton Mifflin, 1985) pp. 751-752.

2. T. Harry Williams, Richard N. Current, and Frank Freidel, *A History of the United States*. (New York: Alfred A. Knopf, 1964) p. 787.

3. *JAMA*, (Dec. 22, 1956) p. 1544.

4. *JAMA*, Vol. 163, No. 11. (Feb. 9, 1957) p. 479.

The AMA and the Cuban Physicians

Following the defeat of the U.S.-supported Cuban forces under dictator, Fulgencio Batista, the pro-communist army of Fidel Castro seized Havana on January 1, 1959. This invasion ended the U.S. 60-year hegemony over Cuba and opened a new, cold war front that would outlast the cold war, itself.[1] It has resulted in struggles between the Cuban and all subsequent U.S. administrations. Many lives have been wasted in such events as the Bay of Pigs fiasco.

Among the many campaign promises made to the Cuban people, prior to Batista's defeat, were "a reduction in medical fees and a wider dispersal of doctors outside Havana, where most of them were concentrated." When measures were instituted to reach these objectives, many physicians ignored them until a total of 259 doctors were expelled from the Cuban National Medical Association (CNMA) in October 1960, for disobeying the enabling governmental directive.

Rather than submit to the enforcement of these and other communist restrictions, from one-third to one-half of Cuba's 6,000 physicians fled the island. While a few went to other Spanish-speaking countries in South and Central America, the majority found a warm welcome in the U.S., principally the greater Miami region of Florida.[2]

The latter group took advantage of the cold war state that already existed between Cuba and the U.S. and were recruited for the American-financed (Bay of Pigs) invasion force that tried, unsuccessfully, to dispose of Fidel Castro and retake Cuba.

Although the Bay of Pigs Invasion was launched early in the Kennedy Administration, it was the brainchild of Allen Dulles, President Eisenhower's director of the CIA. The U.S. operatives assumed that by limiting the invasion force to Cubans, their relatives would rise up during the invasion and overthrow Castro. Then, the communists could be rounded up and sent packing, as happened later on in Grenada.

When the Cuban insurrection failed to occur, Allen Dulles became the sacrificial lamb. He had fared well and was untouchable under the protection of President Eisenhower, having gotten rid of the pesky Patrice Lumumba in the Congo[3] and providing a safe haven for Klaus Barbie in Bolivia, among many other things. His luck ran out under President Kennedy, who fired him after the Bay of Pig's rout. He became the fall guy for the first of many U.S. miscalculations against the redoubtable Fidel Castro.[4]

Representatives of the Cuban refugees and members of the American medical establishment met at Miami's Cuban Emergency Center to plan for a speedy re-entry of immigrant, Cuban doctors into the U.S. medical field.

Dr. Franklin Evans, chairman of Florida State Medical Society's Committee to Aid Exiles, urged the immigrant physicians to take the state licensing examinations that would enable them to work as residents in Florida hospitals and to go into private practice after licensure. This decision had already been approved by the AMA's board of trustees in September of 1961. Quick action by this board led to:

1. Establishment of a committee, under Dr. Gunnar Gundersen, past AMA president, to consider the problems of foreign physicians.

2. Official AMA recognition of the Cuban Medical Association-in-Exile (CMAE).

3. Appropriation of $1,000-per-month to finance the expanded operation of the CMAE.

4. Encouragement of the faculty of the Univ. of Miami's (Fla.) Medical School to assist in post-graduate training, residence and hospital appointments for the refugee physicians. Some former members of the faculty of the Univ. of Havana's Medical School were appointed to the faculty of the Univ. of Miami.[5]

These actions were endorsed by AMA President Leonard W. Larson, who also urged American physicians to try to absorb the refugee Cuban physicians into their practices or other such opportunities.[6]

Author's Note—At that time, few, if any, African American interns had ever been appointed to any approved Florida hospital. Their opportunities for residency training were even less obtainable.

Dr. Evans, assisted by Dr. Robert Boggs, the national chairman of National Committee for the Resettlement of Foreign Physicians (N.Y.), arranged for the Univ. of Miami's Medical School faculty to establish refresher courses for the refugees.

Meanwhile, Dr. Evans and his local group were seeking employment for the refugee doctors as medical technicians in hospitals and clinics, until they could become citizens and licensed. On December 29, 1960, they set up a "broad" 3-month course of study to prepare 300 of the refugees to take the qualifying exam starting in April 1961.

"Our primary aim is to enable these men to function as physicians, to support themselves and their families and, at the same time, contribute to the medical needs of the community," observed Dr. Ralph Jones, head of the Univ. of Miami Medical School's dept. of internal medicine. The estimated $100,000 needed to fund the program was supplied by the ECFMG and several other educational funding sources.

December 12, 1960—Univ. of Miami officials met with 287 Cuban refugee physicians to enroll for the free, 3-month refresher course.

Arrangements were made for Dr. Jose J. Centurion, former professor of medicine at the Univ. of Havana, and governor of the American College of Physicians for Cuba, to serve as liaison officer for the course.

Florida's governor, Faris Bryant, proposed that Florida's state hospitals consider hiring qualified Cuban refugees "to ease the shortage of medical experts in the state hospitals." State comptroller, Ray Green, opined that Cuban doctors may be hired without a Florida license "if no 'qualified' resident doctor is available."

Rep. Dante B. Fascell proposed to Pres. Kennedy that the U.S. government provide financial aid for young Cuban exiles who want to finish their education in the U.S. He reminded the President that cash from the contingency-fund section of the Mutual Security Act could be used.

January 26, 1961—The university's medical school officials were already discussing the possibility of providing tuition for Cuban medical students whose training programs had been interrupted by their sudden departure to the U.S.

Author's note—I was unable to find a similar proposal from any official, governmental, or other agency, offering such financial assistance to African American medical students. Unlike my schoolmates from several other Southern states who were subsidized because of their state's practice of racial segregation, the Floridians, like us Alabamians, were on their own.

Some of the refugees were welcomed to the Milledgeville (Ga.) State Hospital. "Without these additional doctors, the hospital would be far behind in its present schedule in meeting the treatment needs of the patients," observed a grateful Dr. Irville H. McKinnon, hospital superintendent.

When John F. Kennedy won the U.S. Presidency in 1960, he inherited from President Eisenhower an anti-Castro military operation that was well past the point of no return. Dr. Antonio Rodriguez Diaz was among nine Cuban refugees who were alerted for transfer to a rebel (Bay of Pigs) training base. Six physicians were to leave in the first group, with three colleagues to follow soon afterwards.

"All are members of the executive board of the Cuban Medical Association in Exile (CMAE), recently organized to help refugee doctors obtain U.S. medical licenses through a Univ. of Miami refresher program. They are part of an anti-Castro military force that participated in the Bay of Pigs invasion of Havana on April 17, 1961."

According to Dr. Enrique Huertas, the CMAE's president, "The six medics listed at their headquarters at 213 Argon, have all agreed to serve with the volunteer, anti-Castro forces. Only Cubans are accepted."

As the Cuban invasion became a certified disaster, recruitment of Cuban doctors was stepped up and others were being urged to volunteer by Aristides Menendez, the so-called "surgeon general" of Miro Cardona's recently-formed Cuban government-in-exile.

"On April 12, 1961, the U.S. Public Health Service sent a representative to Miami to recruit 50 Cuban refugee doctors to work for the federal government. This is the first phase of a joint government-business drive to put refugee professionals to work in their specialized fields, around the country and in Latin America.

"Most of the doctors are being sought by the U.S. Public Health Service to go to work in the federal American Indian health program in Oklahoma, the Dakotas, and other southwestern states. The jobs are being offered as a result of a request by Abraham Ribicoff, secretary of HEW, after he made a personal survey of the situation."

"Dr. Ralph Jones, of the Univ. of Miami's Medical School, reported that the medical training program had been highly successful in helping refugee Cuban physicians find placement in American health institutions and enter private practice."[7]

According to a Univ. of Miami spokesman, "75% of the Cuban physicians who completed the Univ. of Miami's post-graduate course passed and are qualified to work in this country.

"Their eligibility extends to employment as hospital interns and residents or, to begin their own practices. The University offered to repeat the course, in Spanish or English, at no charge to those who failed.

"They were assisted by English tutors, facilities for simultaneous translation and bi-lingual volunteers. With such help, and Spanish translations of textbooks provided by pharmaceutical companies, the language barrier was breached in record time."

Author's note—For many years, the NMA has tried to convince the AMA that the NMA is a more respectable route into the AMA for African Americans than through its racially biased, local, Southern affiliates. But several senior AMA

213

officials declared, repeatedly, that the route through the affiliates "is the only way to go."

"The AMA bolstered programs to make use of these trained men in their fields. They not only helped to meet shortages of medical personnel in this country, but also assist the displaced doctors to expand their knowledge for the day when they will return to serve their own people in freedom." This was the opinion of many of Miami's refugee physicians.

Some Cuban physicians, who elected not to flee Cuba had other ideas:

March 3, 1962—"Cuban doctors have been a big pain in the neck. Of all the island's professional people, they have been the hardest to convince that the socialist revolution of the past year has been good for the country. The trouble is that many of Cuba's doctors have had backward ideas.

"Before the revolution in January 1959, Cuba had 8,000 doctors, 4,000 of whom were in Havana. The rest were in cities and towns across the country. But none were in the country itself. Our doctors have always been involved in politics and supporters of a corrupt system. As a group, they are reactionary.

"Seventy-five percent of the susceptible population has been immunized against polio; the government's budget for the ministry of public health has increased from $21 million to $100 million; parasitic difficulties and malaria have been eliminated; and within the next two years, between 2,000 and 3,000 new doctors will graduate from our medical schools."

The AMA announced that it has co-signed loans for needy Cuban physicians in exile for more than $50,000. Of the $60,000 pledged to the fund by the AMA's board of trustees, $52,185 has been committed to provide for three months of emergency relief. Repayment at the rate of $50-per-month is expected when the doctor begins employment.

The acceptance of Cuban physicians as equals in Florida's medical community was certified by the installation of Cuban-born, De Pedro J. Greer as president of the Dade County Medical Association in 1974.

In 1981, when Cuba's minister of Health addressed our group, he took a dim view of the AMA's role in "enticing half of our physician population to flee from the most equitable socialist system that Cuba had ever enjoyed." He made many favorable comparisons between their present system with that of the earlier U.S.-financed, Batista regime.

"Medicine that cost up to $12 before can be had for $1.50 today. Twenty-nine new hospitals have been built where none existed before. The number of hospital beds has increased from 10,000 to 21,000."[8] The minister answered many questions about Cuba's health system. Departing, he paused before me, the only African American physician in the audience and asked amidst absolute quiet: "Senor, are you a member of the American Medical Association?"

"Not since they came to the rescue of the Hungarian physicians, during the 1956 uprising," I replied.

"Then you were a member before 1956," he questioned.

"Yes."

"What did they ever do for you?"

I could not think of a single benefit that I had received from my membership in the AMA. He waited briefly, smiled knowingly, and disappeared quickly amid a burst of applause.

The foregoing report is only a partial study of the beginning of a cold war struggle between the U.S. and Castro's Cuba that has brought suffering and death to many Africans and African Americans for more than 35 years and shows no signs of ending.

While Castro's timely interference in the affairs of Angola may still be remembered, his rescue mission to Grenada possibly remains a faint memory of the events of 1983. Castro was the only head of state in this hemisphere to heed a call for assistance from Prime Minister Maurice Bishop of Grenada.

The Cubans and their allies sent in physicians, dentists, nurses, technicians, etc., who helped to raise the level of the public's health enormously. After the U.S invasion of Grenada and their deportation of communists, the public health situation went back to normal.

The presence of Cuban communists in Grenada was intolerable to President Reagan so he decided to invade the tiny island and drive them out. Because he was fairly certain that permission would not be granted by the U.N., the Organization of American States, nor the U.S. Congress, Reagan requested and got the questionable consent of the eight-member Eastern Caribbean Union.

During the invasion, all of the communists were captured and sent back to Cuba, or wherever else they had come from. The public health conditions continued to deteriorate, and a representative from the U.S. Agency for International Development called upon the founder of Project Hope, Dr. William Walsh, for assistance.

Dr. Walsh and I had met in 1967, during my tour of duty aboard the S.S. Hope as chief of ob-gyn in Cartegena, Colombia. He related this story to me in 1990. When I told him of the support given to the Hungarian and Cuban refugee physicians, we both wondered why the AMA did not come to the relief of a U.S.-created medical crisis in Grenada, after such heroic, prolonged efforts in Austria and Miami?

This fount of opportunity through which refugee Hungarian and Cuban physicians and their families poured, and were showered with every opportunity the American medical establishment could provide, has remained open for many years. Through it came assistance from many other, non-medical sources.

In August 1966, Under-secretary of State George Ball proposed to the House Judiciary Subcommittee a bill, which had already been approved by the Johnson Administration, to allow thousands of Cuban refugees to become American citizens—virtually overnight.

Two months later, the subcommittee passed a private bill for doctors that allowed only physicians to become citizens in such a manner and to enter private practice if they had already passed the state board of medicine.

Although this bill initially provided only Cuban physicians unhampered entry and automatic U.S. citizenship, it was soon was quietly expanded to allow all Cubans the same privileges. The selective, anti-Haitian enforcement of this measure by every

U.S. administration since 1966—even when Cuban and Haitian refugees arrived on the same boat—has produced another shameful chapter in the history of U.S. foreign policy relations.[9]

It was only after the flood tide of Cuban refugees threatened the capacities of Guantanemo and the U.S. Coast Guard, did President Clinton threaten to rescind the 28-year law that assured Cubans automatic U.S. citizenship after a year of residence. When that development is coupled with California's recent passage of Bill 187, the Republican's 1994 sweep of both Houses of Congress, and Haitian President Astride's return home to a re-occupied Haiti, the political future of this hemisphere could become very interesting, indeed.

It was reported during "Morning Edition of Public Radio" on February 6, 1995, that Miami's population today is more than 60% Latin American. In many Miami regions, Spanish is the *lengua franca*, especially in Little Havana. If you can't speak the language, you won't be hired, no matter what other skills you offer. This language barrier is increasing tension in the Miami neighborhoods at an alarming rate. Unless relieved, there will be trouble ahead.

1. Gary B. Nash, John R. Howe, Allen F. Davis, Julie Roy Jeffrey, Peter J. Frederick and Allan W. Winkler, *The American People*. (New York: Harper & Row, 1990) p. 908.

2. *New York Times*, (Nov. 23, 1960).

3. Perry, p. 783.

4. AMA, "News." (September 4, 1961) p. 3.

5. *JAMA*, Vol. 178, No. 1. (Octctober 7, 1961).

6. AMA, "News," Vol. 178. (October 2, 1961) p. 5.

7. Editor's note: At that time I was not aware that there was or had ever been any African American medical student at either of Florida's two medical schools nor interns nor residents in any Florida hospital. Insofar as I knew, none of my Florida schoolmates had been admitted to the staff of any first-class hospital in Miami.

8. Lecture given to a delegation of U.S. citizens by the Cuban Minister of health in the fall of 1981.

9. *New York Times,* (December 20, 1993). "In recent years the Governors in California, as well as in Florida, have notified the federal government that they expect reimbursement for welfare benefits paid to immigrants."

Most of the data in this section, "The AMA and the Cuban Doctors," was taken from, or verified by, articles in the *Miami Herald,* a source to which I was given free access.

Detroit's Fourth NMA Convention, 1979

Many changes occurred in Detroit after the NMA's last convention in 1959. For example, the opening session was quite different. Instead of Detroit's Mayor Louis Miriani sending the keys to the city by a subordinate, this time Mayor Coleman A. Young, Detroit's first African American mayor, delivered them, himself. Mayor Young, highly visible throughout the convention, made the delegates feel welcome.

The number of practicing African American physicians in southeastern Michigan exceeded 300 and nearly all the specialties were represented among them. Thus, the medical menu served to the delegates was tastier this time around.

There were still areas of racial prejudice that demanded our attention. Thoracic surgeons Hayward Maben and John Feemster were denied use of the heart pump during open heart surgery, because "as African Americans, they were not expected to attract enough patients to justify its use."

In an effort to get a better idea of the magnitude of the racial problems still in existence, the DMS sent inquiries to about 350 of its members. Unfortunately, only 50 were returned. When contacted individually, some expressed fear of reprisals and others had no problems to report and said nothing.

On March 29, 1977, DMS members voted to purchase the building at 580 Frederick, which had served as Dunbar Hospital, Detroit's first African American proprietary hospital, and as well, the three adjacent lots. The plan was to renovate the building and convert it into headquarters for the DMS and other medically related groups.

Through the efforts of Dunbar's Historical Committee, the Michigan Historical Commission declared the building a historical landmark. With that designation, the renovation had to adhere to a rigid code of choice of materials, workmanship, etc.

Because it was aware of the impending NMA convention to take place in Detroit in 1979, the Dunbar Medical Museum Committee worked diligently to prepare the site. In 1978, Attorney Gregory Reed announced that the IRS had granted tax-exempt privileges to the Dunbar Project and fundraising had begun among the members of DMS and as well as generous donors from the health care field. The drive "to make Dunbar presentable" began in earnest.

With the opening of the opulent Renaissance Center, on the Detroit Riverfront, DMS members and their wives were anxious to show off their hometown.

Dr. Richard O. Brown, president of the DMS, and Alma Rose George, president of the Wolverine State Medical Society, took charge of the convention plans and coordinated an enjoyable three-day event. There were informative medical lectures, tours of automobile plants, and visits to the African American and other museums.

Robert Dawson, M.D. (Meharry, 1943), was chosen president-elect in 1978. A certified ophthalmologist, Dr. Dawson served as a member of Meharry's board of trustees and was awarded the NMA's "Distinguished Service Award" in 1982. He and I had also been classmates at Meharry.

Dr. Dawson presented the NMA's Distinguished Service Award to LaSalle D. Lefall, M.D. (Howard, 1952). Lefall's positions and honors included, but are not limited to: acting dean, 1964-1970; professor and chief of surgery, Howard, 1970-; SE Surgeons Congress, 1970; Institute of Medicine, National Academy of Sciences, 1973; American Surgeons Assn., 1976; president, Society of Surgeons of Oncology, 1978; president, American Cancer Assn., 1979; president, American Cancer Society, 1979; National Advisory Cancer Board, diplomate, American Board of Surgery, 1980; Society of Surgeons; Commission on Cancer; secretary, American College of Surgeons, 1983; Distinguished Service Medals; Medico-Chirurgical Society of the District of Columbia; James Ewing Society of Head and Neck Surgeons; and, more recently, president, American College of Surgeons, 1994.

220

The AMA in South Africa

Steve Biko, a charismatic, but no nonsense, native South African, appeared on the scene when South Africa was in desperate need of indigenous leadership. The traditional leaders of the African National Congress (ANC) and the Pan Afrikanist Congress (PAC) had either been exiled, imprisoned for life, or killed, during the scorch-the-earth policies enforced by South Africa's apartheid government following its rise to power in 1948.

At that time, most of the veteran leaders of the ANC had already served 10 years of their life sentences in the segregated, Robben Island Prison which was located seven miles off the coast of Cape Town. Robert Sobukway, leader of the breakaway PAC was held in isolation at Robben Island Prison for many years following the 1960 Sharpeville Massacre.[1]

Bishop Desmond Tutu had side-stepped the government's efforts to transform him from a man of the cloth into a man of the streets. Mongosuthu Buthelezi, an aggressive Zulu leader, waited for a call from the apartheid leaders who, apparently realizing that they no longer needed to bid for his services, bided their time.

Biko's preparation for leadership included medical studies at a "natives only" medical school and the formation of his Black Consciousness Movement (BCM) party with a pro-black, do-it-yourself agenda. The party prohibited subservience to whites, especially those who were members of apartheid's Nationalist Party.

When several arrests and six months of solitary confinement failed to break his spirit, Biko was arrested for the last time on August 18, 1977 and imprisoned in South Africa's automobile capitol in Port Elizabeth's prison. During his 26 days of non-stop interrogation, starvation and physical torture, no one knew of Biko's whereabouts.

Between alternating interrogations and abusive attacks by the security police,[2] Biko was examined by five prison doctors. None of the physicians could find anything "wrong" with him, and one doctor went so far as to suggest that Biko, a former medical student, was feigning illness. The captive was sent to the prison hospital where a spinal tap revealed bloody spinal fluid.

For reasons unknown at that time, the Port Elizabeth Prison's chief medical officer, Dr. Benjamin Tucker, signed an order transferring the moribund Biko from the southern prison in Port Elizabeth to the "better equipped" Pretoria Prison, 750 miles to the north. Naked, comatose and incontinent, Biko was strapped to the floor of a Land Rover for the 18-hour journey.

When the Security Police arrived in Pretoria with their human cargo, the same floor mat which had served as Biko's bed and stretcher in Port Elizabeth, became his bier in Pretoria. Just before his death, he was examined by another prison physician who was also unable to offer any medical care. The Port Elizabeth physicians had "forgotten" to send along Biko's hospital records from the Port Elizabeth Prison. Shortly thereafter, Biko died on September 12, 1977—untreated and unattended, on a floor-mat of the Pretoria Prison.

Following his death, "Death of Detainees While in Custody of South Africa's Security Police" became a topic for international debates in many parts of the world, including Russia and her satellites.[3] They recalled that Biko was South Africa's 28th victim of police brutality. Despite Biko's fate, the murders in South Africa continued without a pause.[4]

An inquest was reluctantly performed by members of the South Africa Medical Association (SAMA), where it was revealed that Biko had been held naked, incommunicado, and was scarcely fed for 20 days. He was also interrogated and tortured by the Security Police under the command of senior officer, Colonel Pieter Goosen.[5] The savagery of security policemen was common knowledge as noted by Donald Woods, Biko's biographer,[6] and others.

In a *South African Medical Journal*, dated August 22, 1981, the autopsy pathologist estimated that the brain damage which caused Biko's death, was sustained during his prolonged and traumatic interrogation.

None of the five examining doctors ever recorded the presence of extensive head, neck, and facial injuries that were so clearly obvious during the autopsy. Dr. John Gluckman, chairman of the Southern Transvaal branch of the SAMA and a world renowned pathologist, assisted in the autopsy, representing the Biko family.[7]

Of equal importance was the "bloody, mislabeled" spinal fluid which was not revealed until the autopsy report was released on November 9, 1977, seven weeks after Biko's death.[8] The magistrate reviewed the inquest findings and referred the matter to the South African Medical and Dental Council for its final disposition.

The council's members reviewed the report, leisurely, before concluding: "There is no prima facie evidence of improper or disgraceful conduct on the part of the practitioners. No further action on this matter will be taken."

The SAMA concurred: "On the evidence available, we felt that the doctors who treated Biko exercised proper, reasonable skill and care and were not guilty of negligence."

Dr. Brian Lewis, a British Medical Association Council senior member, denounced SAMDC's decision as "disgraceful." Momentarily lost for words, he continued, "The South Africa Medical Association did not have the courage to use the mechanisms that existed for it to pick up the problem and deal with it."

"The ethical requirement of the Hippocratic Oath and the Declarations of Geneva and Tokyo require that the interests of the patient be served above all other considerations. The most clearly applicable document, the 1975 Declaration of Tokyo, offered guidelines for doctors concerning torture and other cruel, inhuman and degrading punishment in relation to detention and imprisonment." It defined deliberate infliction of physical or mental suffering to obtain information or a confession, or for any other reason, as torture.

It also identified the clinically independent alleviation of distress as the doctor's fundamental responsibility. "No motive, whether personal, collective, or political shall prevail against this higher purpose." The Tokyo Declaration is a by-product of the World Medical Association (WMA).[9]

When the SAMA refused to act on these findings, there began a wholesale withdrawal of memberships from the WMA, with which the SAMA had been affiliated, prior to its 1976 withdrawal. The membership, following Biko's murder, fell from 60 to 27 by 1984, the year of the final departure of the British Medical Association.[10]

Medical groups and similar organizations around the world were more horrified by the SAMA's callousness, if that is possible, than they were about the cruelty of the security police and their level of contempt for and intimidation of the prison's doctors.

An international conference on apartheid and health, convened by the World Health Organization's (WHO) regional committee for Africa and held in Brazzaville, Peoples Republic of the Congo, on November 16-20, was opened by Dr. C.A.A. Conium, WHO regional director for Africa. The members discussed the effects of apartheid on health and sought to design a plan of action to protect and promote health for everyone.

Dr. Conium declared, "Health action is political as well as economic. Apartheid has been proven to be, above all, a racist ideology based on the two key elements: the alleged superiority of the white race and the need to safeguard its economic and political supremacy."

"Throughout the world, South Africa is the only country where racism was written into the constitution, the only country where skin color entirely and definitely determine the place of one category of national citizens within the social category."

Dr. Lang, the first prison doctor to see Biko after his arrest, gave testimony that he knew to be false.[11] Despite the inquest's disclosures and findings, all of the doctors, policemen and other prison personnel were absolved of any responsibility for Biko's murder. Minister of justice, Paul Kruger, exclaimed somewhat prematurely, "the case is closed!"[12]

Although the early verdict absolved the doctors and the security police, nearly all of medical societies in the western world were harshly critical of the five doctors' failure to provide proper treatment of Biko, as well as the SAMA's callous disregard for his life.

The medical community was further stunned by the failure of the SAMA and the SAMDC to schedule proper hearings of the case, even if they chose not to censure their members for what appeared to be serious derelictions of duty.

A glaring contrast to this world-wide criticism of the SAMA's actions was the obvious disinterest and inaction of the AMA. A review of AMA publications of that period suggested that, although Biko's murder and inquest commanded international attention from the media and medical community, AMA officials took little notice of it.[13]

The editors and subscribers of the major medical journals in England, Canada, Australia, and the *Journal of the NMA* were among the severest critics of the SAMA. They, unlike the publishers of the *AMA Journal,* kept their readers informed on the many aspects of the Biko case for several months after his murder. Several journals still make occasional references to it, editorially, and in their "Letters-to-the-Editor's columns."[14]

To the contrary, AMA officers, Drs. Robert Hunter, chairman of AMA's board of trustees; Tom Nesbit, AMA president; James Sammons, executive vice-president of AMA; and Joe D. Miller, deputy vice-president of the AMA made an AMA-sponsored visit to the 1979 South African medical convention (less than two years after Biko's murder) "to demonstrate to us," according to their hosts, "the good will that exists between the medical professions of the two countries."[15] Following that visit, the AMA published an "objective" report on the Biko tragedy.[16]

This blossoming relationship between the AMA and the SAMA had begun in 1976, the year *before* Biko's murder, during South Africa's bantu education crisis. At that time, Biko became a marked man when he, among other things, opposed Prime Minister Henrik Verwoerd's all-out efforts to force all

Africans to learn the "Afrikaans," the language of apartheid, instead of English, "to serve their white masters better."

Biko's resourceful resistance to his apartheid oppressors caused many South Africans and some American conservative Republicans to dismiss him as pro-communist and earned for him the animosity of the cold warriors of the western world, especially those in the U.S. Senate.

Charging other African members of the WMA with discrimination, the SAMA withdrew its membership from that organization in 1976,[17] following the prior example of the AMA.

By 1977, the WMA began to feel the financial pinch of the absence of its wealthiest member (the AMA) and negotiations were begun for the AMA to renew its membership. A deal was struck that:

1. Allowed the African continent to be subdivided into three parts, one third of which would be controlled by the SAMA.

2. The AMA accepted the SAMA's invitation and sent a four-man "goodwill" delegation to South Africa. They toured carefully selected medical schools and hospitals in the Cape, the Transvaal, and the Orange Free State, from January 16-26, 1979.[18]

3. The AMA delegation extended a warm invitation to the SAMA's secretary general, Dr. C.E.M. Viljoen, to attend the AMA's next annual convention. The idea was to introduce him to the AMA's membership before touting him for membership on the WHA's Ethic's Committee, as was the case in 1981!

4. Later, at the WMA's 1979 meeting, the AMA paid its membership dues and rejoined with full privileges.

5. Due to the ill-will against South Africa, generated by the Biko murder, AMA officials advised the SAMA to delay seeking re-admission to the WMA until 1981, thus allowing the Biko stench to subside. The first test of the SAMA's readmissability into the international medical community was with the WHO in 1981. The AMA controlled only one vote in the WHO, so the vote to deny the SAMA admission was 29:1.

The next test was within the WMA, where the SAMA got all of the AMA's 36 votes and 41 others, which included those of the immigrant Cuban physicians who had fled to Miami in the 1960s and formed their own Cuban Medical Association, a recognized affiliate of the AMA. Such flaunting of the AMA's political clout cost WMA additional members; defections which proved advantageous to the AMA in 1983.

With this whopping AMA-led majority, the SAMA's severest critics were discouraged from bringing up such penalties as the promise of an apology by the SAMA for Biko's mistreatment and murder and the withdrawal of consultative status from the WMA by the World Health Organization.[19]

News reports of the SAMA's readmission to the WMA carried the full endorsement of the SAMA's Secretary General Viljoen, in whose opinion, "The successful readmission of the SAMA to the WMA could play a significant role in combating the efforts of others to isolate South Africa and might pave the way for similar recognition of other professional groups."

While Dr. Viljoen's opinion did not deter those members who cancelled their WMA memberships, it did gain the attention of the members of the AMA delegation. Now, they felt secure to move more boldly than ever, to complete each item on their pro-apartheid agenda by:

6. Passing an AMA-supported, 1981 proposal that Dr. Viljoen be placed on the WMA's Ethics Committee. The proposal, like the one for the SAMA's readmission, was bitterly opposed but successfully passed at the expense of more WMA membership cancellations.

7. It was during the WMA's 1983 meeting in Venice, Italy, that the AMA, now fully confident of her winning hand, went for broke for apartheid. The SAMA was encouraged to put in a bid to host the WMA's 1985 convention in Capetown, South Africa. This bid, much like their previous 1981 bid to rejoin the WMA, was enthusiastically supported by the AMA.

The WMA's reduced, residual membership made it easier to gain a majority approval for Capetown among the disgruntled members than would have been the case, otherwise. When the delegates headed for home, the 1985 WMA convention's location seemed assured.

Meanwhile in 1980, two significant South African events had surfaced that should have warned the AMA that their pro-apartheid policy had almost run its course:

1. Dr. Wendy Orr, a white female, South African physician, had been assigned to treat anti-apartheid activists who were imprisoned while resisting security police intimidation. She reported that her patients were so severely beaten by the security police that she could not administer to their injuries from prior assaults.

Dr. Orr was the first South African government employee to file an affidavit charging police with the abuse of anti-apartheid activists. Although her affidavit was filed in the first week of October, a hearing was not scheduled until November 26, 1985. Meanwhile, according to Rev. Robert Orr, Dr. Orr's Presbyterian minister father, she was subsequently transferred to a new job that did not allow her to treat prison patients.

Rev. Orr was not sure if this change in his daughter's medical responsibilities was a form of punishment by South Africa's medical establishment (she had joined with 43 relatives of detained activists in bringing action against the security police.) Rev. Orr was also unaware of any "cease and desist" orders to discourage police brutality.

2. Dr. Jonathan Gluckman, a highly-respected, white South African pathologist, reported in 1992 that he had performed autopsies on some 200 prisoners who had died while in police custody. He found evidence that 90% of the victims had been "violently done to death" by the police.

His first effort to stop the murders was to appeal to Prime Minister P.W. Botha, who had been South Africa's minister of defense before being chosen, unanimously, in 1984 as the first executive president of South Africa.

As minister of defense, President Botha had transformed South Africa's military arm into a formidable fighting force, the most feared throughout Africa. His troops had been the enforcers

228

of "Bantu education," with soldiers replacing many of the African teachers in the native schools, beginning as early as the 1960s.

Since the recruits for the South African military and those who became security policemen came from the same pool, it is understandable why Prime Minster Botha turned a deaf ear to Dr. Gluckman's complaints about police brutality.

Dr. Gluckman continued performing autopsies on the victims of police brutality until the more-moderate president, F.W. de Klerk, replaced Botha in 1989.[20] But soon after Prime Minister de Klerk's election, the media asked him to explain why Zulu Chief Mongosuthu Buthelezi's name was on the payroll of Adrian Vlok, South Africa's minister of law and order.

When Prime Minster de Klerk's answer was unsatisfactory, and he refused to call off the security police, Dr. Gluckman went public with his autopsy findings in July, 1992. He declared, "I can't stand it any longer. The lower rungs of the police are totally out of control."[21]

These and other developments in the U.S. and South Africa gave the impression that the AMA's juggernaught of power was invincible.

The long-range goal of this interplay between the AMA and the SAMA was "to gain full acceptance for apartheid medicine in the eyes of the international medical community."[22]

The bid to convene the 1985 WMA Conference in Cape Town was a major item in the AMA-SAMA's scheme for achieving this goal. Fortunately, it did not succeed.

Many of the WMA delegates were caught off guard by South Africa's 1983 invitation and the AMA's sudden support to take the 1985 Convention to Cape Town. This strategy was relatively easy since the AMA had begun dominating the WMA after reinstating its membership.

The AMA further hedged its bets by taking advantage of another unique opportunity to field a winning team. The thousands of Cuban physicians who had found refuge in the U.S. in the 1960s, were organized as a separate body, yet followed the AMA's lead in supporting the WMA's move to Cape Town.

The AMA-SAMA delegates departed from Venice with little knowledge of the backlash that awaited them once their coup became common knowledge. Anti-apartheid protesters were mobilized nationwide. One of the many picket lines was led by Dr. Benjamin Spock, the celebrated pediatrician and veteran street-fighter.[23]

Dr. Spock and 75 other demonstrators, paraded just outside the AMA's Chicago headquarters protesting the AMA's preparations to participate in the Cape Town Conference. "The AMA's decision to send delegates to this October meeting was interpreted as giving direct approval of the South African Government's apartheid policies," Spock said.

"The South African government, as everyone knows, is a terribly racist government. In South Africa, it's a constitutional policy to be racist." While Dr. Spock called on AMA officials to take a "bold position" and withdraw from the conference, the demonstrators shouted:

"Two-four-six-eight, encourage health care instead of hate" and "AMA, you can't hide, we know you are on apartheid's side."

Many anti-apartheid Letters-to-the-Editor and other pertinent propaganda flooded the media, opposing the AMA's "sell out" to South Africa. One such letter appeared in the *British Medical Journal, Lancet,* on February 9, 1985:

Sir, the World Medical Association (WMA) plans to hold its next triennial conference in October 1985 in Cape Town, South Africa. For several decades now, international medical and scientific organizations have refused to hold scientific meetings in South Africa. The AMA holds the largest vote in the WMA and was instrumental in the 1981 readmission of the SAMA to the WMA. The official Journal of the AMA, to which we wrote on this subject on behalf of the Committee on Health in Southern Africa, declined to print this letter; so we turn to the Lancet to air the issue.

The planned break of the WMA with the tradition of avoiding meetings in South Africa is the extension of a policy that is already supportive of the South African regime's medical ethics, and a peculiar objection already supportive of the South African regime.

The re-admission of the SAMA provoked the resignation from the WMA of medical associations in the Netherlands, Britain, Canada, the Scandinavian countries and many others. A major concern of the WMA is medical ethics and a particular objection of the national associations of physicians who resigned was SAMA's refusal to investigate the medical care given to Steve Biko, who died of head injuries while in police custody and received grossly inadequate care from prison physicians.

The AMA, with the WMA, has participated in what seems to be a campaign to rehabilitate, in the minds of physicians, the only regime in the world with a constitution based on racial discrimination.

Signed:

June Jackson Christmas Sophia Davis School of Biomedical Education City College of New York	Arthur Davidson, Member Natl Med Assn Empire State Chapter
James McIntosh, President Committee of Residents and Interns	Victor W. Sidel, Montefiore Medical Center Albert Einstein College of Medicine
Meredith Sirmans, president Manhattan Central Medical Society	Mervyn Susser Columbia Univ., New York

Gerald Thompson
Columbia Univ. and Harlem Hospital, New York[24]

The editors of the *AMA Journal* followed the example previously established by the *Journal of the SAMA*, a few years earlier and ignored pro-Biko propaganda. The SAMA, however, unlike the *JAMA*, did relent and published the following letter in a subsequent issue:

The Steve Biko Case,

To the Editor: I note with incredulity the publication of two letters on the Steve Biko case in the SAMAJ of 15 November 1980.

I find it impossible to understand why two letters expressing a similar point of view were selected for publication when other letters expressing a contrary view were not published. In particular, I refer to a letter sent to you by myself and two colleagues on 24 September 1980. I also find it strange that an important letter, on 24 September, from Professor P.V. Tobias was published in prominent British American and Australian Journals but not in our own Journal.

As a member of the Association, I wish to record a most vehement protest at this biased selection of correspondence on a most important issue. The editor of our Association's journal should not misuse his position by selecting correspondence from a member in order to propagate a one-sided view of this or any other issue.

Actions such as these bring into question the credibility of not only the Editor and the Journal but the whole Association. I have sent a copy of this letter to the Chairman of the Federal Council.

I request, Sir, that you take urgent steps to correct this error of judgement and publish, immediately, a fair selection of correspondence on the subject of the Biko case.[25]

This same group of protestors sent the same letter to the SAMA and it was answered by Dr. Viljoen,[26] the AMA's appointee for the WMA's Ethics Committee in 1981.

Sirs, Dr. Christmas and her colleagues comment on the WMA's plan to hold a conference in Cape Town later this year. Considering the many incorrect statements in this letter, I am not surprised that the JAMA refused to publish it.

...(4) the statutory body required to investigate the medical care given to Steve Biko is the South African Medical and Dental Council, not the SAMA. Independent investigations, such as those done by S.A. Strauss, professor of law at the Univ. of South Africa, by an AMA delegation and by a former chairman of the WMA's Council, and Dr. L.L. Wilson of Australia, proved that the SAMA had done everything within its power to secure as objective as possible an assessment of the ethical issues brought to the fore by the Biko case and that it could not have done more.

(5) The SAMA is a voluntary body open to all legally qualified medical practitioners in South Africa and does not discriminate on the basis of color, race, creed, or political persuasion.

Medical Associates of South Africa
428 King's Highway 428
CEM Viljoen
Secretary General
Lynwood, Pretoria 00801
South Africa

Less than two years before Dr. Viljoen wrote the above letter, and several years *after* an AMA president declared that racism did not exist in South African medical education, the following letter was written by acting dean of the Medical

School at the Univ. of the Witwatersrand, Dr. D.G. Moyes, from Johannesburg, S.A.:

"To the Editor:

The Executive Committee of the Faculty of Medicine of the University of the Witwatersrand has noted with deep disquiet that, according to an official statement made by South Africa's Minister of National Education (and future Prime Minister) F.W. de Klerk, on 30 August 1983, black applicants for admission to the medical and paramedical courses at this university will continue to be required to obtain ministerial permits to accept offers of places in the Medical School.

....We, therefore, earnestly entreat the Minister to reconsider his decision and to free the Faculty of Medicine from all constraints in the free admission of students.

D.G. Moyes, Acting Dean
Univ. of Witwatersrand

After some of the protesters denounced South Africa as a pole-cat country, and an unfit place to hold an international convention, the AMA's Dr. Sammons rushed to South Africa's defense.

Despite the well-known facts about the poor health conditions for Africans in South Africa, Sammons later declared, among other things: "We've been there, and we have no doubt that South Africa's standards of medical care and education are equal to those of the U.S."[27]

The AMA spokesman picked up additional support from Dr. Mardi, WMA president in Portugal. After a two-day tour of South Africa, Dr. Mardi gave his approval, also, for the 1985 Cape Town convention. His praise for apartheid medicine supported Dr. Sammons but did not help his cause.[28]

Dr. Dilizia Mji, a former president of the National Medical and Dental Association of South Africa, was a charter member of the ANC's Youth League in the early 1940s. He took a strong exception to Dr. Sammons' allegations of equality of opportunity and accused him of trying to "white-wash the discriminatory medical practices of the apartheid regime." He also pointed out

233

the great disparity between medical care and training for white South Africans and non-whites.[29]

He recalled the well-supervised, "good-will" South African tour of medical facilities in the late 1970s that avoided the overcrowded, malodorous and violent squatters' camps which scarred the South African countryside.

The tour guides were careful to by-pass Hillbrow's Baragwanath Hospital, where, a delegation from the Transvaal Council reported, "there was one patient under each bed, two in the bed and two on the floor."[30]

My own review of the South African literature of that period tends to support the assessment of Dr. Mji, who has lived there all of his life rather than that of the AMA's Dr. Sammons, after his guided tour of several days.

"The dept. of Medicine of Baragwanath Hospital consists of 470 beds; two wards have been constructed since 1980, adding 70 more beds. In April 1987, two thousand four hundred thirty-nine patients were admitted to the medical units, which gave an average bed occupancy of 166%, or 780 patients per day for 470 beds. That means at any given time, 310 patients were forced to do without a bed.

"I cannot understand the justification for having half of the projected number of beds at the new H.F. Verwoerd Hospital in Pretoria for non-white patients, while the almost exclusively-white Johannesburg Hospital has an unused capacity of over 1,000 beds."[31]

Jet Magazine published articles by the NMA president, Dr. Phillip Smith, and me urging all NMA members to cancel their membership in the AMA.[32] Having already canceled mine in 1956, during the Hungarian Uprising, I collaborated with Danton Wilson, editor of the *Michigan Chronicle*, in the preparation of an editorial that was published on July 13, 1985. Members of the NMA were urged to abandon the AMA because it, among other things, was the major sponsor of Cape Town's WMA convention.

Our editorial was read by Dr. W. Peter McCabe (then president of the Wayne County Medical Society and is now chairman of the Michigan State Medical Society's board of trustees) who sent the following letter to John H. Sengstacke, chairman of the *Michigan Chronicle:*

234

This letter is in response to the article written by Editor, Danton Wilson, 'Black Doctors Urged to quit AMA.' The American Medical Association has notified the Wayne County Medical Society that the WMA has changed the location of its 37th World Medical Assembly, which was to be held October 21-25, 1985 in Cape Town, South Africa. This meeting is being rescheduled, during the same time, in Brussels, Belgium.

The World Medical Association took this action in view of the current unrest in the Republic of South Africa and in recognition of the depressed world economic climate and its effect on national medical associations.

Along with the WMA, the AMA reaffirms its support for the Medical Association of South Africa, which was to host the assembly. The SAMA represents that nation's medical professionals, regardless of their race, sex, color, religion or political persuasion.

The AMA continues to commend the Medical Association of South Africa for its policy of non-discrimination, its actions to bring equality of opportunity for medical and health workers of all races in South Africa and its efforts to provide quality health care for all South Africans.

The National Medical Association and the AMA, in a joint effort, were largely responsible for the change in location.

W. Peter McCabe, President
Wayne County Medical Society.

This Letter-to-the-Editor, although a bit long, was presented in its entirety because it reveals that:

1. The monolithic AMA was moved to action by an article in *The Michigan Chronicle.*

2. Officers of the AMA's affiliates are, also, as careless with the facts, as are their colleagues in Chicago.

3. Unrest and economic depression in South Africa were less severe, in 1984 than 1979, when the AMA sent its "good-will" delegation to South Africa "to study medical practices in South Africa," just after Biko's murder.

A review of the NMA's records do not support the existence of a "joint effort" between NMA and AMA to move the WMA convention to Belgium.

Author's note—Were the pickets, protesters and others who were opposed to the AMA's decision to hold the WMA convention in Capetown, South Africa, totally ineffective in forcing a change in SAMA's venue?

While the jury was out on the decision to hold the WMA's 1985 meeting in Cape Town, I wrote a letter to the Wayne County Medical Society[33] and the Michigan State Medical societies that challenged Dr. McCabe's allegations on the sanctity and benevolence of the AMA and requested documented support for them. This and all subsequent requests have gone unanswered.

Although wholesale resignations from the WMA began soon after Biko's death, the British Medical Association did not throw in the towel until 1984. Their withdrawal statement, issued in January 1984, reflective of the stresses that undermined the integrity of the WMA.

"Further doubts arose over the representative status of the WMA when the Transkei (a native South African dependency) was admitted to membership of our Association which, already included free doctors of Cuba" (who fled to Florida, after Fidel Castro seized control of Cuba, beginning in 1960).[34]

Dr. Mji, like most native South Africans, was violently opposed to the recognition of any of the so-called Bantustans of South Africa as sovereign states, the most advanced of which was the Transkei.

The country that came closest to exchanging diplomatic representatives with the Transkei was Israel. Dr. Mji was visibly upset by outside, "pro-apartheid" interference in the affairs of his country.

In Dr. Mji's opinion and that of other native South Africans, was that the ultimate goal of taking the WMA convention to South Africa was to legitimize apartheid medicine in the eyes of the international medical community.[35] This opinion is shared by many observers—those who don't want to see it come to pass, as well as those who do.

Dr. Mji and other South African physicians are to be congratulated for their efforts, individually and collectively, to provide fuel for the worldwide debates of "Death in Detention in South Africa" in general, with special emphasis on the Steve Biko tragedy.

Three well known South African doctors, Professors Frances Ames, Trefor Jenkins and Phillip Tobias, instituted proceedings against the South African Medical and Dental Council alleging that it had failed to carry out its statutory duty by not holding an open inquiry into the circumstances surrounding Biko's murder.

The litigants, anticipating legal costs upwards of £20,000, asked the public to assist by making deposits to their account in the Standard Bank of South Africa, Hillbrow, S.Africa.[36]

It was only after receiving an application from six additional South African doctors, who also felt their profession had been sullied by the Biko affair, did the Pretoria Supreme Court order the case reopened.

Although Dr. Tucker expressed contrition in his confession and we did not hear anything from Dr. Lang, it must not be forgotten that even Dr. Tucker did not speak up until 14 years after Biko's murder. He was then under threat of a lawsuit by his colleagues and a command order from the Pretoria Supreme Court.

Unlike the earlier, reluctant decision by the Council which exonerated everybody, this time, Dr. Tucker was found guilty of 10 allegations of disgraceful conduct and three of improper conduct. He was suspended from practicing medicine for three months, but the sentence were suspended for two years. Dr. Lang was found guilty of eight allegations of improper conduct and reprimanded. Only after these developments did Dr. Tucker release the following statement in October of 1991, fourteen years Biko's murder:

"On September 12, 1977, after being held three weeks in police custody without charges, Stephen Biko, a leading anti-apartheid activist, died of multiple head injuries. Dr. Benjamin Tucker, who twice examined Biko in prison before his death, was barred from practicing medicine in 1985 by a disciplinary committee of the South African Medical and Dental Council for 'disgraceful' conduct in Biko's death. This week, Dr. Tucker's medical license was reinstated after he sent a letter of apology to the Medical and Dental Council."

Excerpts from Dr. Tucker's letter, which ran in the *Sowetan,* a Johannesburg daily, follow:

Without wishing to traverse all the facts surrounding Biko's death, I realize and appreciate that I failed in my duty toward Biko in accepting certain information as given facts and making assumptions about important aspects relating to Biko's condition, without having made proper inquiries or investigations, thereafter.

In failing to make full and proper inquiries from the patient, himself, from members of the South African Police, and from colleagues about matters relevant to Biko's condition, and failing and neglecting to examine Biko thoroughly and adequately, I was the author of my own misfortune. I compounded these failures by allowing myself to be swayed by security considerations, thus failing to insist on the hospitalization of Biko, all to the detriment of my patient's well-being.

On reflection on the cause of this failure, I came to realize that over the period of 30 years, I had at that time been employed by the state as a district surgeon, I had gradually lost the fearless independence that is required of a medical practitioner when the interests of his patient are threatened.

I had become too closely identified with the organs of the state, especially the police force, with which I dealt practically on a daily basis. In the circumstances of Biko's case, I, too, readily accepted the decisions of the security police, without safeguarding the interests of my patient.

I have spent many years of utter despair and self recriminations at my actions following the recognition and appreciation by me of the part I had played in the events leading to Biko's death. As a result of my conduct, not only my patient's interests suffered, but also those of the medical profession and my country.

Although Dr. Tucker has apologized and received a light tap on his wrists, and Dr. Lang got a lecture before it was back to business as usual, nothing more was said or done, to my knowledge, about James Thomas Kruger, minister of Security Police nor security policeman, Col. Pieter Goosen, who was Biko's main custodian and tormentor during his incarceration while he was in the Port Elizabeth prison.[37]

While Dr. Tucker's confession was still a news item of world-wide interest, I called the confession to the attention of members of the medical establishments in Detroit's Wayne County Medical Society, The Michigan State Medical Society and Chicago's AMA headquarters, all of who had "commended the South Africa Medical Association for its policy of non-discrimination, its actions to obtain equal pay for medical and health workers of all races in South Africa, and its success in providing high quality health care for all Africans.

I suggested to them that since Dr. Tucker had sought, and I hope, found relief from his "utter despair and self-recriminations" for his part in the events leading to Biko's murder, by apologizing, they might begin the same redemptive process for their role in this unfortunate matter for themselves. My first request was dispatched soon after Dr. Tucker broke his 14-year silence, in late 1991. I am still waiting and hoping for the best. It is difficult to imagine a more appropriate pad from which to launch the NMA into a higher orbit during its second century.

On January 20 and 21, 1995, the *Washington Post* published successive articles by Paul Taylor, their foreign service correspondent from Johannesburg, S.A. Both reports discuss an "ugly spat between Mr. de Klerk and President Mandela over immunity from prosecution for crimes committed by South African police and security officers, on both sides, during the era of white minority rule."

It was hoped that this controversial granting of blanket amnesty to all malefactors, black and white, would be the cement that would maintain the integrity of the uneasy ANC-Nationalist coalition. The amnesty measure, passed by former President Frederick W. DeKlerk's government before he lost the election to Nelson Mandela, is a constant bone of contention between the two sides.

This face-off has much in common with the century-long struggle between the NMA and the AMA. It has not been as happy or as-fruitful a relationship as it could or should have been. The NMA is on the threshold of its second century and the world is near the threshold of the 21st century. The decisive, unanswered question remains: Can the two organizations co-exist in a mutually respectable partnership?

The only safe reply is: I don't know. It has never been tried. Our only hope is that the members of the AMA will follow the example of former Secretary of Defense Robert S. McNamara, who on April 9, 1995, admitted that his war against the Vietnemese was "wrong, terribly wrong." That was equally true of his next role as head of the World Bank, from which he provided financial support for, among other things, South

Africa's apartheid regimes.[38] Let us hope that the AMA will not take quite so long.

1. Leonard Thompson, *A History of South Africa*. (New Haven: Yale University Press, 1990) p. 200.

2. Thompson, p. 200.

3. Patricia Oosthuizen, Letter-to-the-Editor, *South African Medical Journal* (15 November 1980) p. 792; Charles H. Wright, *Travesty on the Oath of Hippocrates*, JNMA, Vo l. 70, No. 4 (1978); and C.E.M. Viljoen (Secretary General, Medical Association of South Africa) Letter-to-the-editor, *British Medical Journal* (January 28, 1978).

4. *Sowetan*, (August 14, 1985).

5. *SAMJ*, (August 22, 1981) p. 3.

6. Donald Woods, *Biko*. (New York: Paddington Press Ltd, 1978) p. 139.

7. *New York Times*. (November 14, 1977. See also entry for September 13).

8. *New York Times* (November 14, 1977. See citations for ; September 13 and November 9).

9. Proceedings of the WMA convention, Tokyo, Japan (October 1975).

10. Letter-to-the-editor, Peter Kandela, *The Lancet* (November 2, 1985).

11. *New York Times* (July 21, 1977). Upon being called in, Dr. Lang gave a patently false certificate. Neither he nor his superior, Dr. Benjamin Tucker, made an inquiry of their patient as to the origin of even the lip injury, which they admitted seeing. Nor did they ask the police. Further evidence of governmental control of the medical profession was Dr. Tucker's report that Biko was in "satisfactory condition" when he signed the travel order for the comatose Biko to be transported 750 miles to Pretoria. His medical opinion that Biko should be hospitalized in Port Elizabeth was over-ridden by the local security police chief, Colonel Pieter Goosen. Dr. Tucker deferred to the state's authority and signed the transfer order without protest. Biko's bloody spinal fluid was mislabelled "Stephen Neljo," as a part of the official cover-up. During the inquest, Biko's representatives were not allowed to question the doctors.

12. *SAMJ*. The Steve Biko Case, letter. Vol. 63, No. 21 (May 1983) p. 827.

13. A review of other *JAMA* publications yielded scant reference to the Biko matter.

240

14. Vest Johnson, *Canadian Medical Association Journal*, Vol. 1130 (June 15, 1984).

15. *SAMJ*, Proceedings of the Convention of the South African Medical Association (1979) 55:63.

16. *AMA News* (September 10, 1980).

17. *SAMJ*, SAMA and the World Medical Association, Vol. 69. (1986) p. 1001.

18. *SAMJ*, Proceedings of the Convention of the South African Medical Association, Vol. 1979. (1979) 55:63.

19. *The Lancet*, (February 13, 1982). The World Health Organization (WHO) is governed by the World Health Assembly, which meets each May, and an Executive Board of 30 members whose 69th session was held in Geneva in 1982. While nominated by member countries who compete for the privilege, board members sit in their own right as individuals, expert in one or other area of public health.

20. *Eastern Province Herald*, "Botha Has All The Cards." (South Africa: September 6, 1984).

21. *Time* (June 7, 1993).

22. British Medical Association Press Statement (May 1, 1984).

23. United Press International (March 23, 1985).

24. *The Lancet* (February 9, 1985).

25. B.A. Bradlow, Professor & Head of the dept. of hematology-pathology, *South African Medical Journal*. (South Africa: January, 10, 1981).

26. *Journal of the SAMA*. (February 9, 1985) p. 542.

27. *SAMJ*, Vol. 63:21 (May 1983) p. 829.

28. Dilza Mji, M.D., *The World Medical Association in South Africa*. (The Baywood Publishing Co., Inc., 1985) p. 351.

29. Dr. Mji, a contemporary of Mandela, was one of the 100 young Africans who gathered in Bloemfomtein in 1944 to form the elite ANC's Youth League that replaced their elders with more activist policies. He was chosen executive secretary of the ANC Youth Group. He was swept up by the security police in 1956, arrested, and charged with treason during a trial that lasted for four years before he and 156 other defendants were exonerated in 1960. Dr. Mji was chosen as president of the NMA of South Africa when South African's native physicians became alienated from the South African Medical Association by its gross mismanagement of

the Steve Biko affair. They saw a common cause in the origin of our National Medical Association in 1895 and their founding of the National Medical and Dental Association of South Africa in 1978.

30. *Rand Daily Mail,* (May 24, 1976).

31. *SAMJ*, Vol. 73:2 (April 1988) p. 437.

32. *Jet Magazine* (Johnson Publications, July 1985). While President Smith advised writing letters of protest to the AMA, I advised cancellation of membership by all NMA members. In the earlier report concerning Dr. Spock, he concurred with other protesters and added: "The AMA's decision to send representatives to the October meeting of the World Medication Association in Cape Town infers indirect approval of the South African government's apartheid policies. The South African government, as everyone knows, is a terribly racist government. In South Africa, it's a constitutional policy to be racist." Dr. Spock called on the AMA to take a "bold position" and withdraw from the conference.

33. *Detroit Medical News* (October 14, 1985) p. 12.

34. *South African Medical News* (April 3, 1983).

35. British Medical Association Press Statement (May 1, 1984).

36. *The British Medical Journal*, Vol. 289 (November 17, 1984) p. 1378.

37. Woods, p. 9.

38. *New York Times*, (April 9, 1995).

Michigan's African American Medical Trailblazers of the Twentieth Century

Edgar B. Keemer, Jr., M.D. (Meharry, 1936), began the private practice of medicine in Detroit in the early 1940s. His specialty was abortions, although it was illegal to perform abortions at that time. He reported having performed 50,000 abortions without a death or serious complication during forty years of practice.

In 1956, he was convicted of a conspiracy to perform abortions and sentenced to two-and-a-half to five years in prison, but was released after 14 months on a special parole. His conviction was set aside in 1976 and he returned to Detroit and resumed his abortion practice.

During the 1955-56 Montgomery Bus Boycott, Dr. Keemer and his wife donated a station wagon to the movement for the duration of the protest. A photograph on page 181 of his widely read book, *Confessions of a Pro-life Abortionist,* shows Dr. Keemer in the Selma to Montgomery March in 1965.

These events suggest how strongly Dr. Keemer felt about a person's rights: civil, human, and otherwise. His 235-page book, published in 1980, makes his position clear.

A review of *Confessions of a Pro-life Abortionist*

Dr. Keemer's most enduring contribution, as one of Michigan's African American medical pioneers, is described in his *Confessions.* This interesting and informative autobiography was published at his own expense.

The author begins by establishing his position that a woman's right to control her own body must not be violated by financial, political, legal nor any other impediment to the exercise of her freedom of choice. From his first "illegal" termination of a pregnancy in 1971, to his last, Dr. Keemer's position that he was rendering a necessary and valuable public service to women remained steadfast.

On more than one occasion, Dr. Keemer heard the word "murderer" hurled at him by angry anti-abortionists. His response was "each fertilized egg must undergo evolutionary changes before it becomes a human being, as it has done over millions of years. But in the current, emotion-shrouded debate, how often does one hears the clear, demonstrable, scientific facts? When is it admitted, for example, that in the metamorphosis of the six-to-eight-week embryo, there is a striking resemblance to the lower forms of animal life as they go through the transition from fish to amphibian."

After considerable meandering along this pathway, Dr. Keemer raised a crucial question that everyone answers to his and her persuasion: "Is the careful and compassionate doctor who helps a woman with a desperately unwanted pregnancy to solve her problem with safety, a murderer or pro-life?"

Despite wholesale arrests of staff and patients during office hours, harassment from the FBI, attacks from many anti-abortion groups, and fourteen months of maximum security imprisonment, Dr. Keemer insisted that his abortion practice was neither medically, nor morally, wrong.

Vindication of his pro-abortion position finally came on Monday, January 23, 1973, after his second well-publicized arrest. He described the event, many times over:

"This was the picture; the backdrop included a mass arrest at my office. Several of us are awaiting trial on another serious felony charge. The recent defeat of our Michigan proposal at the polls, and on the other side of the coin, the patient's countersuit against the prosecutor and the police department were all cooking at the same time. With this background comes the morning of January 22, 1973. The U.S. Supreme Court ruled 7-2 that first trimester abortions were legal and the state had no authority to interfere with that right.

"Nobody else seemed to notice, but I am sure that I was three feet off the ground, floating, weightless. This was a true high, the high of self-satisfaction—the high of reality."

He said that his first thoughts were of the patient: "Now, no patient will have to endure a degrading psychiatric consultation and pretend she is crazy in order to not bear a child if she so desires."

Dr. Keemer continued performing abortions for the remainder of his medical career, and with some appreciation. He was named Citizen of the Year (1974) by the Detroit Chapter of the National Association of Social Workers; special awards came from The National Abortion Federation; the City of Detroit; and Meharry Medical College.

Joshua Williams, M.D

"The theory that state, county and municipal authorities tolerated or encouraged aggressive acts against black physicians in Georgia during the '50s and '60s is probably incorrect. A different experience in Georgia, when compared with that of other black physicians elsewhere, may well be a reflection of more militant action on the part of the Georgia's African American physicians," says Dr. Williams.

"The NAACP branch had been inactive for some years during World War II, until 1952. As a part of a mutual agreement to strengthen unity during the war effort, the whites pledged to, likewise, place the KKK in mothballs. Something sparked Georgia's African American citizens to call for reactivation of the NAACP, so I attended the reorganization meeting. When no one among the traditional leaders would accept the responsibility to lead the organization, I agreed to accept the leadership, if the Search Committee could not find anyone else. Two weeks later, I was informed that I was it.

"The accomplishments of my administration were:

"1. As a native son, I made invalid the claim that only 'outside agitators' were dissatisfied with the way things were.

2. All officers were self-employed or employed by other blacks and relatively protected from economic sanctions by whites.

3. We challenged the use of the City Auditorium for public meetings by the KKK.

4. We began taking measures to force the city to desegregate the recreational facilities, including the golf course.

5. I refused to surrender our list of NAACP members to the Attorney General of Georgia.

6. We achieved desegregation of the civilian, industrial area of the Warner-Robins Air Command.

7. We began legal action against the Bibb County Board of Education to force its compliance with the Supreme Court's *Brown v. Board of Educ.* decision of 1954.

8. We grew from zero to over 500 members; the whites believed we had thousands.

"A brief description of what was significant about these eight accomplishments is warranted. The first two are self-explanatory.

"Number 8 was based on reliable information given to me by whites. The importance of No. 3 was the existence of a city ordinance which forbade the wearing of masks by anyone except on Halloween or in attendance at a masquerade ball.

"We knew that among the klansmen were policemen, insurance salesmen, service station operators, grocers, clerks, ministers and sundry other persons, who conducted business among blacks. They would have to arrive at the auditorium unmasked, carrying their robes, since they could only legally, place the hood over their heads in the auditorium. Six of us stood on the steps leading to the entrance to recognize and record as many as we could.

"Then, we tried to attend the 'public invited' klan meeting, insisting to the police that the usual section reserved for coloreds, on other occasions be accorded to us on this occasion. After an entreaty from the chief of police and the understanding that one favor deserves another, we left. I think that the chief kept his word.

"The Georgia Legislature passed a law that membership in certain organizations would disqualify those persons for jobs in which state money was part, or all, of the salary. Black teachers were particularly apprehensive—several were secret members of the NAACP, a disqualifying organization.

"I was telephoned by the newspaper reporter, as soon as the bill was passed, and asked what would I do when the attorney general demanded the list of members of the Macon (Ga.) branch of the NAACP. My reply was: If I have time, I'll burn it! If not, I'll eat it. So he will be searching through the ashes or my excreta!

"My threat to burn the record was published in the *New York Times.* The attorney general never fulfilled his mandate. The desegregation of the city's golf course was easy, but for an unlikely reason. I asked for a conference with the mayor on the matter of recreational facilities in general, and the golf course, in particular. I was not then and never have been a golfer.

"There followed meetings with the organization of white golfers who had, up to this time, been the financial supporters of the golf course. The mayor feared that even if a few blacks were allowed to play on the course, the white golfers might start a private club or join an existing one.

"There was a case pending in Atlanta, filed by two black doctors, on the same issue. The city attorney had already advised the mayor and city council that the plaintiffs would win. Politically, the mayor and council didn't want to be perceived as jumping the gun and surrendering before a decision was rendered which they could use as the reason for their capitulation.

"Suddenly, one local black tried to get the city to buy his farm on which to build a golf course for African Americans. A group of African American golfers organized to petition the city to allow them use of the existing course on a segregated basis, one or two days per week.

"The city accepted, as did the white golfers. After a month, the white golfers petitioned the City to drop the color bar and allowed all golfers to play every day.

"A young air force officer, a 1952 graduate of Howard Univ., was flying tankers for refueling planes in flight. We became friends while he was stationed at the Warren-Robins Air Base, and he was made aware of wide-spread practices of racial discrimination in the military.

"In the area of the military base where air force personnel carried on their activities, there were no obvious signs of the practice of racial discrimination. However, down in the area where the civilians worked, the rankest kind of segregation was practiced, overtly and constantly. Lt. James Groves, an air force officer, was informed of the real situation on the base and he arranged to get a pass and conducted a tour of the region for me.

"I saw 'white' and 'colored' signs on toilets, drinking fountains, wash facilities and in the cafeteria. Segregating partitions divided the races everywhere. These signs and dividers had been installed by white civilians. Compliance was assured by white civilian supervisors and ignored by the commander general.

"Groves and I recorded everything we saw. I requested and received an appointment with the special assistant of Defense, an African American, with an office in the Pentagon and gave him a copy of my report. He ordered the base photographer to send pictures of every location about which I had complained and found the photographs true to my report. He ordered the signs and all restrictive partitions removed and follow-up photographs were made.

"When I returned to the Pentagon, a few weeks later, he presented me with a new set of pictures. Upon my return to Macon, a visit to the to the air force base confirmed the absence of all signs and partitions, but African Americans were, still sitting where they had always sat—on their side of the now invisible curtain!

"After the land-mark school desegregation case, I was shown on television telling members of Macon's Bibb County Board of Education to comply with both the spirit and the letter of the law. This was seen as a threat to the very foundations of the Southern social structure. My prior telegrams and letters to the Board of Education, asking for a meeting to discuss plans and preparations for compliance with the Supreme Court's decision, had all been ignored. But the "Letters to the Editor," describing

248

how blood would flow in the streets and why dissidents should leave the state, all met with editorial favor.

"At that same time, I was meeting secretly with two white newspaper reporters who would frequently provide me with insightful information about various whites who could influence the course of events. I knew it helped to moderate the tone of the printed text, when the action of the NAACP was described or predicted.

"By now, I had talked personally with Walter White, executive secretary of the NAACP in Savannah, and Atty. Thurgood Marshall, in my Macon home and had become a devout and dedicated NAACP 'character.' About two-thirds of my waking hours were spent in the practice of medicine and one third with the NAACP, except for my recreational activities on weekends.

"As the Board of Education's resistance to change became more violent, the national office of the NAACP called for an escalation of efforts to force integration. Finally, we presented the board with a petition signed by 30 to 50 parents, requesting action to implement the Court's decision to integrate the schools.

"The newspapers printed the names and addresses of all of the petitioners on the front page. Harassment began immediately; most of the petitioners denied that they knew what or why they signed the directive. However, enough of them, including a school teacher, stood fast to make the petition valid. It became the rock on which we made a stand.

"A young white man, a dancing teacher, telephoned and asked to see me in my office. He had been a former patient. During the office conversation, he warned that local telephone operators were eavesdropping my telephone. He knew some women who had been solicited to monitor my phone calls.

"His report was accurate. I was able to prove that I was being monitored. If I did not receive any calls at night, the telephone operators called off and on all night. Most of the time they would say nothing; at other times, the female voice would say 'leave town nigger' or 'nigger your name is mud', etc.

"I did leave town, on weekends, to get some uninterrupted sleep. Lt. Groves sat with me nights, when I felt particularly apprehensive. As each automobile passed my home, I had my rifle aimed at the driver's side.

"The murder of Dr. Tom Brewer, in Columbus, Ga., brought home the awareness that this struggle was no friendly contest. Further, other leaders, like Dr. Brewer, would likely be the focal point of attack by some white fanatic. It would help, tremendously if the leader had a surprise for the would-be assailant.

"Meanwhile, I was informed that the status of my being essential, which had deferred me from active military duty in the Korean War, was no longer valid. I knew that if I left Georgia for two years in the military, I would not return. The major activity now was to raise money for the suit against the Board of Education. Finally, my successor had to be chosen and added to the NAACP.

"During the final years, 1954-1956, the City and the County launched an effort to build a new hospital. The old practice was to grant staff membership to County Medical Society members. I was either president or secretary of the Macon Academy of Medicine, Dentistry and Pharmacy, an affiliate of the NMA composed of six African American physicians, four dentists and one pharmacist.

"We would not endorse or recommend the proposed, new hospital to black voters, unless certain demands were met:

1. We must be granted equal staff membership in the new hospital.

2. Employment opportunities for black nurses and paraprofessionals.

3. Internships must be available to African Americans.

4. The academy members must be allowed to review the hospital plans before they are submitted to the voters.

"Immediately, we were given full membership in the Bibb County Medical Society. A question arose about handling the Society's four dinner meetings each year. The main problem was not with the Society but with the proprietors of the establishment where the meeting's were held. His license to operate a business could be lost if blacks and whites ate together under the same roof, even with a segregating partition between them. Their solution was to serve the white members dinner. After the dishes and tables were cleared away, the African American members were allowed in and only then was the meeting was called to order."

Due to the constant threat of violence at work and in his home and the possibility of being drafted into the military for service in Korea, Dr. Williams collected his family and resettled in Detroit in 1956. He brought with him valuable civil rights experience that he put to good use on many of Michigan's battle fronts, especially as president of the DMS and as editor of the *Wayne County Detroit Medical News.*

C. Arnold Curry, M.D. (Rush Medical College, 1973)

Following a medical residency at Henry Ford Hospital and fellowships in hematology at Wayne State Univ. and the Univ. of Mich., Dr. Curry began the private practice of hematology in 1978 with appointments at Harper, Hutzel, Samaritan and Receiving Hospitals.

In 1984, Dr. Curry incorporated Caraco Pharmaceutical Laboratories, Ltd. where he is a registered investigator for Phase II drug studies for the National Cancer Institute at the Detroit Medical Center. His involvement in the investigative work of the Caraco Corp. has fulfilled a childhood ambition "to put something back into the community." Caraco's $10 million, four-acre complex is located at Research Park in Detroit's inner city.

"Detroit is my city. Except for my medical school years, I have lived here all my life." Dr. Curry expects Caraco to forge a leadership position in the industry by using the following strategies:

"Producing a broad line of quality medications that are available to the consumer at affordable prices; continually improving efficiency in operating through advanced technology, improved procedures, and expanded capabilities; and conducting research for new, innovative and worthwhile products.

"Caraco Pharmaceutical Laboratories has the support of my terrifically supportive wife, Cara and two sons, the older of whom, Mark, is employed by Caraco."

Recently, Dr. Curry announced that Caraco Pharmaceutical Laboratories was hale and hearty. Not only had it survived the "lean and mean" times of the past ten years but had generated sales of nearly $2 million last year.

The economic forecast for Caraco Pharmaceutical Laboratories has shown significant improvement within the past year. The reordering of priorities in the health care industries is a factor in this improvement. One such priority is the cost of drugs. Its reordering requires the wedding of efficiency and economy, which means, among other things, a wider use of generic drugs in all areas of medical care.

Since Caraco Pharmaceuticals' original purpose was to manufacture and distribute generic drugs, it seems well positioned to share in this multi-billion dollar market. Chase Pharmaceutical was a major supplier of generic drugs to the industry until it went out of business recently. Caraco has become a supplier to many of Chase's customers for the drug "Nifedipene" and large orders for this and other products are being filled.

Caraco's facilities are located at 1150 Elijah McCoy, just southwest of the New Center area near downtown Detroit. My tour, conducted by Tom Hicks, was impressive. The $10 million plant and its modern equipment are a significant departure from the "mom and pop" operations of yesteryear.

Walter Evans, M.D. (Univ. of Mich.) cert. surg. 1977

Dr. Evans is rumored to wield the fastest scalpel in town. Others will challenge that distinction and add that speed isn't everything. When he is designated as our premier collector of fine art and rare books, these erstwhile naysayers nod their heads in silent agreement.

When Dr. Evans was asked what launched him on this exciting and expensive course, he said:

"Throughout my childhood in Savannah, Ga., and Beaufort, S.C., I became familiar with the names and teachings of many of our black leaders, both at home and at school. People such as Langston Hughes, W.E.B. Dubois, Mary McCloud Bethune, Paul Robeson, Booker T. Washington, Frederick Douglass and a number of others were household names to me.

"However, when the family moved north to Hartford, Conn., where every teacher and counselor was white, I did not hear of a single achievement by an African or African American. In fact, I was encouraged by the counselors to seek work in one of the factories in and around Hartford in spite of my having one of the highest grade-point averages in the school that I attended.

"It was at Howard Univ. (after a 3-year stint in the U.S. Navy in the mid-1960s) that I, again, became aware of black achievers. It was also a time of great social unrest in the black communities and on college campuses throughout the country. For those who wanted to be involved, there was no better place to be than Howard Univ., in Washington, D.C.

"Speakers such as Dr. Martin Luther King, Adam Clayton Powell, Jr., Stokley Carmichael, LeRoi Jones, H. Rap Brown and so many others were frequent visitors to the campus. Sterling Brown, a truly great poet and later, a close friend, was a fixture on that campus. How could one not be involved? Yet, my involvement at that time was only superficial. Chemistry, biology, and physics consumed the lion's share of my attention, during those fervent days.

"Although I was a frequent visitor to art galleries and museums in the U.S. and Europe, my introduction to blacks as artists came, surprisingly, rather late. In the late seventies, I met with Shirley Reid, director of a Detroit art gallery, who encouraged me to purchase a Jacob Lawrence portfolio of prints—the John Brown Series.

"Shortly thereafter, I met Romare Bearden and invited him to my home in Detroit, where a large reception was held in his honor. The reception was so successful that I later hosted receptions for such other black luminaries as Elizabeth Catlett, Gwendolyn Brooks, John Henrik Clark and most recently, Oliver W. Harrington.

"My collection of the works of these and other artists, writers, and historians has grown exponentially. Scores of museums have sought loans from this collection. Currently, an exhibit of approximately 75 pieces from this collection has been on tour for three years and has bookings through 1996.

"This exhibit includes paintings and sculptures by Robert Scott Duncanson, Edward Mitchell Bannister, Aaron Douglas, Romare Bearden, Elizabeth Catlett, Charles White, Richard Hunt, Archibald Mottley, and Henry Owassa Tanner.

"I have introduced two books recently published by the Univ. of Mississippi Press on celebrated cartoonist Ollie Harrington, who created 'Bootsie.' This long-forgotten cartoonist and warrior for civil rights was forced into exile in Europe during the McCarthy Era. He became a hero of mine when I saw one of his cartoons published in an obscure magazine edited by a close friend.

"I have also collected a number of his original cartoons which are now on tour. He has been brought back from Berlin on several occasions and, like Nelson Mandela, has picked up where he left off pre-exile, before 1951.

"My goal is not just to collect art, literature and documents from our rich cultural past, but to preserve and share that which I have learned and collected with others in hopes that it will bring them as much pride, joy and understanding as it has brought to me."

The Walter Evans collection of fine art is now a firmly-established group of works that has been well-received in many museums throughout the country.[1]

---

1. The following is an exhibition schedule for the Walter O. Evans collection:

June 1-Aug. 31, 1995	Kalamazoo Institute of Arts	Kalamazoo, Mich.
Sept. 4-Nov. 2, 1995	Lowe Art Museum, Univ. of Miami	Coral Gables, Fla.
Nov. 4-Jan. 19, 1996	Taylor Museum, Colorado Springs Fine Arts Ctr.	Colorado
Jan. 31-April 1, 1996	Hofstra Univ. Museum	Hemstead, N.Y.
April 3-June 30, 1996	Art Museum of Western Virginia	Roanoke, Va.
July 1-Dec. 31, 1996 (ten.)	Historical Society of Western Penn.	Pittsburgh, Pa.

Matthew's Disciples

After the Civil War, two formerly enslaved men, Isaiah T. Montgomery and Benjamin Green, were able to convince officials of the Yazoo and Mississippi Valley Railroad Co. to deed 30,000 acres of their snake-infested, swamp-land over to them. The land was cleared, inhabited and grew to become the all-black city of Mound Bayou, in the heart of the Black Belt of the Mississippi Delta.

Within this community was established a benevolent social organization, the Knights of Tabor, with a history that extended back into the period of enslavement. Its principles were morality, temperance, freedom and Christianity. Stress was placed on self- reliance and maturity.

The Mississippi section of the Knights of Tabor, beginning near the end of the 19th century, started a medical insurance, prepayment plan to cover the medical and hospital fees of the neighboring, share-cropper subscribers. At its peak, the number of participants reached 40,000.

In the middle 1930s the plan's managers began to consider building a hospital to care for illnesses of the target subscribers. The group raised $100,000 from the funds of the Knights and Daughters of Tabor and built a hospital that opened in 1942. Subscribers to the Hospitalization Insurance Plan paid a small, regular membership fee and were guaranteed outpatient and 30 days of hospital care, which included medical care, drugs, surgery, X-rays and laboratory fees. This program was one of the earliest managed care plans in the nation.

Hospital income was supplemented by financial drives among the subscribers and by payments from the government for the care of non-registered patients. Although the medical needs of the African American community exceeded the medical facilities available, they were exceedingly better than they were before the hospital was built. Before that, the patients were forced to accept inadequate, segregated facilities in the often-crowded basements of hospitals in small, nearby Mississippi towns.

In quest of nursing and medical personnel to staff the hospital, a delegation of Knights and Daughters of Tabor visited Matthew Walker M.D., chief of surgery at Meharry Medical College, to seek his assistance in finding a competent medical staff. Too busy with faculty obligations to leave Meharry, Dr. Walker sent Dr. T.M. Howard, a Meharry graduate who was practicing in Nashville.

Dr. Howard went to Mound Bayou, but a rift developed between him and the Taborians. He was soon employed by a rival faction and began to practice under their auspices. The Taborians returned to Nashville and reopened their discussions with Meharry and Dr. Walker.

Although he was busier than ever, Dr. Walker, through Meharry, did provide surgical residents on a rotating basis sufficient to meet their needs. Thus began nearly 30 years of a symbiotic affiliation between the Taborian Hospital and the surgical department of Meharry Med. College.

During that period, all of Meharry's surgical residents, and many in the surgical specialties, rotated through the Taborian Hospital for some, if not all, of their surgical training. The affiliation agreement included medical residents and students as well, with Walker and his staff making regular visits, especially for the most critical operations. It is estimated that during the life of the Meharry-Taborian agreement, "Dr. Walker completed his duties at Meharry and drove down there at least 200 times."[1]

The relationship prospered and each resident spent at least 4-6 months at Taborian Hospital providing competent surgical care to many patients from the surrounding areas. At the same time, the Meharrians were exposed to a rural practice, unlike that seen in Nashville and other urban centers. Moreover, the experience prepared them for managed-care programs of the future.

The Taborian Pre-Payment Plan reimbursed Meharry for a portion of the services provided, but the major beneficiaries were the patients who received first-rate, respectable medical

256

care and their caring doctors who profited, unforgettably, from their training.

In 1958, Dr. Walker's surgical trainees formed the Matthew Walker Surgical Society "for the promulgation of his ideals and the advancement of surgical knowledge." My research of Dr. Walker and his protegees led me to the Matthew Walker, Special May 1979 issue of the *NMA Journal,* which names the 65 residents for whom Dr. Walker was primarily responsible.

The names of three of Detroit's most prominent surgeons, Drs. Waldo Cain, Garnet Ice and Hayward Maben were listed as members of the MWSS. Dr. Ice died before this book was begun, but Drs. Cain and Maben, easily recalled and readily agreed to talk about "their years spend at the feet of the master."

Dr. Cain was among the first group of surgical residents to become one of Matthew's Disciples and stayed on for additional time as "staff," at Mound Bayou. All three Detroit physicians were denied surgical residencies in their home town, but were welcomed by Dr. Walker to the facilities and experiences offered by Meharry Medical College.

Matthew's Disciples

My own memories of Dr. Walker from my student days at Meharry are not very distinctive. At that time, the idea of a career in surgery was not very high on the agenda of many African American physicians. Few, if any, had become certified as surgeons and the chances for doing so seemed remote in the early 1940s. Persistent rumors about Dr. Walker's surgical skill, his dogged discipline and humble humanity have not only persisted, but grown as his "disciples" carried his surgical gospel into the far corners.

Soon after I began to write this book, it became apparent that Dr. Walker had to be included. His name and image became increasingly interwoven with the fabric of the NMA, in general, and with that of Meharry Medical College, in particular.

After a long and productive surgical career, Dr. Walker retired in 1973, twenty-five years after taking the reins of the department from the unforgettable Dr. "Big" John

Hale in 1945, and was succeeded by Dr. Louis J. Bernard, one of his trainees.

Another grateful trainee was Dr. Dorothy Brown, chief surgeon at Riverside Hospital, a member of the surgical staff at Meharry and, a former member of the Tennessee state legislature. At his funeral, Brown recalled: "despite the protests of many of his colleagues, he trained me as the 'first black woman surgeon.' Dr. Walker had confidence in me, even when I could not get accepted anywhere else. One of the mandates of my professional career has been not to disappoint, nor let the chief down."

The 65 residents who received all, or nearly all, of their training under the supervision of Dr. Walker, began with Dr. Asa Yancey in 1948, and ended in 1978 with Dr. Jerry Word. An additional forty received a portion of their training under his supervision.

Dr. Yancey recalled that "Dr. Walker brought documented, accredited education in general surgery to Hubbard Hospital and Meharry."

Dr. Cobb, although editor emeritus at the time, returned to write: "Dr. Matthew Walker was born in Waterproof, La., on December 7, 1906. His father was a pullman porter and his mother worked as a domestic employee. His parents moved to New Orleans when he was small. He received the B.A. degree, with honors, at what is now Dillard University in 1929.

"Meharry Medical College awarded him the M.D. degree, with honors, in 1934. He served an internship the following year and entered into surgical pursuits for the remainder of his career. His wagon was already hitched to a star." Dr. Walker served as president of the NMA in 1954-1955. Five years later, the NMA presented him with its highest honor, the Distinguished Service Award, during the NMA's Detroit, convention in 1959."

The Influence of Dr. Matthew Walker on the Practice of Surgery in Detroit, Michigan

Aside from Dr. Walker's visit to Detroit in 1959 to receive the NMA's Distinguished Service Award, I found no other evidence that he had made any other visits to this region. Yet his influence was quite strong due to the presence and practices of three of his

Detroit disciples—Waldo Cain, Garnet Ice, and Hayward Maben. Their testimonies, in word and deed, to his competence and compassion, are essential to this Centenary Report.

Waldo Cain, M.D. (Meharry, 1945), had fond memories of "one of the world's great human beings."

"During my senior year in Meharry (1944), I was not sure what my primary medical interest was, nor where I should spend my internship. Applications were requested from St. Mary's and Receiving hospitals in my hometown, Detroit. I did not know that St. Mary's Hospital, which had opened in 1879, had never appointed an African American to its staff; and Receiving Hospital had appointed only two since it opened in 1915. Although my first desire was to return home, I did not get a response from either hospital. My interest in surgery did not begin until my internship, following my rotation through surgery. My initial goal was to become a gynecologist, but not an obstetrician. At that time, Dr. Walker had become chief of surgery, but he still controlled gynecology.

"Dr. Charles Drew, chief of surgery at Howard University, often served as visiting surgeon at Meharry during my rotating internship. I was accepted to both surgical residencies. Having had the opportunity to observe and work with both men, I chose Meharry and Matthew.

"Then, too, there was the rumor that in order to make it on Dr. Drew's service, a resident had to be 'light, bright, and damn near white.' So I went with Matthew, a decision I never regretted.

"There are so many facets to this discussion that it is a difficult subject to document. Matthew's influence created a sense of pride and responsibility, respect and fairness in all of us who were trained by him. For me, he was the most fair-minded, objective, and rigorous of task masters. He was awe-inspiring in his surgical abilities, and yet, the salt-of-the-earth type in his humanity. He taught by example as well as by exhortation.

"Whether or not it was intended, he gave us an immediate sense of pride in having been trained and educated in a black institution, and to emerge with the ability to compete with those from major institutions throughout the nation and globally.

"He left me with a feeling of responsibility to share with my colleagues, older and younger, what I had learned, and the medical responsibility to continue to learn and teach. He urged all of his residents to seek university affiliations, both for learning and teaching. Matthew taught and lived respect and opportunity for all people, without regard for gender, age or race.

"I was the first of his 65 trainees to practice in Detroit. I was in the first group, beginning in 1951, followed by Garnet Ice (1952) and Hayward Maben (1963). We have tried to transfer this sort of compassion to residents assigned to our services, in university hospitals and elsewhere.

"I am sure that Matthew did not ask me to perform his thyroidectomy because he thought I was his best product. I believe he chose me because he thought I was the only one, at that time, who had not been trained outside of Meharry. He wanted the world to know that his product, alone, was as good as those who had been trained elsewhere.

"The sense of responsibility that he imparted to me was a major factor in my serving as a receptor for Dr. Billy Kyle, surgeon, for two years in order for him to become eligible to take and pass his specialty board for surgery. Billy's successful completion of his board gave me a great personal satisfaction.

"Each of us—Cain, Ice, and Maben—at one time or another was chief of surgery in one of Detroit's smaller hospitals. I think that the standards we set as department heads changed greatly the prior practices in some of the minority hospitals. The caliber of surgery improved, and the incidence of unnecessary or 'exploratory' surgery declined.

"Our influence has not been limited solely to the black community; but all of us have participated in the formal training of residents in many of Detroit's major hospitals. We encounter former trainees at various scientific meetings who remind us of the valuable lessons learned, while on our services. These lessons were taught to us by Matthew Walker.

"When Garnet and I came to Detroit, Matthew Walker's influence was felt in the black hospitals whenever we exerted whatever persuasive pressures we could to curtail the practice of surgery being done on people who had an abdominal scar and abdominal pain, on the pretext that the scar caused the pain.

"There was also a common practice of operating on people with abdominal pain, who did not have a scar, with a diagnosis of 'chronic appendicitis.' I thing that Garnet and I had a great influence on curtailing and finally stopping that practice.

"I have never regretted the choice of Matthew Walker and Meharry as the sources of my surgical training."

Dr. Garnet Ice, like Dr. Cain, was trained in general surgery. Unlike Dr. Cain, Dr. Ice graduated from Detroit's Wayne Univ. Medical School in 1943, at a time when surgical residencies could not be had by African Americans in Detroit at any price. Fortunately for Dr. Ice, Dr. Walker offered him a helping hand as readily as he did the Meharry graduates.

Hayward Maben, M.D., thoracic surgeon. Maben's relationship with Walker began in the spring of 1949, as he was completing his first year of surgical training at Detroit's Receiving Hospital. He was looking for another site to complete his residency training for thoracic surgery because of racial harassment in Wayne Univ.'s program.

"I called Dr. Walker, explained my situation to him, and he agreed to accept me into his program at Meharry at a second-year level in July. Prior to calling Dr. Walker, I had a conference with Dr. Charles E. Johnston, chief of surgery at Wayne Univ. and Receiving Hospital, regarding my future status as a resident.

"I had been originally accepted into Wayne's surgical program by Dr. Nicholas Gimble, the assistant chief, while Dr. Johnston was on a sabbatical leave in Japan. During Dr. Johnson's absence, Dr. Gimble had accepted three African Americans into the program. When Dr. Johnson returned, he was quite upset that African Americans were being trained in his department and one had even become board certified.

"Dr. Johnson called me in for a conference and tried to get me to transfer into orthopedics or urology. I asked him if he was dissatisfied with my work. He admitted being satisfied with my work, but he thought that I would be unable to withstand the rigors of Wayne's surgical program. He suggested that if I'd go into one of the surgical specialties, I would do rather well as a leader in the black community.

"I told him that I was not interested in the specialties. He countered that he was not certain that his program could afford me at the second-year level because of the financial problems within the department.

"Then, I began to look around for other places to go. I talked to Dr. Ponka at Henry Ford Hospital by phone, explaining that I was looking for another place for my second year of surgical training. He told me, verbally, that there was an opening at Ford. When I submitted the application, Dr. Ponka called and apologized. He said that he was told that Ford Hospital's by-laws stated that African Americans could not serve on any clinical service at Ford Hospital. This was in the spring of 1959. He apologized and assured me that such a policy did not reflect his personal beliefs.

"Waldo (Cain) suggested that I call Dr. Matthew Walker, and he accepted me into a very good program at Meharry. When I reached the fourth-year level, Dr. Walker told me that he would like to send me to the Univ. of Arizona to study cardiac surgery. I declined, because I did not want to become obligated to return to Meharry. During my third year, I had decided not to return to Detroit to do general surgery, but to seek a more specialized service that offered patients a form of surgery not immediately available to them.

"Pediatric surgery seemed the way to go, but a residency could not be found throughout the country. Then I applied to various hospitals for thoracic surgical training. Hines Hospital in Illinois had a very good program.

"Dr. Walker had invited Dr. Charles B. Puestow, chief of thoracic surgery at Hines, to come to Meharry and give the Hale-McMillan lecture in the spring of 1963. He asked Dr. Walker if I would be a suitable person to be accepted into the Hines program. A few weeks later, I got a letter of acceptance in to the Hines program, beginning on July 1, with a six-month period to begin at Chicago's Presbyterian-St. Luke's Hospital in their cardiovascular departments.

"I later learned that Dr. Walker told Dr. Puestow that Meharry needed a cardiac surgeon and the Hines people expected me to return to Meharry to set up a department of thoracic surgery.

In the spring of 1965, when I was chief resident, I returned to Meharry and discussed the matter with Dr. Walker. Walker admitted telling Dr. Puestow that I would return to Meharry to increase the possibility of my getting the Hines appointment.

"He realized, however, that Meharry did not have the finances to afford a thoracic surgical department. I realized that Dr. Walker had gone out of his way to assist me. At that time, there had been only four certified African American thoracic surgeons in the entire country. When I took the board in the fall of 1965, I became the 5th, and the 6th was a doctor from Howard Univ. who was tested with me."

Several months later, Dr. Maben continued his inetrview:

"After finishing my training in thoracic and cardiovascular surgery in Chicago in 1965, I returned to Detroit, but did not immediately pursue hospital privileges. Aware of Detroit's racist climate, I didn't want to apply for privileges in major hospitals without having received my surgical board certification. So I spent the next few months preparing for my boards, which I passed in August 1965, twenty years after graduation.

"Applications were sent to nine different hospitals in the Detroit area: Harper, Grace, Hutzel, Sinai, Mt. Carmel, Highland Park General, Providence, St. Joseph Mercy, and Children's hospitals. My only favorable response came from Children's Hospital where I was given an appointment in their cardiovascular surgery department without any problems.

"However, I was warned by Children's Hospital's cardiac surgeon, who was doing most of the work there, that they would not refer any surgical cases to me if they could help it. I got no favorable responses from the other hospitals. My surgery was done at the Boulevard General and Burton Mercy

Hospitals in Detroit, and later at Outer Drive and Sumby Hospitals, downriver.

"In May 1966, during the DMS's annual 'Clinic Day,' while Dr. Josh Williams was the DMS president, reporters from the *Detroit Free Press* were present and wanted to know what was the purpose of the DMS and why was it necessary to have a black medical society because we had an effective Wayne County Medical Society.

"They were informed that the black physicians had problems that the Wayne County Medical Society was not addressing, including problems regarding hospital privileges. The reporters asked for examples of black doctors who could not receive adequate hospital facilities. My name was mentioned.

"I received calls from the *Free Press* and verified my earlier allegations. Subsequently, an article appeared in *The Detroit Free Press* and *Detroit News*, stating that a board-certified African American surgeon had been denied privileges at most of the major hospitals in this area. The matter received considerable, temporary publicity in the news media, but it was ignored by the Wayne County and Michigan State Medical Societies.

"It was shortly after this that I received a telephone call from HEW officials in Chicago, who expressed an interest in this problem and subsequently visited all the hospitals in the area that had denied me privileges to see if they were in violation of Medicare laws in Articles XVIII and XIX.

"Complaints were sent to the Michigan Civil Rights Commission and the WCMS to see if the society, with which I held membership, would intervene on my behalf. I was told by Elsie Kohelde, the long-time secretary of the WCMS, that "you must not 'rock the boat.'" I was told that HEW would conduct a federal survey of the discrimination problem, not only in my instance, but in other areas of hospital activity. This was done about the same time.

"Harper Hospital, in 1967, was the first major hospital to grant me surgical privileges. However, a year passed before I learned that my privileges did not include the use of the heart-lung machine. I spoke to Dr. Day, chief of thoracic surgery at Harper and he denied knowing anything about the discrimination.

"He had assumed that all of my privileges which I requested were based upon my training and would be granted. Upon finding that such was not the case, he washed his hands of the matter. However, I subsequently learned that the chief of surgery, Dr. William Carpenter, had arbitrarily denied my privileges without having informed me. I did not learn of this problem until I attempted to board a patient for a procedure involving the heart-lung machine and was denied privileges.

"A subsequent inquiry was made and I was told that I would have to have someone who did have privileges govern me. The interesting thing was that there were doctors at that time who were given privileges to use the heart-lung machine at Harper Hospital who had not received any specific training in this area, but who were given privileges because they, as I, were board-certified in thoracic surgery. The quality of cardiac surgery being done at Harper Hospital at that time, in my opinion, was very poor; unqualified people were then performing open-heart surgery.

"Thus, the privilege to use the heart-lung machine was denied without having someone scrub with me. I was also told that the reason for this is not that I did not receive adequate training, but it was because there were no black cardiologists to refer patients to me. They didn't want to have someone doing occasional open heart surgery at Harper Hospital.

"When HEW investigators contracted me regarding this problem, I was told that they had investigated all of the hospitals in the area and were assured by all that they had all of the thoracic surgeons that they needed. They assured HEW that if any new thoracic surgeons were added to the staff, I would receive consideration. However, nothing really happened.

"Two years later, I became a staff member at Highland Park General Hospital mainly through the pressure from the black activist organization there at the Highland Park Caucus Club, which exerted pressure on Highland Park officials to have me granted privileges at that institution.

"In order to be in compliance with HEW's dictates, Sinai Hospital offered me privileges, four years later, but denied me use of the heart-lung machine. When asked the reason for denial of these privileges, the chief of surgery stated that it was, again, the question of race. Since there weren't any black cardiologists to refer patients to me I was unlikely to get any referrals from white cardiologists in this area.

"In the early 1970s, I was able to get on the staff of Grace Hospital, only after making it known to members of the board of trustees there that I was going to institute a suit against the hospital. Once this was known, I had no problems gaining staff privileges at Grace Hospital.

"In 1981, I received a call from the local head of the Civil Rights Division of the Justice Department wanting to know if I were willing to sue Harper Hospital in regard to open heart privileges, And, if I did so, they would be glad to act as a 'friend of the court' on my behalf.

"The local head of the Civil Rights Division stated that if John Feemster, Detroit's other certified African American thoracic surgeon, and I were willing to sue the hospital, he would play an active role. However, I did not pursue this course of action since several attorneys were unwilling to take the case on a contingency basis. Moreover, if I were to win the case, it would obviously be necessary after having been out of cardiac surgery for 15 years to seek further surgical training. So I elected not to pursue the matter any further.

"That, in summary, is a brief of my professional status with the hospitals in this area. I subsequently did get on the staff of Providence Hospital. Dr. Remus Robinson used his personal influence to gain surgical privileges for me at Providence Hospital in 1970.

"I confirmed that Ford Hospital did have a staff by-law that prohibited hospital appointments to African Americans until the 1960s. When the Ford Hospital administration needed more land for the expansion of their current site, city officials forced them to do what the Medical Center was forced to do—integrate! This was done grudgingly and without any significant support from the medical establishment."

266

The net result of Walker's influence on surgical practice in the nation has been, to say the least, awesome. Only three of his 68 full-time disciples, and none of the 31 part-time trainees, practiced in Detroit. All of them completed their surgical training between 1948 and 1978.

Even if the Detroit experience is only a partial reflexion of Dr. Walker's surgical legacy, it provides us all with a model of what one man can do, if properly motivated. It is also a story that must be told, preferably by someone who was there.

There must be several physicians, among the many Matthew's Disciples still around, who are capable of undertaking this interesting project. Certainly, Matthew must be our most illustrious alumnus. A well-researched, interesting story about him could, if properly managed, become a bestseller that could improve Meharry's cash position enormously.

1. James Somerville, *Educating Black Doctors*. (Birmingham: Univ. of Alabama Press, 1983) p. 124.

   Meharry also continued to reach out to the impoverished people in Mississippi. Two dozen surgical and obstetrical students were sent annually to Taborian Hospital. "In the first 20 years of the affiliation agreement, Dr. Walker, himself, made the trip between Nashville and Mound Bayou more than 200 times."

Matthew Walker, Sr., Surgical Residents (1948-1978)		
1948	Asa Yancey	Atlanta
1949	Edward Bennett	
1950	George Hilliard	
1951	Waldo Cain	Detroit
1952	Frank Perry	Nashville
1953	Charles Brown	Los Angeles
1954	John Jackson	Lakeland
1955	Dorothy Brown	Nashville
1956	Webster Brown	Portland
1957	Junius Cromartie	Dayton
1958	Louis Bernard	Nashville
1959	John Blasingame	Atlanta
1960	Nehemiah Cooper	Monrovia

1961	Edward Brown	Nashville
1962	Warner Meadows	Atlanta
1963	Allen Harvey	Winston-Salem
1964	William Andrews	Tampa
1965	Charles Brown	Nashville
1966	Robert Harris	Houston
1967	Thomas Turner	Los Angeles
1968	George Bugg	Los Angeles
1969	Clinton Battle	Clarksdale
1970	Avery Parnell	Houston
1971	Yerng Terng Hseuh	Nashville
1972	Wendell Blake	Lakeland
1973	Ira Thompson	Nashville
1974	James McGriff	Nashville
1975	Kosit Priebrjrivat	Belleville, Ill.
1976	William Garrett	Fort Worth
1977	Will Feston	Seymour Johnson AFB, NC
1978	Frank McCune	Jackson, MS

Surgeons who received a portion of their training from Matthew Walker, Sr. (1948-1978):

Walton Belle, Richmond; Joseph BoBo; Earl Cullins, Jacksonville; Kenwars Dadmarz, Teheran; Richard Ewing; Mallippa Gowda, Fayetteville; Andree-elen Gunther, Nashville; Yong Ho Parks, Elbin, NC; Garnet Ice; Fred Jackson; Todd James, Natchez; Wesley King, Los Angeles; Phillip Lavizzo; Fritz Lemoine, Clarksville; Hayward Maben, Detroit; James McCleod, Dothan; William Moses, Louisville; Pakala Nithyananda, Nashville; Julius Pryor, Montgomery; Milton Quigless, Raleigh; Edward Reed, Memphis; Fred Robey, Houston; Adebayo Samuels, Brooklyn; Edgar Scott, Chattanooga; George Simpson, Miami; Robert Smith, Pine Bluff; Cyril Spann, Columbia; Seri Thitathan, Alexandria; Danny Thomas, Tacoma; David Todd, Nashville; Edward Verner, Newark; Charlotte Walker, Nashville; Charles Wiggins, Nashville; Jerry Word, Nashville.

African American Firsts in Medicine, in Michigan

Physicians who have blazed trails into the hostile territory of medicine have been as creative and as courageous, if not more so, as any other pioneers. Despite the illusion of white supremacy and the constancy of racial bias, the men and women of this group have been provoked, but not deterred, in their quest for the best of their profession.

We pause to herald their achievements, realizing that this society too often only sees us as victims rather than victors. Their experiences are unique and can warn us of dangers to be avoided, friends to be cultivated, and diversions to be ignored. Read carefully, the experiences of some of Michigan's African American physicians who had the courage to be first.

With no claim for accuracy or completeness, I offer this list as a small sample of what is available to the diligent student, nuggets in a minefield of ignored achievements that are awaiting your further exploration.

Allergy-Immunology

Marva Jenkins Morris, M.D. (Meharry, 1965), was certified in allergy and immunology in 1987. At the outset, this residency was closely associated with pediatrics and did not provide sufficient training for A-I certification. Candidates were accepted under a "grandfather clause" that summed up the total of their experiences to reach the level of qualification required for specialization.

Fellowships that were established primarily at pediatric hospitals have blossomed into full residencies that now provide adequate specialty training. While Dr. Morris is still Detroit's only certified African American allergy-immunologist; there are two others in the region.

Anesthesia

Willard Holt, M.D. (Meharry, 1962), was the first African American in Detroit to be certified in anesthesia (1968). He is the director of respiratory care at Riverview Hospital. Because of his publications on pulmonary care, Dr. Holt was admitted to the American College of Chest Physicians in 1969.

He was the first medical director for the School of Nursing Anesthesia at Mount Carmel Hospital; and, was president of Mount Carmel's medical staff from 1972-1974. The first African American to be asked to serve as an examiner for the American Board of Anesthesia, Dr. Holt did so for two years. From 1967-1978, he also served as an examiner for the American Board of Respiratory Therapists.

Dermatology

Robert Heidelberg, M.D. (Howard, 1965) cert. dermatology, 1972. Clinical asst. prof. Wayne Staff Univ., Grace and Children's hospitals).

Emergency Medicine

Emanuel Rivers, M.D. (Univ. of Mich., 1981; M.P.H., 1981; cert. emergency medicine, 1987; inter. med., 1986; critical care med., 1991). He is on emergency medicine staff of Henry Ford Hospital.

Family Medicine

Amos Taylor, M.D. (Howard, 1960; cert. family practice, 1973-1993 and regularly renews his certification every seven years, as required). Staff physician at Grace and Sinai hospitals. He is also certified for capitation and quality assurance review.

Internal Medicine

Allison B. Henderson, M.D. (Meharry, 1937; cert. int. med. 1945), was the first African American to be certified in internal medicine in Detroit. Like all other early African American medical specialists, he was forced to seek his specialty training outside Detroit. He served a rotating internship and a residency in pathology at Cleveland's City Hospital in Ohio. Following

270

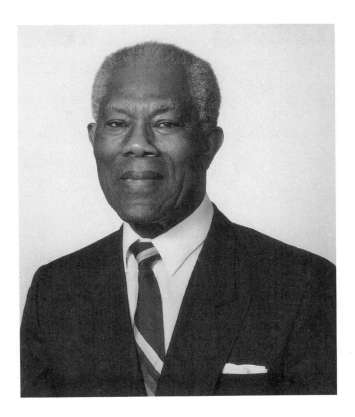

Lionel F. Swan, M.D., Detroit's first NMA president, 1967.

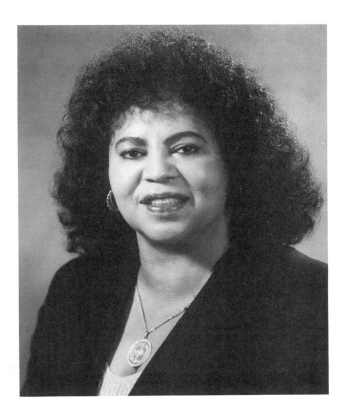

Alma Rose George, M.D., was Detroit's second NMA president, and the NMA's third female president in 1991.

Lonnie Bristow, M.D., NYU, 1957; cert. int. med. His rise to power, in AMA began in 1987, as Altern. Del. and continued through Hse of Del. and Bd of Trustees to the presidency of AMA in 1995.

Tracy Walton, M.D., became president-elect of the NMA in 1994, and will preside during the Centenary Session in Atlanta, 1995.

Ambassador Andrew Young, former mayor of Atlanta, invites them to his home town.

William Anderson, D.O., was elected president of the American Osteopathic Association in 1994. The event was heralded by the establishment of a $25,000 fund in his honor.

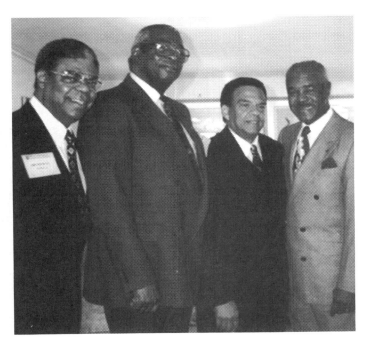

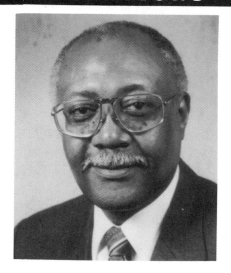

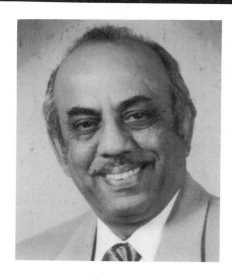

James W. Patton
President
and Chief Operating Officer

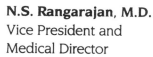

James W. Patton
President and CEO

N.S. Rangarajan, M.D.
Vice President and
Medical Director

THE WELLNESS PLAN

Comprehensive Health Services, Inc.
6500 John C. Lodge, Detroit, Michigan 48202
(313) 875-4200, Ext. 5212, Fax: (313) 875-5366

Presiding officers of The Wellness Plan, Detroit's first Health Maintenance Organization.

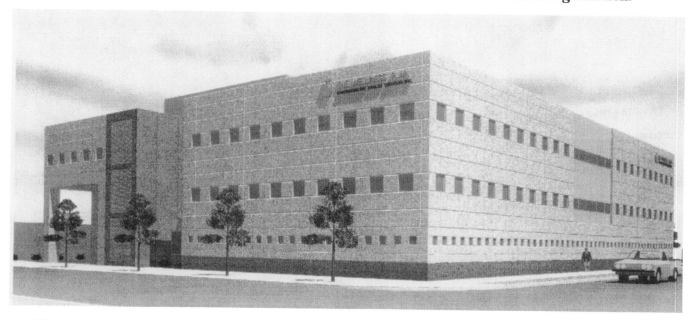

The most recent addition to The Wellness Plan is this $7.5 million medical center at West Grand Boulevard and the Lodge expressway. It is scheduled for occupancy during the summer of 1995.

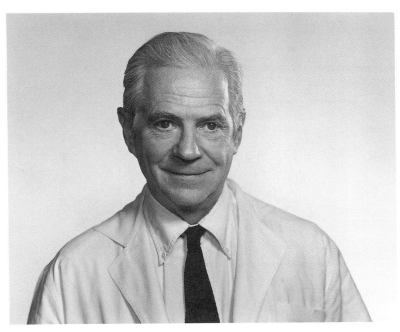

Charles Stevenson, M.D., Johns Hopkins, 1934; cert. obg., 1941; professor of obg. at Wayne State University, 1948-1972; chr dept. for 15 years. He appointed Addison Prince the first African American to serve an obg. residency in Michigan in 1951.

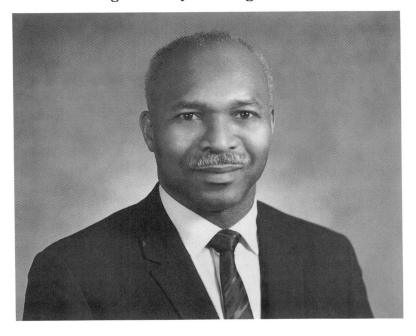

Addison Prince, M.D., Wayne, 1944, was the first African American to be given a residency in obg. in the state of Michigan, in 1951 by Dr. Charles Stevenson, during the early part of his tour as director of the department of obg. After successfully completing his residency in 1954 and passing the certifying board as a specialist in 1958, Dr. Prince was able to realize his potential as a physician and a man by: (1) earning a M.P.H. degree from the Univ. of Michigan in 1974; (2) serving as consultant to the Prescad program, 1972-1976, (3) being appointed to the Governor's Commission to Review and Revise the Public Health Code, 1978, and (4) accepting a position on the Michigan Board of Health, 1978-1986.

The Wellness Plan - 20 Year Performance
Members/ Revenue/ Net Income/ Hospitalization

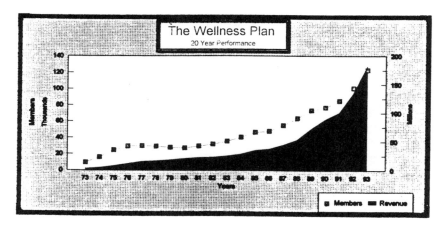

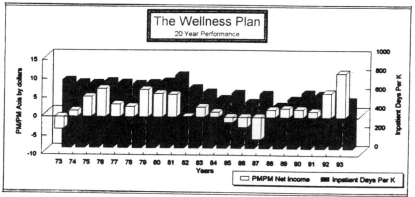

Growth curve performance review for The Wellness Plan during its first 20 years, 1953-1973.

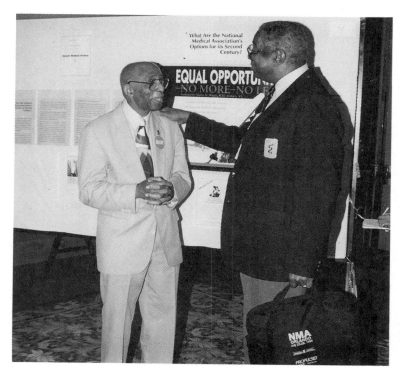

Tracy Walton, M.D., as NMA's president-elect (1994), visited the book display of Charles H. Wright, M.D., during the 1994 NMA Convention in Orlando, Fla.

further post-graduate training at Detroit's Trinity Hospital, Dr. Henderson was inducted in the U.S. Army.

His prior academic training earned him an army rank of "clinical pathologist," which enabled him to do research in malaria in Liberia, and sickle cell disease at the Tuskegee Army Air Force Base in Alabama. From this research flowed many papers on a wide variety medical subjects into national and international journals and lectureships at many medical centers.

In 1969, Dr. Henderson's DMS colleagues chose him as the Physician of the Year. In 1972, he became the first and only Michigan physician to win the NMA's Distinguished Service Award for his pioneering research in tropical diseases and aerospace medicine. As owner-director of Dexter Laboratories, Henderson served his colleagues and patients well with the latest in diagnostic tests and clinical studies, until his death in 1978.

Marjorie Peebles Meyers, M.D. (Wayne Univ., 1943), was the first African American woman to graduate from Wayne's Medical School. After an internship at Receiving Hospital, she was chosen to and became the first African American resident in internal medicine in 1944. In practice, she was a member of the area's first interracial medical practice group with Drs. A.B Henderson and Eugene Schafferman.

Unlike her European American classmates, who were readily given unfettered hospital appointments immediately after their residency training, Dr. Meyers' patients were admitted to Woman's (Hutzel) Hospital, indirectly, under the names of two European American colleagues, Drs. Schafferman and Nathaniel Brooks, until she passed the first part of her medical specialty board in 1949. She became a fully-certified internist in 1950.

Dr. Meyers recalled "only after passing the first part of the specialty board did Mr. Lichtwardt (Woman's Hospital administrator) pull out my staff application and make me a 'junior attending.' Meanwhile, all of my white classmates had been readily accepted for appointment to the full staff and granted direct admissions privileges immediately after their residencies."

Lawrence Lackey, Sr., M.D. (Kansas, 1952), although a board eligible internist, chose to blaze his trail as a geriatricist in the southwestern suburbs of Detroit. Over the years, his practice increasingly reflected his affinity for and interest in the elderly.

With the assistance of hospital officials, a department of geriatrics was established at Sumby Hospital and operated by Dr. Lackey and the medical staff. Dr. Lawrence Lackey, Jr. informed me that although there was no specialty board for geriatrics at that time, his father had been "grandfathered" into various organizations that served the same purpose.

Obstetrics Gynecology

All of the medical specialties were difficult to achieve for Michigan's African American physicians, but none encountered quite the levels of racial rejection and hostility as did obg. As early as 1930, the Michigan State Medical Society expressed some awareness of the "peculiar amenability of improved maternal and infant morbidity and mortality rates to improved public health practices. Education, sanitation, and control of milk supplies are promptly reflected in the lives of young children."[1]

Despite this admitted awareness, neither the Michigan State nor the Wayne County Medical Soc. did anything to increase the pool of African American physicians (obstetricians-gynecologists and pediatricians) who were especially trained to carry out those measures that would be "immediately reflected in the lives of young, African American children."

Even those African Americans who were born in Michigan and attended Michigan's colleges were not readily acceptable in Michigan's medical schools. Early on, residencies were not available in Michigan for African Americans at any price, especially in obg.

The first African American to be certified in obg. in Michigan was **Lewis F. Boddie**, M.D. (Meharry, 1938). Following a residency in St. Louis, he was cert. obg., 1949. After nearly five years of practice in Detroit, Dr. Boddie found a more favorable climate in Los Angeles. He is now retired and doing rather well in the "City of Angels."

For the next nine years following Dr. Boddie's certification, all of Michigan's certified, African American obg. specialists were forced to seek their training outside the state. Even after an adequate training and board certification as a specialist, he or she was never sure of a staff appointment. They often had to run the gauntlet of a staff of biased European American physicians and/or a complacent board of trustees.

This list of other obg. residents trained outside Michigan included, but may not be limited to:

1. **William Goins**, M.D. (Wayne Univ., 1941)—Although a graduate of the Detroit school system, including medical school, he was not accepted as an intern or resident in Detroit's hospital community. He served an internship and an obg. residency at Homer G. Phillips Hospital in St. Louis, Mo., and was cert. in 1950.

2. **Arthur D. Harris**, M.D. (Wayne Univ., 1946)—He served an obg. residency at Homer G. Phillips Hosp. and was cert. 1952. He practiced in Detroit.

3. **Charles H. Wright**, M.D. (Meharry 1943)—was unable to get a residency in obg. and did general practice (1946-1950) before closing his Detroit office and returning to Harlem Hospital (N.Y.) for an obg. residency. He was admitted to Woman's Hospital in 1953 to practice ob-gyn. and was certified in 1955.

4. **Ethelene Crockett**, M.D. (Howard, 1945). After three years of general practice, she closed her office and served residencies at Sydenham (N.Y.) and a third year at Herman Kiefer Hospital. She was cert., 1955. Dr. Crockett preceded me in closing her general practice office and seeking an available residency elsewhere. New York's Sydenham Hospital could offer her only two of the required three years of training. By the third year, Dr. Charles Stevenson was chair of the obg. dept. at Wayne Univ. and she was able to complete her residency and

273

qualify for the certifying board examination, which she took and passed in 1955.

5. The selection of **Charles Summers Stevenson**, M.D. (Johns Hopkins, 1934; cert. obg. 1941), as professor and chairman of the dept. of obg. at Wayne Univ. (1948-1972) came, like "a bolt out of the blue" and challenged the 100 years of pervasive racism that was prevalent throughout Detroit's medical establishment prior to his appointment.

Dr. Stevenson faced a stubborn, deeply-rooted brand of racial bigotry when he began during his 24-year tour in 1948. By this time, only Dr. Boddie, among Detroit's African American physicians, had satisfied training requirements, for obg. specialization.

In 1951, when **Dr. Addison Prince** applied to Wayne Univ. to become Detroit's first African American obg. resident, he had been out of medical school for seven years; three of which (1943-1946) were spent in the Army Medical Corps. His 14-year journey from medical school graduation in 1944, to board certification in 1958, included a variety of other, unstructured medical programs that were not required of his European American classmates. Some of these appointments were salaried; others were not. Some appointments were in Detroit and others were not.

After his residency at Wayne Univ. and board certification, he was able to serve the community in many ways: M.P.H. Univ. of Mich., School of Public Health, 1974; consultant to the Prescad Program 1974-1976; appointed to the Governor's Commission to Review and Revise the Public Health Code. 1976-1978; member Michigan Board of Medicine, 1978-1986.

While considering the format for this book, my thoughts went back to my own residency in New York when Branch Rickey, manager of the Brooklyn Dodgers and Jackie Robinson (with Rickey's help) broke through the color barrier of major league baseball. Despite the snubs and insults to Rickey and the racist attacks on Robinson, those men remained steadfast and won a battle for racial justice. Suddenly, it occurred to me that Drs. Stevenson and Prince had much in common with Rickey and Robinson.

My only request to Dr. Stevenson, now retired in New Hampshire, for information about Dr. Prince, went unanswered for nearly a year. Early in 1994, however, the following message and a personal letter[2] flew over my transom:

"The appointment of Dr. Addison Prince as an assistant in the residency training program of the department of obstetrics and gynecology at Detroit's Wayne State Univ. Medical School was one of the most satisfying things I was able to accomplish in my 24 years as professor and 15 years as chairman of that department.

"Dr. Prince was a rotating intern at Detroit Receiving Hospital in the year of 1951-52 and he had interested Dr. Charles G. Johnson, professor and chairman of the department of surgery, there, to work out a special rotation for his 12 months as an intern. This program was to include more than the usual three months of general surgery, because Dr. Prince thought that eventually, he wanted to become a general surgeon. He also persuaded Dr. Johnson to arrange for three months in the department of obstetrics and gynecology, because he also thought he might like to consider some training in this dual specialty for his life's work, rather than straight general surgery.

"Dr. Johnson spoke to me about Dr. Prince in late December 1950, stating that Prince was doing very careful and reliable work on the surgical service and that he believed I would find him a satisfactory intern when he rotated to the gynecology service the coming January 1st (1951).

"During the first week of January, I encountered Dr. Prince at our Friday Afternoon Grand Rounds and Patient Examining Clinic. There, Dr. Prince, when it was his time to present a patient, related the history, physical and laboratory findings on the patient he was presenting. It was the best verbal report by the interns all afternoon. I noted the care with which he spoke and the clear thinking that was evidenced as he, step-by-step, reviewed the differential diagnosis of the case, as he perceived and judged it. Also, the way he stood by the woman as she lay on the examining table and spoke gentle and reassuring words to her while I

275

did the abdominal and vaginal examinations, was a fine example of a concerned physician.

"Later in the month, I had the occasion to instruct him in performing the minor surgical operation, the dilatation and curettage; and during this process he showed a good knowledge of the pelvic anatomy and properly determined the size, mobility and position of the uterus. I was well impressed with him as a person and by his apparent potential for becoming a good gynecologist.

"In September 1951, Dr. Prince called my office and asked if he could come and speak to me. I saw him right away that afternoon. He said he would like to apply for a position as junior resident in the training program of the department of obstetrics and gynecology at Herman Kiefer and Detroit Receiving hospitals, starting the next July (1952). Right on the spot, I told him I would give him the job he was requesting. He smiled, broadly, and said nothing for a few seconds, and then, in a soft and restrained voice, he spoke two words—thank you.

"He didn't need to speak any more; he was radiating his happiness. I instructed him to pick up an application blank at the Gynecology Service Nursing Office, fill it out and leave it for me. This he did the following day.

"Addison reported for duty at 7 a.m. on July 1st and was eager to get to work. Having already spent three months on the service as an intern, he 'knew the ropes' and helped to indoctrinate the other, new residents.

"He developed right along with the first-year resident group, did his work with great thoroughness and showed his traits of thoughtfulness and serious consideration in all the patient care matters that came up for his decisions and handling. He appeared to have more maturity than the other residents, in his class and was more reserved and courteous, in general, than they were. He served as a stabilizing force in the group; and a head nurse once referred to him as 'a wise old man.'

"The patients loved him. He was just as gentle and thoughtful to the unschooled, poor, black woman, newly arrived in Detroit with several children from Mississippi whose husband came seeking a job, as he was to a poor, white, native Detroit woman.

"He set an example for the medical students and other residents for the proper, respectful and gentle handling of women patients. Once a nurse had placed a woman on the examining table in the pelvic examination teaching clinic; and Addison was the presenter and attending staff physician. He would not approach the patient to do a pelvic examination until she had been properly and thoroughly draped to his satisfaction. He always showed respect for a woman's natural modesty.

"In the out-patient clinic, Addison patiently wrote down the brief 'history' note, pelvic examination findings, his diagnosis and what prescription, if any, he gave to the patient. He also carefully described to her just what treatment measures she should take for herself. He did all of this before going on to the next case. Although he did this methodically, he did it as rapidly as possible; because we had to 'put through' the clinic 70-80 patients on most mornings, between 8 a.m. and 2 p.m., with only two residents and two interns doing the entire job, and with the supervision of one member of the visiting staff.

"The attending gynecologist had to examine and review difficult-to-diagnose patients with the resident and medical students. Several of our visiting staff men remarked to me that when Addison had examined a patient and written out his note on her record, they could trust his findings and treatment with complete confidence.

"In the operating room, Addison worked very carefully and accurately in all of his dissections; and, after I had scrubbed with him through the 10 or 12 most common major operative procedures on the gynecological list, I conceded he had the necessary talent and would surely go on and develop into a good surgeon. He also fell in with my insistence that he keep the field dry and never close the abdomen until the operative site was absolutely dry.

When he completed the 3-year training program, I felt that he had readily learned all that we tried to teach our residents before we sent them out in the world of private practice or teaching.

"Addison succeeded well in practice, just as we all expected. His patients loved and trusted him completely. He

277

was able to instill confidence and trust in his patients, almost without speaking more than a few words, which was right in line with his taciturn make-up.

"His great wife was a wonderful teammate for him and she stood by him and aided him in every way a good wife can. The wife of one of his good friends once said to me 'they are two of a kind, completely devoted to each other and, obviously enjoy going through each day together.'

"After graduation from the program, Addison volunteered to do assigned teaching in the obg. department's student teaching program. He practically never failed to show up and was punctual for all the teacher's meetings to which he was assigned. He had a very orderly mind and went carefully through all the didactic parts of the syllabus to which he was assigned.

"He always asked for questions and patiently answered them the best he could. He read all the journals carefully that came to the department and to which he subscribed. When he took the written exam for the American Board of Obstetrics and Gynecology, he found that he was well-prepared for it. He went through it and the subsequent oral exams the next year successfully.

"He was among the first 'blacks' to gain this diploma in our country, which gave me real satisfaction as I know it did for him and his wife.

"I never heard a white woman complain that she did not want Dr. Prince to examine her because of the color of his skin. This certainly was because of his gentlemanly manners, demeanor and his very respectful approach.

"It was truly sad when I heard of Addison's tragic drowning when thrown from a native canoe in the very turbulent surf off the north coast of Timor in the Indonesia area. But, at the same time, I realized that this round-the-world trip for his wife and himself was the realization of a long-held dream and it symbolized the great success that he and she had made of his professional and their personal lives together. It was a great celebration of it for both of them. Addison will be greatly missed by his family, his colleagues and, especially, his patients."

Dr. Prince's immediate African American successors in the Wayne program—Drs. James Robinson, Ed Turner, and Ed Nash—were also beneficiaries of the Stevenson influence. Only 11 years were required for Drs. Turner and Nash in 1966; nine years for Drs. Julius Combs and Charles Vincent, two years later, to achieve board certification after graduation.

Dr. Stevenson's courage and generosity are so highly appreciated that he was asked, and he agreed to tell me in his own words, about this significant event. Dr. Stevenson's years at Wayne State Univ. will always be remembered by Michigan's African Americans. They began just before Prince's 1951 appointment and continued until his departure in 1972.

By that time, the racist traditions of the past were deeply disturbed and the doors of opportunity, although far from ajar, were no longer sealed. We owe a debt of gratitude to our great benefactor, Dr. Charles Stevenson.[3]

Ophthalmology

The first of Detroit's African American physician to limit his practice to a specialty was **Lloyd Bailer**, M.D. (Northwestern). I am not sure if or when he received specialty training. From the outset, he limited his practice to Eye/Ear/Nose and Throat, especially the eye.

His wife was converted to Christian Science and, in deference to her, he eventually abandoned the practice of medicine altogether. He first tried his hand at real estate and when that proved unprofitable, he began to work for the Ford Motor Co. as an assemblymen. He was soon transferred to the plant's chemical section where they made glass, rubber and steel.

Sometime later, Dr. Bailer left Ford's assembly plant and began to work as an oculist at a downtown optometry shop near Hudson's department store.

George W. Morrison, M.D., a Barbadian, graduated from Canada's Dalhousie Univ. in 1921, and blazed the ophthalmology trail in Detroit. He was certified in 1956 and became the staff ophthalmologist, first at St. Joseph's Mercy Hospital and later, the chief of ophthalmology at Burton Mercy Hospital.

Orthopedics

John McCollough, M.D. (Univ. of Mich., 1970), became Detroit's first African American certified orthopedist.

Otolaryngology

Burton Phillips, M.D. (Meharry, 1944., cert. otolaryngology 1951). He began his three-year residency in EENT at Homer G. Phillips Hospital in 1945 and did post-graduate study in otolaryngology at the Univ. of Wash.-Seattle in 1948-1949. He began a private practice in Detroit that, at that time, included ophthalmology. He was on the staffs of Burton Mercy, Grace, Providence and Receiving hospitals.

Pathology

John Burton, M.D. (Meharry, 1941), was certified as Detroit's first forensic, African American pathologist in 1955. He served as Wayne County pathologist in Eloise, Mich. and instructor in pathology at the VA Hospital in Allen Park, Mich. (1952-1955).

Pediatrics

Natalia Tanner Cain, M.D. (Meharry, 1945), became Detroit's first certified African American pediatrician in 1951. Her pediatric career began with a year's residency at the Univ. of Chicago in 1946. Despite their entreaties to stay longer, she returned to her alma mater and completed her residency at Meharry's Hubbard Hospital.

Dr. Tanner returned to the Univ. of Chicago in 1950 to serve a pediatric fellowship. In 1951, she passed the American Board of Pediatrics, the first African American in Michigan to do so. She did the same in the Academy of Pediatrics that same year in 1951.

In 1952, she entered private practice in Detroit, with an affiliation at Children's Hospital of Michigan, beginning in 1953. Her highest aspiration was to continue a professional pediatric career she had successfully launched at Meharry Medical College and the University of Chicago.

Although she was a board certified pediatrician and a fellow of the American Academy of Pediatrics prior to coming to Detroit,

280

Dr. Tanner's rejection by her Detroit colleagues because of her race and sex, was a true reflexion of the era:

"I came to Detroit in 1952 with aspirations of continuing my previously established professional career. These aspirations were quickly thwarted by obstacles of gender and race, when I elected to establish a private practice with a special interest in adolescent medicine.

"Children's Hospital, in 1951, still had segregated wards for black 'clinic' children and white 'private' patients. No black resident had ever received pediatric, residency training at Children's Hospital.

"I was told that there was no money for a faculty position, even though my credentials, qualifications and recommendations were unquestioned and came from some of the most powerful leaders in pediatrics, nationally and internationally.

"As a recourse, after my former chief from the University of Chicago called the power-that-be, at Children's Hospital of Michigan, I was offered a fellowship in pathology and hematology, a consolation position. The Detroit Pediatric Society accepted my application for membership in 1951, but no acknowledgement was made of it by the society. After nine months, I was informed that the application had been misplaced and to reapply. I did and was made a member in 1952.

"The Michigan Chapter of the American Academy of Pediatricians ignored my presence at the first meeting in 1952, even though I was a full fellow transferring from the Illinois Chapter. I acknowledged my presence to the chair. From 1983 to 1986, I was elected as the first female and black person to serve as their president.

"After 10 years in Detroit and as a staff member of Children's Hospital of Michigan, the chairman of the department of pediatrics at Wayne State Univ. recognized my talents and teaching ability and saw fit to appoint me as a clinical instructor. I then rose through the ranks and in 1992, was elected to full, clinical professorship, 39 years after joining the staff.

"All of these experiences have left a bitter imprint of racism and gender discrimination which I will never overcome, but these experiences have contributed to my being a stronger individual, able to deal with all the issues."

Arthur Thompson, M.D. (Meharry, 1942) cert. ped. 1956, was the first African American medical officer in the U.S. Navy (1943) and the first African American resident at Detroit's Children's Hospital in 1952. The U.S. had just entered World War 2, but had not yet completed its special arrangements for an expanded segregated, military fighting force.

Dr. Thompson completed an internship and the first year of a pediatric residency before volunteering for the Army Medical Corps in 1944. Just before induction, he learned that the Navy was accepting African American medical officers for the first time. He withdrew his application for army training and was accepted as the Navy's first African American medical officer. This apparent change in the Navy's policy of racial segregation was neither voluntary nor real.

During a White House conference in October 1941, just before Dr. Thompson's graduation, Secretary of the Navy Frank Knox had reaffirmed his official, naval policy: "Negroes would be recruited only in the messman's branch."[4]

During the Japanese attack on Pearl Harbor on December 7, 1941, two months later, Third Class Messman, Dorie Miller, aboard the Battleship Arizona, raced up on deck from his mess hall station, seized the machine gun of a disabled European American and became a man, for a moment.

With everyone else incapable of ordering him back down into his quarters below deck and, despite his lack of training for the job at hand, Messman Miller, in a flash, was transformed into Machine Gunner Miller. Although Dorie claimed six Japanese Zeroes that Sunday morning, the navy brass decided to reduce the figure to four. It was difficult for them to defend their claim of "white supremacy" when Dorie was the first and apparently, the only American hero, at Pearl Harbor.

Messman Miller's bravery, and the awarding of his Navy Cross, fueled a nationwide tide of protests against the Navy's policy of racial segregation that forced Navy Secretary Knox to sing a different tune on April 7, 1942, exactly four months later: "Negro volunteers, henceforth, will be accepted for general services as well as for mess attendants."

So it was under the "Dorie Miller Dispensation" that Lt. Arthur Thompson helped to end the Navy's policy of racial discrimination, while its policy of racial segregation remained intact. Lt. Thompson, among many other things, was denied service in the Officers' Club at the Great Lakes Training Station and other naval installations wherever he served.

On May 7, 1942, Fleet Admiral Chester Nimitz awarded Dorie Miller the Navy Cross "for distinguished devotion to duty, extraordinary courage and disregard for his own personal safety."

Despite the meaningless praise by Fleet Admiral Nimitz, Secretary of the Navy Knox and President of the USA, Franklin Delano Roosevelt, Dorie Miller's fortunes did not change. The Japanese finally settled their score with him on November 25, 1944, nearly two years after earning the Navy Cross at Pearl Harbor. Miller went down with his new, torpedoed ship—the Liscomb Bay—still a messman.[5]

Lt. Thompson J.G. was assigned only to African American units upon being inducted into the U.S. Navy. One of his camps was the "Robert Small," in honor of the enslaved South Carolinian who stole a Confederate ship and delivered it to the Union forces during the Civil War.

When Dr. Thompson was invited to attend "a wetting down party,"[6] a medical admiral advised him against "making waves." He didn't attend. Later on, his superior medical officer ordered Lt. Thompson's unit to deny that a flu epidemic was then sweeping the base in Oahu. When Lt. Thompson supported the statement that there was indeed an epidemic, the Admiral ordered him to Guam, charged with the "inability to control his men."

The Navy was still segregated when the war ended and Thompson resigned his commission. Since his prior pediatric training had not been sufficient to qualify him as a pediatrician and a pediatric residency was not available to African Americans, even if they had just returned from combat duty overseas, Dr. Thompson became a general practitioner for nearly six years.

In the meantime, he was allowed to volunteer his medical service at the Northend Clinic, operated by Sinai Hospital. When he did seriously seek a residency at Children's Hospital years later, Milly Reece, Children's Hospital's administrator was neither impressed by Lt. Thompson nor his military record, and refused him a residency.

John Dancy, executive director of the Urban League, tried to help Dr. Thompson by referring him to Bill Norton, administrator of the Congressman Couzens' holdings. Norton surveyed the local scene and offered to find a pediatric residency for Thompson in Marquette, in Michigan's Upper Peninsula. Dr. Thompson thanked him but expressed the hope that a residency could be found a bit closer to home.

Meanwhile, practicing pediatricians Drs. Irv Posner and Lou Heidelberg allowed Thompson to work voluntarily in their North End pediatric clinic once or twice per week. Thus, he was able to sharpen his pediatric skills while waiting for a residency to show up.

"Without my knowledge, a group of pediatricians led by Dr. Paul V. Wooly, chairman of pediatrics at Children's and head of pediatrics at Wayne Univ. Medical School, threatened to resign from the hospital if they did not accept me. I later learned that Nate Shapiro, of the Cunningham Drugstore chain, threatened to report the hospital to the union if they did not give me a residency. My friends prevailed.

"My residency began in January 1952, six years after leaving the Navy. Miss Reece never forgave me for forcing the issue. Nor did she speak to me during the first year of my residency. She did become friendly after a SID tragedy in my family, and even visited my home.

"In retrospect, it was a unique situation being the first black resident at Children's Hospital. I guess we had a lot of problems then that we were not aware of at that time. Early in my residency, I was put on what we called a 'white' ward. After the first month, I was assigned to a 'black' ward, or, at least, a mixed ward. But, they had two separate wards, one was for older kids and one for newborns, to which only white patients were assigned."

A comparison of Dr. Tanner's comments and experiences with those of Dr. Thompson reveals that they refer to the same institution, Children's Hospital of Michigan. While Dr. Tanner was well-qualified and sought access to available medical resources to bring better service to her patients, Dr. Thompson sought access to available training resources so that he could qualify as a certified pediatrician.

Despite the high infant morbidity and mortality rates so widely rampant in the communities where they practiced, both physicians endured racist oppression from those in charge.

It was brought to Dr. Tanner's attention that Dr. Wooley, her chief, was exerting pressure on the Children's Hospital staff on Dr. Thompson's behalf. Although she did not know Thompson at that time, she had serious doubts if any comparable events were then taking place on her behalf.

Dr. Thompson reported that the wards became gradually integrated during the last year of his residency, in 1956, the same year when the other Medical Center hospitals were beginning to face mounting threats of closure from the DMS, the NAACP, the Urban League, Senator Phil Hart, the Cotillion Club and sundry other civil rights groups that opposed the racist practices throughout the medical establishment.

Dr. Thompson's two firsts were: African American naval medical officer and pediatric resident at Children's Hospital. These experiences extracted from Drs. Cain and Thompson reflect a terrible toll in pride, patience and perseverance.

Physiatry

James A. Raikes, M.D. (Howard), was certified in physical medicine in 1968. He has retired from Sinai Hospital's Rehabilitation Institute and moved to Delaware.

Psychiatry

Sidney Bernard Jenkins, M.D. (Howard, 1951), became Detroit's first certified African American psychiatrist in 1957. He was the director of the Psychiatric Division of Wayne County Gen. Hospital in Eloise, Mich., 1963-70; gen. supt., Det. Mental Health & Drug Treatment Center, 1970-73; asst. prof. (Wayne State Univ.) asst. clin. prof (Univ. of Mich.).

Public Health

Virginia Mesa, M.D. (Chicago, 1982) cert. in public health, and was chief of the department in Genessee County, Mich., until April 1995. She is now medical director of Orange County, Fla., which includes Disney World, Epcot Center, and an Orlando health department with several hundred employees.

Roentgenology

Robert I. Greenidge, M.D. (Wayne Univ., 1915; cert. X-ray 1941). After several years of general practice in Detroit, and with no residency available to him, he closed his office to do post-grad studies in X-ray at Cook County Hospital (Chicago). These sporadic courses went on for many years and at great cost and inconvenience to him.

He persisted, was certified by the American Board of X-ray in 1941, and inducted into the American College of X-ray in 1943. Yet, during the 25 years that he practiced after becoming certified, Greenidge was never admitted to the staff of any certified hospital, even Detroit's TB hospital, Herman Kiefer.

As chairman of the X-ray departments at the small, segregated Dunbar/Parkside and Fairview Hospitals, operator of a private chest clinic, the Eastside Medical Laboratory (located at 4839 Beaubien), and through several serious TB epidemics in Detroit, Dr. Greenidge was credited with having read more chest films than anyone else in the entire state.

Harold Perry, M.D. (Howard Univ., 1948), led the way in oncology cert. X-ray therapy, 1955; int. 1948-49; asst. res. and res. in X-ray therapy at Freedmans Hospital in Washington, D.C.; fellowship at Memorial (N.Y.) and other hospitals in Cincinnati and Dayton. Came to Detroit's Sinai Hospital in 1966; clin. prof. radiation, oncology (Wayne). Retired, 1994.

Detroit's First African American General Surgeon, Alexander Loudin Turner (1884-1944)

Dr. Turner, M.D. (Univ. of Mich., 1912), was born in Macon, Georgia in 1884. He entered the Univ. of Mich. in 1906, and emerged in 1912 with a B.S. and M.D. degrees since internships were not available to African American physicians. Instead, Dr. Turner did post-graduate work in surgery at Howard Univ.'s Medical School.

He returned to Detroit and opened a private office at Gratiot and St. Antoine. Due to his surgical skill, his growing European American patient clientele and his frequent use of European American physicians as consultants, the medical establishment recognized Dr. Turner's economic potential.

Early in his medical career, Dr. Turner was granted admitting, and eventually surgical, privileges at Woman's and Grace Hospitals, becoming Michigan's first African American physician to be given full admitting privileges in a Detroit general hospital.[7]

He apparently confined his practice to Woman's Hospital and is not well-remembered, even by those few physicians who have survived his period. Those who are able, recall his flamboyant life style which included Lincolns and Pierce Arrow automobiles, driven by chauffeurs who waited during ward rounds and surgical operations; an obedient Doberman Pincher and Dr. Turner's loud boast: "I can still catch on the Class A baseball team."

Dr. Turner was financially successful from his largely white, private practice and envied by his colleagues because of his unique admitting privileges at Woman's Hospital.

He was the first of three African Americans to be attacked by an enraged white mob when he purchased a house outside the black ghetto and tried to move into an upscale neighborhood.

In June 1925, Spokane Avenue in Detroit's Tireman area was a "no man's land" for African Americans. "Several thousand" of Dr. Turner's would-be, white neighbors greeted him at his new home with a hail of stones and bricks. They broke every window in the house and tore the tiles from the roof. The policemen were amused, but immobilized.

After "one stormy day" of attempted tenancy, Dr. Turner sold the property at a loss and fled the neighborhood to 3410 W. Warren Ave. This area, although predominantly white, was inhabited by eastern European immigrants who were less hostile to African Americans than those in the region from which he fled.

Although Dr. Turner remained in private practice for some years after the racial assault, he was never the same afterwards. His private practice and business in his drugstore gradually declined.

Attorney Kermit Bailer recalls friendly visits with his father, Dr. Lloyd Bailer, to Dr. Turner's home in the "meadows" near Mount Clemens. They traversed the Clinton river in Dr. Turner's Chris Craft boat.

Eventually, Dr. Turner retired to Ravenna, Ohio, where he died on August 12, 1944, at the age of 61. A review of his death refers to him as being a member of Hutzel Hospital's Ob-gyn dept. Yet, the scant public references to him say "surgeon." The fact that he did an appendectomy on Kermit Bailer's brother during his youth reflects the breadth of his medical skills.

No matter the designation, he blazed a trail through the thicket of racism that left a spoor for Remus Robinson, Waldo Cain, and Garnet Ice, just to name three of his fairly immediate successors in the field of surgery.

Atty. Kermit Bailer bemoaned the fact that Dr. Turner is better remembered for his fearful flight from a white mob, one day in June of 1925, than for his many contributions to the health and well-being of this community during more than 25 years of private, surgical practice in Detroit.

Remus Robinson, Jr., M.D., Detroit's first, certified African American surgeon, is described by his widow, Maribodine.

"Remus Robinson, Jr., was born in Birmingham, Ala. His father, Remus Robinson, Sr., was an immigrant from Bermuda and a Dartmouth College graduate. His mother was LillyBelle Hill Robinson, the daughter of a farmer and fruit and vegetable merchant. She was a graduate of Alabama A & M College. His father was a full professor in the English department at Tuskegee Institute. Remus was in the ninth grade at the time of his father's death. In 1918, his mother sent him North for a better education. In Detroit, he lived with his aunt and uncle, Drs. Daisy and David Northcross, owners and operators of the Mercy General Hospital, Detroit's first hospital for blacks. Remus and his cousin, Bill Goins, both worked and lived in the hospital for a short while, before striking out on their own.

"Remus lived in rented rooms, worked, and went to the Detroit Public Schools. He graduated from Detroit Central High School in 1921 and attended the (Detroit) City College. While at City College, he supported himself by working midnights at the U.S. Post Office. Upon completion of the two years offered at City College, he transferred to the Univ. of Mich. and enrolled in the Medical School. He earned his undergraduate and medical degrees simultaneously, in 1930.

"By 1938, he had developed his golfing skills sufficiently to win the Negro National Amateur Golf Championship, the first of over 75 Championship Flight Golf awards he would earn.

"In 1934, he married Maribodine Busey Robinson of Columbus, Ohio, a graduate of Ohio State Univ. After marriage, they settled in Detroit and had three children. His wife was a full-time participant in his medical practice and also acted as office manager, medical technologist, X-ray technician, and triage nurse.

"After his graduation, Remus, a student in the top 10% of his class, was selected to serve his internship at Detroit Receiving Hospital. Upon presenting himself for duty, he was rejected because he was black. He vowed, at that moment, that he would never forget nor forgive, and if he ever got in a position to do something about such an attitude and action he would. He did.

"Fortunately, he was able to get a training assignment at St. Louis Hospital #2, the precursor of Homer G. Phillips Hospital. After completion of his rotating internship, he spent three years in surgical training and was promoted to chief surgical resident. It was during his third-year of residency that the classification of third-year surgical resident was eliminated due to budget limitations. Dr. Robinson agreed to work without pay for the experience, because it allowed him to qualify as a fourth-year resident and earn a salary.

"He returned to Detroit in 1934 and opened his medical practice in the Michigan Avenue corridor. He applied to Grace Hospital for staff privileges. In spite of his four years of surgical residency he was assigned to the courtesy staff. His admission letter stated that they would be happy to admit his white patients (only). He also became a staff member of Parkside and Martin Place Hospitals and several smaller proprietary hospitals.

"He regularly attended Grand Rounds at the Univ. of Mich. Hospital. Dr. Coller, chairman of Michgan's dept. of surgery, asked why he had not written for his 'Boards.' At that time specialty boards were usually written only by physicians affiliated with medical schools. Upon replying he had no university affiliation, Dr. Coller replied 'that can be arranged'—which, in turn, was done immediately. For three years, Remus carried a special assignment at the Univ. of Mich. Hospital and his own private practice at the same time.

"The first part of the board certification, at that time, was a supervised practicum, i.e., his special assignment. The second part consisted of an oral and a written examination. His examiner stated the indications and asked Robinson for his diagnosis. Robinson stated 'the supporting evidence and information, which, if correct, indicates the diagnosis should be ulcerative colitis, but do you know, I have never seen a case of it.'

"The examiner was astounded and impressed, and stating that Robinson's response was correct, further added 'that pathology (at that time, 1945) does not appear in your race.' He shook Robinson's hand and complemented him on a brilliant diagnosis, announcing he had decided not to proceed with additional problems.

"Robinson also achieved certifications as: fellow, American College of Surgeons; fellow, International College of Surgeons; diplomate, International Board of Surgeons; and diplomate, American Board of Surgeons.

290

"Despite his newly-won board certifications, Grace Hospital did not elevate him to full staff status. When Providence Hospital invited him to join their staff with full staff privileges in 1945, he accepted. During his tenure at Providence as a senior attending surgeon, he aided in upgrading Providence's intern-residency programs. The first two residents assigned to him are now faculty members at the Univ. of Toronto's Medical School. He received 'Physician of the Year' awards from both the Michigan State Medical Society and the Detroit Medical Associates.

"Remus Robinson realized that positive impact at the policy-making levels in agencies, organizations, and institutions that form the city's civic health and welfare infrastructure was necessary to bring his people into the mainstream of the total community. He understood that it is necessary to institutionalize the policy of equal access to opportunity, if the needs and concerns of his race were to be realized and obtained.

"As a member of the Detroit Medical Center board of directors he was able to initiate and institutionalize a policy of equal opportunity for member institutions in all aspects of their operations, patient care, employment, and procurement. This opened the way for training opportunities, jobs, staff privileges, and access to hospital beds by blacks. His participation in human rights organizations had the sole purpose of ending discriminatory behavior towards blacks.

"Remus Robinson was an active member of 'Serve Our Schools,' a coalition of 18-20 multicultural, multi-ethnic, multi-professional organizations interested in improving Detroit's public schools. In 1951, he was asked by this group to be a candidate for a seat on the Detroit Board of Education. He lost this election by a very small margin.

"In that same election, Board Member Patrick McNamara, became the U.S. senator-elect and resigned from the Detroit Board of Education. McNamara requested, and the board appointed, Remus Robinson to fill out his unexpired term. Two years later in 1953, Remus was drafted to run for the same seat by the same organization and won. Robinson served as a board member of the Detroit Board of Education for 17 consecutive years until his death in 1970.

"As a member of the Board of Education, he sat, ex-officio, on the board of directors of the Detroit Public Library. The library board needed a new chief librarian. Their custom was to conduct a nationwide search and import their selection for service. Robinson suggested to the personnel committee that they consider promoting from within. The suggestion was approved and Robinson had created a competitive opportunity for a seasoned local branch librarian, Mrs. Clara Jones, an African American, to rise into the leadership of a major library system. The first minority chief librarian in Detroit was thus selected as a result of his efforts and foresight.

"Detroit City College began in 1917 under the auspices of the Detroit Board of Education and grew into a full-fledged university. By 1954, the responsibility of managing and operating a growing university with 30,000 students had become unwieldy, financially burdensome, and distracting from K-12 concerns, so it was decided to explore a state affiliation for the university.

"In 1956, the Detroit Board of Education shifted Wayne Univ. into Michigan's higher education system. Upon it's affiliation with the state in 1956, it became Wayne State University. Until the next general election was held (in two years), the board of education members acted as the transition board of governors of Wayne State Univ. For two years Remus Robinson was simultaneously president of the Detroit Board of Education and chairman of the board of Wayne State Univ. After the general election, the transition board was dissolved and he was able to focus his full attention on the concerns of running a K-12 system.

"He enjoyed his tenure at both institutions thoroughly as it provided an opportunity to actualize his lifelong dream of being an agent for change in both institutions. He had attended both high school classes and college classes in the Old Main building of Wayne State Univ. and keenly understood the positive impact of education on underprivileged children."

Hand Surgery

Jeffrey Hall, M.D., (Univ. of Mich., 1985). After a residency at Detroit's Henry Ford Hospital, Dr. Hall went on to become the first African American in Michigan to be certified in hand surgery, in 1993. Premedical preparation included a bachelor's degree in chemical engineering, also at Michigan, before beginning his medical studies.

Neurological Surgery

Alexis Canady, M.D. (Univ. of Mich., 1975. cert. neuro-surgery 1984). After serving an internship at Yale's New Haven Hospital, she was appointed to a residency in neurosurgery, in Minnesota Hospitals, 1976-81; fell. (Children's Hosp. of Philadelphia and instr. in Neurosur, Penn.) 1981-82. She was appointed to the staffs of (Henry Ford) 1982-83; ped. neurosurg. (Children's Hosp. of Mich., 1983; William Beaumont Hospital, Royal Oak, Mich., 1984; cl. instr. in Neurosurg. (Wayne State Univ., 1985); and is now dir. neurosurg., Children's Hosp. of Michigan.

Orthopedic Surgery

John McCollough, M.D. (Univ. of Mich., 1962), the first African American orthopedic resident to be trained in Toledo, Ohio, and the first orthopedic surgeon to be certified in Michigan (1970).

Thoracic Surgery

Hayward Maben, M.D. (Meharry, 1945; cert. surgery, 1964; thoracic surgery, 1965; res., Detroit Receiving Hospital, 1958-59; Meharry, 1959-63; Rush, Presbyterian, St. Lukes hospitals, Chicago, 1963-64; res. 1963, chief resident thoracic surgery 1964-65, both at Hines VA Hosp., Ill.; assoc. surg., Harper Hosp.; Cl. asst. prof. of surg., Wayne State Univ.) A more complete statement is found under "Matthew's Disciples."

Urological Surgery

When racial segregation denied **Dr. Chester Ames** the right to become a certified urologist in 1930, Detroit's African

American community was forced to wait for more than 30 years until **Howard O. Gray**, M.D. (Wayne Univ., 1945) was able to find a hospital (Wayne County) that would accept him as a urological resident and a private hospital (Detroit Memorial) that would admit him to its staff.

It wasn't until 1963 that Dr. Ames' goal of becoming a certified urological surgeon was finally achieved by Dr. Gray. Despite the passage of time, Dr. Gray was not readily accepted as a resident nor welcomed to the staffs of the university-affiliated hospitals. Still, he persevered and prevailed.

According to Freddie Guinyard, Joe Louis' close associate and my main source of much of the information on Dr. Ames, the disappointed urologist drifted away from the specialty for which he had been well-trained, and became a general practitioner and Joe Louis' private physician in 1934.

Dr. Ames was ringside at every one of Joe's professional fights, except the first one in 1934, when Louis knocked out Joe Cracken in the first round. He was present during both Schmeling fights, and all others, until his sudden death in 1941. An autopsy revealed that death was due to a heart attack. No doubt, an inquest would have revealed that Dr. Ames' heart was also broken.

Charles Vincent, M.D. (Wayne State Univ., 1958) cert. obg., 1966), is foremost among Michigan's African American physicians who have sought and occasionally found public office from a medical standpoint, but never politically. Among the many reasons listed for Dr. Vincent with the Firsts of Michigan's African American Physicians are:

As early as 1981, and again in 1983, Dr. Vincent was chosen as "Physician of the Year" by his colleagues in the DMS. They elected him to serve as a member of their board of trustees and eventually, as their president.

In addition to serving as director of ob-gyn at Detroit Receiving Hospital and director of gynecology at Hutzel Hospital, Dr. Vincent was chosen as Wayne State Univ.'s Outstanding Faculty Member in 1968 and 1981, and Alumnus of the Year in 1986 and 1991.

As a member of the Michigan State Medical Society and the AMA, and serving on several county and state committees, Dr. Vincent has made the deepest penetration into the medical establishment of any other of Michigan's African American physicians.

It was during the California meeting of the AMA's board of trustees, February 7-11, 1995, that some of us became aware that Dr. Vincent had been appointed to the membership committee of the AMA, the first such appointment for an African American during the entire 147-year history of the organization.

He knew that downsizing of medical schools was on the agenda and that Meharry and Morehouse Medical Schools are particularly vulnerable. Despite his chronic illness, Dr. Vincent, a co-chairman of the committee, felt compelled to attend.

His condition worsened during the session; and he returned home to spend several days in ICU before his condition stabilized. Fortunately, the committee had completed the major portion of its agenda before illness struck. My prediction is that we have not heard the last word from Dr. Vincent who has been a "politician all my life."

Not content with his extraordinary professional achievements, Dr. Vincent has sought on two occasions, but failed to gain, a seat in the U.S. Congress, as a Democrat in 1990 and as a Republican in 1992. He is certain that he could have done better as an independent, the second time.

Urology
Chester Cole Ames, M.D. (Wayne Univ., 1926) was Detroit's first African American intern (1926), resident (1927), and faculty member (1930). According to Hutzel Hospital's former chief urologist, Dr. Frank Bicknell, the practice of urology first began at Receiving Hospital with Dr. Ames as the first resident.

At the end of his residency, Dr. Ames was appointed to the Receiving Hospital faculty of the new department. In spite of this auspicious beginning, Dr. Ames, only because he was African American, never got appointed to the staff of a private hospital and never became a practicing nor a certified urologist. Eventually, he abandoned his specialty altogether to become a general practitioner and fight physician for Joe Louis.

Other Non-Medical Firsts by African Americans in Michigan History

Dr. William G. Anderson, President, Am. Osteopathic Assoc.

The question of where to place Dr. Anderson did give me some brief pause. Although a surgeon, he was not a first surgeon. But since he was a surgeon long before he was elected president of the American Osteopathic Association, he should feel comfortable among them.

"In 1961, the town of Albany, Ga. was completely segregated, with no evidence of change in sight. Fortunately, my prior relationship with Dr. Martin Luther King would become a factor in the effort for change. Although there had been a successful boycott in Montgomery, Ala., six years before, integration had not yet reached Albany, 40% of whose 50,000 citizens were African American," states Dr. Anderson.

"A biracial committee was formed to study the city's rapidly rising racial tension. The committee met with the mayor and city council but did not discuss any of the main racial issues. When Dr. William Anderson, Albany's only African American physician, asked why the race matter was not on the agenda, the mayor replied: 'there was no common ground for agreement; and we chose not to address the subject.'"

Dr. Anderson departed the meeting, dissatisfied with the intransigence of the city's administration. He slept fitfully that night and met the *Albany Herald* at the door. In large, black print, the headline read: "Local Doctor Storms Out of Council Chambers; Demands an End To Segregation." The doctor's address and telephone numbers, printed on the front page opened the floodgates of hatred that was unlike anything he or his family had ever experienced.

The threats and hate calls began within minutes of the delivery of the first newspaper, continued all day, and well into the night. By nightfall, with no abatement in the volume nor virulence of the calls, and no evidence of police protection during the day, the doctor gathered up his wife and small children and fled into the night.

Soon afterwards, members of the Student Non-Violent Coordinating Committee (SNCC) came to Albany and started a voter registration drive. Despite the efforts of the European American community to thwart SNCC's efforts, many voters were registered.

Federal observers were ordered into Albany to make sure that the next election would be honest. Despite arrests for "demonstrating with out a license, distributing literature without a permit and other forms of intimidation," the voting was more democratic than Albany had ever had before.

Later, Freedom Train Riders came to Albany, to test the Supreme Court's ruling against segregation in interstate travel. The Riders entered the "white-only" train station and were promptly arrested. During a mass rally that night, the Albany Movement was organized and Dr. Anderson, already identified as a leader, was elected its president.

Beginning the next morning, a series of mass demonstrations followed by mass arrests began which would continue for many days. The demonstrators began boycotting buses, stores and restaurants. By the end of the week, there had been 1,100 arrests, 700 of whom were still in jail.

Dr. Anderson, inexperienced in dealing with bail bondsmen and not having any money anyhow, called his old friends, the Revs., Martin Luther King and Ralph Abernathy. They had already become veterans of the civil rights movement and they could surely offer him professional advice. Rev. King showed up, despite extreme fatigue from other recent confrontations, and addressed four community gatherings his first day in town.

"Dr. King was stimulated by the determination and fearlessness of the town's people; he seemed to grow stronger with every appearance. No one could have been in the presence of those people and not sensed the energy that was being generated.

"That night, Rev. King made a commitment to Albany and was there almost constantly for the next several weeks as waves of people packed the jails, as a strategy of protest. Coretta Scott King came to her husband's rescue during the melee of the demonstrations and was arrested and thrown in jail like everybody else."

The time spent leading the movement, demonstrating and imprisoned caused major disruptions in Dr. Anderson's family and professional lives. His wife and children suffered through and survived the threats and inconveniences of that period. "Looking back, it seems like the rites of passage through a racist system in quest of justice and freedom."

"Soon, with the city and county jails bulging with protesters and the financial burdens caused by the movement, the city fathers began to rethink their positions. Recognizing that the protesters were gaining the upper hand, the city officials offered to negotiate on our original proposal: to establish a bi-racial committee to study segregation and how to end it.

"We agreed to come out of jail and stop the demonstrations and boycotts. We kept our part of the bargain, but they never did! By the time we realized the city officials were not going to be true to their word, the movement had been undermined."

Anderson came to Detroit in 1963 to begin a surgical residency and to continue the struggle for freedom and justice as a private practitioner, as he had carried on in the South. For many years, he has been involved with the Mich. State College of Osteopathic Medicine and has served as a trustee of the Des Moines College of Osteopathic Medicine, his alma mater.

On July 18, 1993, Dr. Anderson was chosen president-elect of the Am. Osteopathic Association, the first African American to hold that office. The announcement was greeted with a standing ovation by his peers. Two long-time colleagues and friends, Drs. Richard Brown and Jan Janower, donated $25,000 to the AOA Hospital Building Fund in Dr. Anderson's name.[8]

Since taking over the office of president of the American Osteopathic Association (AOA), in July 1994, Dr. Anderson has

298

blazed a trail of African American leadership to the highest office in several, national medical organizations.

Only a few months after Dr. Anderson's rise to power in AOA, Dr. Lonnie Bristow was chosen to direct the affairs of the American Medical Association. Dr. Joe Thompson was elected as president of the American College of Physicians, Dr. LaSalle Lafall was named the President of the American College of Surgeons, Dr. Barbara Ross Reed (Diana Ross' sister) was chosen dean of the Ohio Univ. College of Osteopathic Physicians and, of course, Tracy Alston became president of Meharry Medical College.

Dr. Anderson was interviewed, in late February 1995, about mid-term of his presidency. He was asked about the concentration of power in the hands of African Americans, which disturbed some members of the press:

"How did it happen that so many of you were chosen for top positions, at one time?" they asked.

Dr. Anderson's reply was, "A coincidence that is not likely to recur for a long time, unless we work at it."

"Is there any one else in the pipeline, behind you?"

"No, and that's one of the things that I regret. Dr. Bristow and I talked about that during our recent meeting of African American Leaders of Health Care, at Meharry, when Dr. John Moffet was installed as president. In Orlando last July, Lou Sullivan and I got together and decided to bring more African Americans into the organizational structure of the national bodies. I have appointed African Americans to positions on our bureaus, councils and committees, where they have never served before.

"Bristow shared with me a diversity of sensitivity programs that has been adopted by the AMA. Let's face it. You get there on merit, yes, but they don't know your merit if you don't get a chance to display it."

The Origin of Health Maintenance Organization (HMO)

Thomas A. Batchelor, M.D.(Wayne Univ., 1945). Of the many contributions that Dr. Batchelor made to the evolution of the practice of medicine in Detroit, none surpasses the

299

establishment of Detroit's first Health Maintenance Organization. Formerly known as Community Health Association, it is now known as The Wellness Plan. Dr. Batchelor recalls those early years:

"When Walter Reuther, president of the UAW, convened an advisory group in 1951 to determine the feasibility of developing such a revolutionary form of medical practice, Judge Wade McCree, Max Osnos, and I were invited to attend the meeting at the Whittier Hotel, with overflow attendance. After lengthy deliberations, an overwhelming majority voted in favor of the establishment of a Community Health Association (CHA).

"An immediate alarm spread throughout the medical community, and in Wayne County, to avoid participation in the 'development of socialized medicine.' Despite many road blocks, the program was launched in the leased facilities of the Metropolitan Hospital Clinics.

"I was offered practice privileges in this hospital complex. Max Osnos, president of Sam's Cut Rate Stores, was elected president of the board of directors and Judge Wade McCree was elected to the board. Dr. Ethelene Crockett soon joined the team and was appointed to the obg. staff with full privileges.

"The principal community organizers were Walter Reuther and Millie Jeffries, officials of the United Automobile Workers of America (UAW). Since I had played such a vital role in bringing HMOs on-line in Detroit, and because I was the former medical director of CHS, I was asked to relate how HMOs came to Detroit."

The second veteran and still active member of CHSD's founders is James Patton, now The Wellness Plan's (TWP) executive vice president and chief operating officer. He joined as the organization was taking shape and was asked to recall what went on from his management perspective after he came aboard.

While the two reports do not agree in every detail, both address the issues of the need for growth, the ability to change and the will to survive.

Community Health Associations in Michigan

Thomas A. Batchelor, M.D., makes the following observatons about the development:

"Early in my medical career, I was introduced to the national officers of this new organization; some of whom had attended national meetings and assisted in setting up Community Health Associations elsewhere and were appointed as consultants in other parts of the country. Once your name got on a roll, appointments to other committees followed as a matter of course.

"From these vantaged positions, one gained much insight into what was happening, in the field and nationally. Thus, my influence was maximized by meeting with these different groups.

"In short order, I began to understand what was going on, especially when I was appointed as a consultant to the surgeon general. We searched, diligently, for alternatives to hospital care. Anybody who had such alternatives would submit them to the Project Review Committee for further study and action. Our working budget was $23 million.

"Since our organization was a clearing board, we had the opportunity to review all of the suggestions that came in. This produced a sense of camaraderie that led us to our first venture: providing public renal dialysis centers, strategically placed, throughout the U.S.

"The experience gained from the operation of such centers was refined into an HMO policy that was adopted nationwide. We studied applications and did site visits to determine the feasibility of the proposals. I visited Chicago, Berkeley and Atlanta. Other committee members visited different sites. We met at designated spots to discuss our findings before deciding to refinance, cut back or cancel a program.

"This oversight group, of about 12 people, provided close surveillance over the operation. Our first project was funded at Northwestern University (Chicago) and the second one was at Emory University (Atlanta, Ga.). The scope grew until dialysis centers consumed 17% of our $4.5 million budget. Eventually, the centers were turned over to Medicare.

"We then began to centralize this activity by merging hospitals located in the same areas. Southwest Detroit Hospital was at that time one product of the merger. It was

301

recommended that we merge the hospitals along Detroit's East Jefferson corridor, including the one in Grosse Pointe. The only new ones built were South Macomb and St. John.

"I was placed on the Greater Detroit Area Hospital Council and my voice, seeking more hospital mergers, was more amplified from that position than before. We made a constant effort to determine the amount of resources offered in the various regions and to measure the frequency with which new ideas were presented.

"As should be obvious, politics are the major influence that got me on those various committees. Then, there are medical politics that help in other ways. I was elected chairman of the medical sector of the Wayne County Medical Society (WCMS) on a county-wide ballot. It gave me the opportunity to see what was going on and the chance to have some impact on it. Eventually, I was able to serve on the State Council of the Michigan State Medical Society.

"I was also appointed to various committees of the American College of Physicians and paid my dues by serving on them. Then, I was elected regional councilor for Southeastern Michigan's three districts that led to my being chosen as councilor for the American College of Physicians, which gave me direct contact with the American Board of Regents of the American College of physicians.

"Through this relationship, I became involved with the establishment of internship and residency programs and made closer contact with the Joint Commission. This was the agency through which I was able to establish an approved residency for six people at Kirwood Hospital. I ran the residency program when the hospital was on Davison and Petosky, until 1969, when I moved on to the Model Neighborhood Program.

"As a member of the Greater Detroit Area Hospital Council, I was usually the contact person for an opinion on anything that was going to happen in the hospital building and certification areas. This council had the responsibility to certify a hospital that they knew would be participating at a cost-plus-3% or non-participating at $15 per day/per diem. We made that decision.

"It was there that I ran into Francis Kornegay, then head of Detroit's Urban League and we got the game going. Francis convinced his Urban League buddies and other related agencies; and I convinced my buddies in such areas as hospital administration and other physicians.

"Together, we were able—through general, not medical politics—to mobilize a joint force for action. The superstructure was run by the Metropolitan Fund which provided funding for research grants to determine whether it is appropriate to think of the southeastern Michigan government in terms of a transportation or disposal system or as a hospital industry.

"Such decisions as these were made by the Metropolitan Fund Committee run by Ken Matheson from the downtown Book Building. It was funded by a $10 million grant from the Ford Foundation, the UAW, the Ford Motor Co, Detroit Edison, Michigan Consolidated Gas Co. and Bell Telephone. Judge Wade McCree and I were included, although the real authority extended back to Walter Reuther, who really called the shots.

"The other group was called the Greater Area Detroit Hospital Council which controlled the United Foundation, the Greater Area Detroit Hospital Council, Blue Cross/Blue Shield and the Detroit Medical Center.

"Jerry Cavanagh was the mayor then and I was Wayne County commissioner. That was one of the reasons I was co-serving with Walter Reuther, who announced that he was in with me. Actually, I was appointed the medical consultant to Wayne State Univ. But, the real action began after I was appointed to the Board of Health.

"Wayne State appointed me as medical consultant because they were looking for a way to become involved in the community in some fashion. The opportunity occurred in President Lyndon Johnson's Partnership on Health program, which allowed each community to plan for its own future. Throughout the country, block grants were offered through HUD, so, my consultancy allowed me to represent the total university. Through it, I dealt with Ed Cushman, the first vice president (then president of Wayne State Univ.).

"I was asked to help to develop a medical program for the university. Then, the Model Neighborhood popped up with a funding source. They started a residency in the Model Neighborhood, devising their own plan for health care.

"Dr. Ethelene Crockett, working with the Health Council in the Model Neighborhood, kept a record of what was being requested in terms of health care. Her notes became the frame-work around which Comprehensive Health Care was formed. It became the nucleus around which the program was developed for Model Neighborhood.

"Ed Cushman asked me to go along with Dr. Ernie Gardner, dean of the medical school, and make a bid for this program with this format. Other people were bidding, but we got the nod for Wayne University through the Health Council. It was my job to hold it for the university until such time as they could take it over.

"Everybody supported this move, except Dr. Tommy Evans, chief of Wayne State Univ. Medical School's dept. of Obg. We had expected Tommy to go along with us, so our plan required three full-time equivalents—two of which were offered to Dr. Evans. Tommy demanded all three on Friday, the last day for decision-making.

"Tommy would not agree on a compromise but did promise to call back before the deadline. I had already told the university's representatives that whether I heard from him or not, I was going to proceed on Monday.

"As an official of the Detroit Medical Center, Dr. Robert Mack, an internist, was designated to let me know before Monday morning what Tommy's final decision was.

"Sunday night, Dr. Mack reported that he had been in contact with Tommy and that Tommy and Dean Gardner wanted to talk with me. I got a call shortly thereafter. The dean said that he had been talking with Tommy and had finally convinced him that it would be in the university's best interest to go along with the program. Gardner handed Evans the phone: 'Tom (Batchelor), I still have some reservations, but I'll still go along for you to make the pitch.'

"So, on February 16, 1970, at 8 p.m. (my birthday), they gave me the contract and a letter of credit for $850,000 from the Health Council. I went over to talk with the manager of the Professional Plaza, showed him my letter of credit, told him of our spatial needs and asked for his help. He showed me the space above the Big Boy restaurant, at Woodward and Alexandrine.

"He offered, 'I can't do any remodeling, right now, but you can have it.' We didn't discuss price or anything else. I moved on to the next issue. 'Have you got some old furniture that some doctor might have left when he moved out?' He did provide some office furniture that was sufficient to get the program going.

"The next move was to secure medical equipment and personnel. I called the deans of the various colleges of the university and told them of our needs. When I promised them that my call would be followed by one from Mr. Cushman, I got their full attention.

"Within a week, I had all of the needed directors. Meanwhile, we were receiving equipment that was shipped from display areas in conventions throughout the country, especially from Chicago. The ophthalmologists had just completed a demonstration from which they took the equipment off the floor and shipped it to us by air.

"We were able to pull in all the people we needed and began to enroll patients like crazy. Everyone who lived in the Model Neighborhood area was eligible. We went closely by the map-designated corners and followed the zip codes very closely. The patients came from Lafayette Park and from skid row. We had everybody coming in to get health care. We grew like Topsy.

"Max Osnos appeared in his limousine and went right to the heart of the problem: 'Tom, I hear that you need some space. Here are the keys to the London Inn. Pay us when you can. I know what you are trying to do. We have worked in so many things together. This is old politics coming back. Everything in there is yours.'

"We went over there and started moving the next day. We began selling off furniture, television sets—everything. We

305

were instructed not to sell the mattresses, so we gave them away. Then, we started remodeling and billing those patients who had any kind of private insurance.

"Sylvester Angel, the director of the Model Neighborhood Agency, decided that while we were doing fine, it was one of the few programs that worked. He thought that we should be able to get sufficient money from HUD to pay off the balance of the mortgage.

"It was only then that the price of the building, $1.25 million, became a pressing issue. Sylvester's responsibility was to round up the money to complete the purchase of the London Inn. He, Max Osnos, and several other investors including our lawyer, Stanley Kirk, and our representative from the near-by Commonwealth Bank, Donald O'Connor, met us at the London Chop House to close the deal. At the last minute, Atty. Kirk noted that the check could not be cashed until Tuesday, four days later.

"Unfortunately, the owners insisted on closing the deal, then, on Friday. O'Connor called the directors of the Commonwealth Bank by phone and they agreed to loan me the $1.25 million for the week-end, interest-free.

"The next move was to try to get out of the Model Neighborhood area. Some of us thought that it was too restrictive to ever become fully operative. They wanted to go to the open community. They got a deal that not only included medicaid but other population groups as well. Angel said that he could not go along with this planned expansion. He seemed to fear losing control of the group.

"Our differences of opinion were aired before the Detroit Common Council. But, they refused to act and passed it on to Mayor Gribbs who passed it back to Angel and me. We called each other a few names; Angel threatened to terminate our contract.

"I alerted my staff that night. We got some big trucks and hauled all the movable equipment to the Home for Unwed Mothers at Florence Crittenton, which we acquired over the phone from Mr. Allen. He gave us permission to move to Florence Crittenton's fourth floor that night.

"We remained at that site and continued to expand. We bought a clinic on Schaefer from Manny Sklar, but we soon outgrew that space. One day, Max Osnos called me to come to the Gold Key Inn and he introduced me to Sam Garrison and his son, owners of the Pontchartrain.

"As they were being introduced, Max told them what we had done at the London Inn and expressed hope that we could do the same at the Gold Key. I made it clear that we did not know what it would cost to operate at this new site.

"The Garrisons agreed to accept the $3,000 per month that was being paid to Florence Crittenton for the Unwed Mother's Home, 'until you can do better.'

"We moved into the Gold Key Motel at 6500 John C. Lodge and West Grand Boulevard in one night. It became, and still is, our central office. We left Sylvester Angel with the remainder of the operation at the London Inn."

James Patton, exec. vice-president of CHSD, also known as The Wellness Plan, picks up the narrative here and continues from management's perspective:

"We began as a Model Neighborhood Agency, with two entities:

1. The Health Council, that marketed, enrolled and did system analyses.
2. The Model Neighborhood Comprehensive Health Program (MNCHP) that delivered or provided medical care.

"The council enrolled members only in well-defined neighborhood areas which was a well-defined geographic area and, obviously, the MNCHP provided care to those particular enrollees. Dr. Batchelor, president of MNCHP, organized a multi-specialty medical specialty group, which included Drs. Waldo Cain, You Win Tsai, Charles Vincent, Ethelene Crockett, and others to provide medical care to the membership.

"The membership grew at such a rapid pace that the original space at the former London Inn on Woodward Ave. was made available and subsequently purchased by the Model Neighborhood Agency for its two health contractors. All operations of MNCHP and the Health Council were moved to this new location. The rapid growth and the inability to hire administrative people outside of the model neighborhood created a strained relationship with the model neighborhood agency. So throughout the time we were associated with Model Neighborhood, the relationship was strained and a rather stormy relationship existed.

"This was a direct result of MNCHP's inability to provide reports of medical quality/quantity and financial data to the program, sufficient to extricate itself from this impossible situation, which was the inability to employ people who could perform the tasks that were needed to satisfy the model neighborhood agency's requirements. It decided to pursue a strategy of engaging talented consultants: the first consultant was Ellis J. Bonner, who was consultant to Thomas J. Batchelor, M.D.; I was the second consultant.

"Bonner's primary role at that time was to obtain a medicaid contract that would permit the MNCHP program to expand throughout the city. Bonner accomplished this late in 1971 and early 1972. It was the first prepaid medical plan with the Michigan Department of Social Services.

"In 1972, Patton was engaged as a consultant pending justification of employment, since he was not a Model Neighborhood resident. The purpose for his engagement/employment was to straighten out the administrative mess. Based on the relationship problems that already existed and the many moves described above, this was obviously not an easy task.

"Over time, we were able to satisfy the administrative concerns of the Model Neighborhood Agency. During 1972, the medicaid enrollment was quite successful. Conversion and enrollment of medicaid recipients reached 3,500-4,000 members. MDSS and MNCHP would have to be regulated. Unfortunately, the State of Michigan had no vehicle to regulate a 501(c)3 organization.

"It was decided that a new corporation would need to be created and placed under Acts 108 and 109. The only entity functioning under these acts was Blue Cross/Blue Shield. Comprehensive Health Service (CHS) was incorporated. The medicaid contract was negotiated and transferred to CHS. Subsequent to the transfer of the contract, CHS used medicaid funds to purchase a small clinic at 18400 Shaefer Road in Detroit. It was the belief of management that expansion out of the

Model Neighborhood area was essential if the program was to survive.

"Needless to say, these two incidents, along with other administrative problems, brought the wrath of the Model Neighborhood Agency down on MNCHP and everything around it. The end result was that MNCHP was thrown out of the facility at 3455 Woodward Ave. along with 20% of its membership, mostly new medicaid enrollees.

"MNCHP moved back to 3750 Woodward Ave., from which it had originally come, and provided care to those medicaid recipients who continued their affiliation. The administration moved to the Schaefer building, where many stormy battles continued for a fairly long time. When we began to enroll for the Schaefer Clinic, we were again forced to move. This time, we moved to the unwed mother's home at Crittenton Hospital in Detroit.

"During these various moves, we lost about two-thirds of our enrollees and nearly one-half of our staff. Fortunately our staff was more stable. The ground was shaky, indeed. It was anticipated by many observers that CHS would slide into the lake any day. We obviously survived some very tumultuous times. Enrollment was re-built and things began to improve.

"Early in 1974, the former Gold Key Inn, located in the New Center area near John C. Lodge Expressway, was acquired. In mid-1974, the clinic at 3750 Woodward and the administrative offices at Crittenton Hospital were also moved to the New Center Plaza's Gold Key Inn. Enrollment had grown to approximately 10,000 members at both centers.

"Although membership continued to grow at a steady pace, CHS continued to struggle. Losses reached $150,000 per month. Although the financial situation went from bleak to desperate, CHS never missed a payroll.

"Physician care was provided by the multi-specialty physician team for the New Center Plaza and the Priver Group, from Sinai Hospital, which provided physicians for the Schaefer Center. CHS supplied nurses and other support personnel to both centers. In late 1974, the Priver Group

309

came to a meeting of the CHS board with the intention of taking over the CHS operation.

"Needless to say, the insurgents' plan was defeated and they withdrew their physicians without notice. You can imagine the problems this created for CHS, which was contracted to provide medical care for 3,500-4,000 members.

"The multi-specialty group at New Center moved very swiftly and effectively to fill this void by deploying physicians from their unit and by engaging other physicians on a session-by-session basis, as a temporary measure. Over time, they were successful in recruiting an adequate number of physicians to staff both centers.

"During all of this turmoil, numerous changes were taking place. There were numerous discussions with MDSS and the Insurance Bureau about the inadequacy of the payments being received. At this same time, disagreements with the medical group began to surface about their role and a different payment schedule for their services.

"We were not making great progress at the state level but discussions continued. The medical group's concerns were every bit as, if not more, important than the financial returns. Either one, and certainly both, could sink the organization.

"With regard to emerging medical problems, Joanne Wallace, then on our administrative staff, recommended contacting Mr. Avram Yeddida, an employee of the Kaiser Permanente Group since its founding stages and was still employed there as a consultant.

"According to Yeddida, 'the Kaiser Permanente Group had gone through the same woes and throes between the administration and physician components.' So, there was no need for us to reinvent the wheel.

"Yeddida proved to be wise, judicious and studious in his approach to CHS' problems. He was successful in convincing the physician group that the financial information was accurate and an increase in their pay would not be in the best interest of the group in view of the losses that were occurring.

"As we look back, this problem was moved to another day in the future. It must be assumed that MDSS internalized our arguments regarding inadequate payments. Since late in 1975,

310

CHS has received a check for $2,000,755 to make up for underpayment in prior years.

"We knew that this check would make us whole and we could go on from there, without the financial impediments that had prevented creativity and innovation. It was now possible and probable to talk with the medical group about a different kind of payment arrangement.

"Discussions ensued between the administration and the medical group. Yedidda was brought back to finalize the agreement on a principal of understanding between the parties. This was done, successfully, over a period of time.

"The final contract required CHS to pay the physician's group a capitation fee for each patient, each month, whether the enrollee required services or not. In this arrangement, the physicians were responsible for providing or arranging for all physician services. Capitation negotiations, as usual, were contentious and argumentative.

"During the first two or three years, we managed to come to a satisfactory agreement. The 1980 negotiations were particularly tough in that the medical group demanded an unreasonable capitation and the freedom to do private practice. After many months of less than satisfactory negotiations, the administration decided to meet with certain leaders in the medical group to discuss a more affirmative plan for providing physician services. These leaders bought into the plan, and CHS proceeded to implement it. The original contract with the entire medical group was terminated on October 31, 1980.

"At the same time, offers of employment were issued to all physicians who CHS wanted to retain. Very few, if any of the physicians left the group with the exception of those who were not invited. To this date, the centers operated by CHS are the staff model, that is, the physicians are employed by CHS."

With the able leadership and assistance of Dr. Rangarajan, the new medical director; the medical group and the administration now enjoy outstanding relationships. In the mid-1970s, CHS was licensed as an HMO by the Insurance Bureau and the Michigan

Department of Public Health. It was federally qualified as an HMO by Health, Education and Welfare, a.k.a. Health and Human Services.

The CHS membership continues to grow. The company is solvent and the quality of care is very good. Over the years, CHS has either built or renovated additional centers in and around the City of Detroit. Some 600 people are employed.

Dr. Rangarajan mused, almost inaudibly: "From the humble and, sometimes, tumultuous beginnings, CHS and its people have made very large contributions to this community. Among them are:

1. **Project How**—Over five years ago, TWP's Dr. Richard Henderson, chief of adult medicine, spearheaded Project HOW (Health on Wheels) which provides health care to the uninsured and underinsured at neighborhood churches throughout the city. Since then, Dr. Mark Kesishian, asst. vice president and associate medical director of TWP, and many other doctors in the area, have committed time to serve the community's needs. TWP also provides medical supplies and necessary laboratory tests for patients of "Project HOW."

2. Research TWP is involved in two critical research efforts that will have an impact on the delivery of health care

   2.1 In conjunction with the Michigan Cancer Foundation, we are a part of a physician effort to improve the mammography testing for women.

   2.2 The NIH and TWP are participating in a project that will determine the best, most cost-effective medication for lowering blood pressure.

   2.3 Our physicians are increasingly involved with medical students, interns and residents. Programs are in place where the future doctors will have the opportunity to work in a supervised capacity in the TWP facility and see, first hand, the city's needs. This service includes optometry, nursing and pharmacy students as well.

   2.4 TWP is involved in a collaborative effort with the Dept. of Public Health in two schools which provide immunizations and hearing and vision tests. Through visits to other schools, TWP brings safety, personal hygiene, hope and determination with its instructional fun characters "Wally Well Apple," "Safe Way MacIntosh" and "Granny Smith."

3. A Community Commitment

   3.1 TWP has an "Adopt a Senior Citizen Home" program in which employees of TWP take local, senior citizens under their wing. About 3,000 families participate in the WIC nutritional program at all five of TWP's centers. Currently, there are over 1,000 private physicians in this network, providing care to 62,000 members. In the early 1990s, CHS decided to do business as The Wellness Plan. It was believed that this name is more representative of what we are all about—preventive health care.

TWP has, as of September 1, 1994, a total membership of 123,000 and a gross revenue of $183,711,015 (as of December 31, 1993). With over 91,000 public-sector members, TWP is one of the leading public sector, prepaid, managed-care programs in membership size, financial health and the quality of service delivered. Our lengthy experience in successfully managing an enrolled population, through continuous quality improvement and utilization reviews, makes TWP most-suited to provide similar services anywhere else in the country.

During the summer of 1994, ground was broken for the construction of a $7.5 million health care facility that will provide patients an even higher quality of medical care than they have enjoyed in the past. This four-level facility is scheduled for occupancy in July of 1995.

As indicated in his narrative, Patton describes "many stormy battles that continued for a fairly long time....Throughout these vibrant years, CHS has never wavered from its mission, i.e. 'quality care under reasonable cost to all segments of Detroit's citizens.' In fact, the quality of the care provided by CHS has attracted national, state and local attention. For example:

1. Traffic to our shop reached new heights during President Clinton's efforts the reform the health care delivery system in 1994.

2. In 1992, GHAA proceedings of an analysis of outcome of our 5,000 deliveries for CHS enrollees at Hutzel Hospital, over a four-year period, revealed that the perinatal mortality of CHS enrollees was almost one-half of the perinatal mortality in the rest of Detroit's Wayne County.

3. With a new headquarters building replacing the facilities at 6065 John C. Lodge, in July of 1995, we expect to do much better.

By the early eighties, remedial changes proposed by the consultants to the staff were implemented and a new professional team took to the field for CHS. The main player on this new team is N.S. Rangarajan, M.D. (Univ. of Madras, India), a former member of the Wright, Bentley partnership, who was appointed medical director in 1979.

With very little prior training in medical management, the benefits of his administration were soon apparent. During the 15 years of the Rajan administration, the membership increased from 28,000 to 123,000 and revenue rose from $21,115,230 to $183,711,015—a direct function of good management in a largely Medicaid HMO.

Proof that this economic turnaround is not being paid for with patient-care dollars was published in an article by Charles Wright, M.D., chief of obg.; T. Hershel Gardin, Ph.D., a director of corporate development at CHS; and Carla L. Wright, M.D., physiatrist in Milwaukee, Wisconsin.

The article, published in the *American Journal of Obstetrics and Gynecology,* proved that infant morbidity and mortality figures in CHS' predominately medicaid clientele compared favorably with those in Detroit's suburbs.

The publication attracted a host of doubters, including Dr. Louis Sullivan, then secretary of HEW and various members of his secretariat among whom wondered, a few years later, if the results could be replicated. They were, several years later. Nearly all inquirers wanted to know how had CHS produced such results with a medicaid clientele? Dr. Rangarajan's answer was uniformly simple, "Caring medical management."

Dr. Rangarajan's valedictory speech, after 20 years at the helm of medical management of CHS, reflects a commitment to people as a way of life:

"From the humble beginning of temporary 'shelters,' CHS has grown in the last 22 years to the present status of one of the major health organizations in Detroit and Southeastern Michigan. CHS owns and operated four health centers, three of them full service centers and has contractual relationships with over 1,000 independent care providers, here in Michigan and elsewhere. The anticipated revenue for 1995 will be in excess of $250,000,000. The East Area Health Center, built in 1993, comprised state of the art construction and our renovated Northwest Health Center provides dignified, aesthetic ambience for its Detroit clients. The new, state-of-the-art Wellness Plan facility will be open to patients during the summer of 1995."

Throughout these vibrant years, CHS has never wavered from its mission, i.e., "quality care under reasonable cost," to all segments of Detroit's citizens. In fact, the quality of care provided by CHS has attracted national, state and local attention. For example:

1. An article published in the *American Journal of Obstetrics and Gynecology*, assured the skeptics that good medical care can be a profitable venture.

2. In 1992, GHAA proceedings of an analysis of outcome of our 5,000 deliveries for CHS enrollees at Hutzel Hospital over a four-year period revealed that the perinatal mortality of CHS enrollees was almost one-half of the perinatal mortality in the rest of Detroit's Wayne County.

3. The services and accomplishments in the care of medicaid patients were the reason behind the visits by Gail Wolinski and Sec. Louis Sullivan.

4. Former president George Bush mentioned CHS as an example of a well-managed health care system for the underprivileged in his budget statement.

5. Many of our senior management officers have been requested to participate in national committees and rash focus, involving quality of care.

6. Several collaborative projects are underway, i.e., with the Michigan Cancer Foundation, to reduce preventable cancer morbidity and mortality.

7. Several teaching affiliations with the health care institutions and schools are underway.

While emphasizing quality, CHS was efficient in providing and controlling costs of services such as:

1. Days: 1,000 was reduced over 20 years.

2. Patients' length of stay was reduced.

3. Special programs, like reduction in cases of hypertension, asthma, lead poisoning in children and other high risk illnesses, now receive special attention.

Medical Ethics

Alvin Bowles, M.D. (Wayne State Univ., 1973, cert. I.M., 1976), is one of Michigan's foremost medical ethicists. While there is not a specialty board for this discipline, advances in medicine are demanding that one be created. Meanwhile, Dr. Bowles is responding to an increasing number of calls from his colleagues to assist in deciding medical ethical issues of increasing importance.

Woman President of DMS and NMA

Alma Rose George, M.D. (Meharry), is a surgeon who grew up in Mound Bayou, Mississippi. Her father practiced family medicine in the town's Taborian Hospital, through which Meharry Medical College's surgical residents rotated when Dr. Matthew Walker was the chief of surgery at Meharry.

This hospital, reportedly one of the first U.S. managed care institutions (see section on Matthew's Disciples), provided Dr.

George with a rich and varied experience upon which she built her professional career in Detroit.

Dr. George became the first female president of the DMS in 1979. It was during her presidency that the DMS purchased the building that had been Dunbar Hospital (1918-1928) to prevent its demolition for "urban renewal." Today, the building serves as the Dunbar Hospital Memorial Museum and DMS headquarters where Wilburn Phillips, former exec. director of Home Federal Savings & Loan Association, assisted with paying off the overdue mortgage of $34,934.

Dr. George also went on to become the third female and the second member of the DMS to become president of the NMA in 1991, preceded by Edith Irby Jones, M.D. (Texas, 1985), Vivian W. Pinn-Wiggins, M.D. (Virginia, 1989), and Lionel Swan, M.D. (Howard, 1967), respectively.

Georgia A. Lewis Johnson, M.D. (Univ. of Mich., 1955), was the first African American woman to be named to the medical school faculty at Michigan State Univ. She has served as a board member, Capital Area Comprehensive Health Planning Association and as chairperson, advisory committee to Community Health Services.

Medical Examiner

Thomas A. Love, Sr., M.D (Univ. of Mich., 1930), was affiliated with the Medical Examiner's office during his medical practice in Detroit. He began his training at the Univ. of Mich. in 1926 and earned a Master's degree in Psychology before transferring to the Medical School in 1930. Tom helped to earn his keep by taking care of his landlady's grounds and working at the ice factory for $10 a month.

He and Dr. Remus Robinson were medical school classmates. Another classmate of his was Bernise Yancey of Atlanta, Ga., who was electrocuted while handling a piece of x-ray equipment during his internship at the Homer G. Phillips Hospital in St Louis, Mo.

Dr. Love was the first African American physician to be hired in Detroit's Medical Examiner's office—a political, civil

317

service, salaried job. Love took courses at the Detroit College of Law to improve his understanding of the legal aspects of the work and wrote many papers related thereto.

He expanded the scope of his involvement with the criminal justice system, especially first offenders. He was generally interested in infant mortality, but more particularly in crib deaths. Dr. Love had planned to continue his studies abroad while accompanying his wife, Josephine, to Europe, but he fell ill and died in 1966, just five weeks before their scheduled departure.

Mrs. Love kept her appointment, spending two years in Cambridge, England at the Institute of Independent Studies, which was then extended to another year in Paris. While there, she fulfilled the obligations of a Radcliffe Harvard scholarship and returned in 1969. She teamed up with Gwen Hogue to launch Your Heritage House Museum, a cultural landmark in the Detroit community.

Dr. Tom Love, Sr. began the private practice of medicine in Detroit in 1933. His hospital work was confined almost exclusively to Woman's (now Hutzel) Hospital. His son, Tom Love, Jr., M.D. (Univ. of Mich.) practices psychiatry.

Migration Southward

Harry Montgomery Nuttall, M.D. (Univ. of Mich., 1904). Unlike other African American physicians, Dr. Nuttall migrated to the South after graduating from medical school and established a practice in Greenville, Ala., because the African American citizens of Greenville offered him more inducements to stay than did the people of other towns.

His practice was, for the most part, rural, African American. White patients would only call at night, so that neighbors would not see him entering their houses.

He visited nearby towns in Alabama and met other physicians who eventually moved to and opened offices in Detroit. Among them were Drs. "Bam" Morton and Alf Thomas, Sr.

Dr. Nuttall met and married Susie Naola Lee, and raised four children during his 14 years in Greenville. Life was not easy for the Nuttalls in Alabama. Vandals bombed his drugstore and he received several threats against his life.

His fortunes changed, somewhat, when industrialist, Henry Ford offered a salary of $5 for an 8-hour day of labor and free railroad passes to get there.

Even Dr. Nuttall's daughter did not know how her father gained control of the distribution of the train tickets to Detroit. Dr. Nuttall passed them on to an African American postman, with the names and addresses of the persons who had agreed to come to Detroit.

The tickets were delivered quietly, and the escapee caught the next train in the next town north of Greenville. Dr. Nuttall helped many improvished cotton-pickers to flee from the ravages of the boll weevil to Detroit's automotive assembly lines. Dr. Nuttall continued distributing train tickets even after he moved to Detroit.

Dr. Nuttall had rented a hotel, on Bagley St. near Grand Circus Park, that was operated by his wife's mother, and provided temporary housing for many of the Greenville migrants until they were able to find permanent places to live in the city.

Eventually, Dr. Nuttall moved his practice to Detroit to catch up with many of his patients who had preceded him. His medical practice was service-oriented. He made house calls, by horse and buggy, often as far as twenty miles away, whether the patients could pay or not.

He is remembered as a breeder of fine horses and Doberman Pinschers.

Charles F. Whitten, M.D., M.D. (Meharry, 1945) spent five years in general medicine (Lackawana, N.Y.) and two in the military (Japan and Korea), before embarking upon an academic, medical career. This began with a year of advanced study in pediatrics at the Univ. of Penn. Graduate School of Med., followed by a two-year residency in pediatrics at the Children's Hospital of Buffalo (N.Y.), and a one-year fellowship in pediatric hematology at Children's Hospital of Michigan. His first academic appointment was instructor in pediatrics at

Wayne State Univ. School of Med., while serving as chief of pediatrics at Detroit Receiving Hospital. In that capacity, he was the first, and as of 1993, the only black physician to serve as department chief in a Detroit hospital.

At Wayne State Univ. School of Medicine, he rose through the ranks and upon retirement, his titles were: distinguished professor of pediatrics and associate dean for curricular affairs (a post he held for 16 years). Currently, he is semi-retired and holds the title of distinguished professor of pediatrics emeritus and associate dean for special programs.

This brief discussion cannot do justice to the enormous productivity of Dr. Whitten's 51-year medical career. But we can highlight several endeavors that made a difference in the lives of those he served, at home and abroad.

In 1960, Dr. Whitten joined with Drs. Robyn Arrington, Horace Bradfield, Ethelene Crockett, Charles Wright and the Hon. Charles C. Diggs to form a trustee board for the African Medical Education Fund which offered financial aid to any qualified African or African American medical student who agreed to provide medical service to Africans in their native land.

During AMEF's 25 years of operation, Dr. Whitten was in charge. He corresponded with the 50 student-recipients from 13 African countries and with the medical faculties with which they matriculated. After a quarter century of successful operation, when the medical education climate in Africa was vastly improved, Dr. Whitten oversaw the orderly closing of the fund and the distribution of its assets between the Dunbar Medical Museum and Detroit's Museum of African American History.

Sickle cell disease is another major area of Dr. Whitten's many human concerns. During his fellowship in pediatric hematology, he was appalled by the extent to which the needs of individuals with sickle cell disease and their families were unmet as compared with those of other chronic diseases. His concern about sickle cell disease crystallized into a life-time determination to improve the quality of life of sickle cell patients.

In 1971, Dr. Whitten enlisted the support of other concerned citizens to form the Sickle Cell Detection and Information Center.

Currently, the organization owns its 18-room office building, has a staff of 22 people, and a budget of $1 million. With the assistance of a board of directors and staff, Dr. Whitten has developed the most comprehensive community program in the country and a unique, state-wide network of social services providers.

Also in 1971, Dr. Whitten obtained funding for and organized a meeting of representatives from 13 other community sickle cell organizations to create the National Association for Sickle Cell Disease (NASCD). The association now has over 80 member organizations. He served as the national president for the next 20 years and although confronted with public apathy, a chronic shortage of funds and other obstacles, he has brought clarity, leadership, and a real sense of purpose to NASCD.

Dr. Whitten developed a wide variety of educational materials, designed training programs, and trained sickle cell trait counselors for the member organizations, the VA hospital system and for organizations in the Bahamas and Virgin Islands. His format for sickle cell trait counseling has become a model for the field.

As the leader of NASCD, he played a major role in the resolution of social, ethical and legal issues related to the implementation of sickle cell screening which was the first national screening program for a genetic disease organization.

In 1973, Dr. Whitten also organized Wayne State Univ.'s Comprehensive Sickle Center, one of only a few such centers in this country. He served as its director from 1973 to 1991, during which time the NIH awarded over $16 million to the center, making it the recipient of the largest grant support in the history of Wayne Univ.

Dr. Whitten is most revered by the medical community because of his post baccalaureate program for black medical students, which he established at Wayne State in 1969. In the late 1960s, U.S. medical schools became more receptive to the admission of black students. Dr. Whitten, though, perceived that there would not be a sufficient number of "qualified" black medical students to fill the available slots. He also believed that there were scores of black students who had the intellectual ability to complete a medical school education, but due to educational and financial disadvantages that had been imposed on them, their academic performances did not reflect their medical school potential and thus they weren't admitted. Based upon this, he believed that a year's remedial and enriching program could render many of them medical school matriculants with excellent potential for success.

Wayne State's administration approved Whitten's concept and plan and in 1969, five individuals were selected to participate in the newly-created, post baccalaureate program. The demanding year of courses in basic sciences, introduction to the freshman medical school curriculum, academic skills development and personal adjustment counseling was free of charge, and the students received a small, monthly stipend.

Eligibility was limited to disadvantaged black residents in Michigan, who had applied and been denied admission to a school of medicine because their prior academic performance placed them in a high risk category for failure. Upon successful completion of the year and completion of all course work with a "B" average, the students were guaranteed admission to Wayne State's medical school.

After six years, the program was doing so well that the School of Medicine offered slots for five additional black students. Currently, the post baccalaureate program admits 14 individuals and has expanded to include other minority, disadvantaged students.

As of the graduating class of 1994, one hhundred forty-three black graduates of Wayne State Univ. entered through the post baccalaureate program. The "Whitten Scholars" helped boost Wayne into second place among the 125 U.S. medical schools (exclusive of Howard and Meharry) for the number of black graduates during the past decade.

In 1991, as a tribute to Dr. Whitten, the WSU School of Med. established a $500,000 "Charles F. Whitten, M.D, Post Baccalaureate Endowment Fund" to expand the program from 14 to 16 students. The fund has been fully subscribed (pledges and

322

contributions). It is a pleasure to report that graduates of the program have pledged/contributed over $240,000 to it. Three graduates have pledged $18,000, and one of them has completed her contribution.

Dr. Whitten has been a dedicated community "servant" as evidenced by his involvement in many organizations and committees at the local, state and national levels. In addition to chairing or serving on a number of university and local, community committees, at the same level, he has chaired the Mich. Dept. of Pub. Health Advisory Committee, the Genetic Disease Committee, the Task Force on Infant Mortality and he co-chaired the Expert Committee on AIDS.

Nationally, he has served on the committees of the American Academy of Pediatrics, the Veterans Administration, the National Academy of Science, the National Institutes of Health and has been the vice president of the American Blood Commission.[4]

In the corporate sector, he served on the board of directors of the Gerber Corporation for 21 years, and the National Bank of Detroit, for five years. Currently, he is also on the board of trustees of Comprehensive Health Service (The Wellness Plan).

Dr. Whitten's academic credentials include over 40 publications in medical journals, co-authorship of a book, five chapters and six presentations at national pediatric research meetings.

---

1. Charles H. Wright, M.D., T. Hershel Gardin, Ph.D. and Carla L. Wright, M.D. "Obstetrical Care in a Health Maintenance Organization and a Fee-For-Service Practice: a Comparative Analysis," *American Journal of Obstetrics and Gynecology,* Vol. 149, No. 8. (August 15, 1984) pp. 848-856.

2. April 23, 1994

Dear Charles Wright,

I'm grateful for the opportunity you have given me to put down in writing my recollections of Addison Prince, one of my best and most satisfying residents I ever worked with. I'm sorry for the long time it has taken me—writing it and getting it on to you. I hope I'm not too late for your publication. Addison was really a great man and his wife, a fine and strong woman. If she is still alive, give her my best regards and also a xerox copy of my signed manuscript (even though my typing is so poor.)

Your letter was very interesting. I'm glad you are compiling brief biographies of the leading African American of this era, as it is something that should be done. Recognition should be given where recognition is due. I really enjoyed my visit to Detroit last June; and Betsy and I speak of it frequently as we recall what a heartwarming celebration it was. I'm so proud of the great advances the department of ob-gyn is making, and it is clear that Dr. Cotton knows what he is about. I got a great kick when I read about the great accomplishment he and his colleagues achieved when they clamped the cord of the "deceased runt" twin in that pregnancy operatively, without precipitating the onset of labor and came out of it with a subsequent labor and the delivery of a healthy and mature other twin. It came from our "little old department!" that you and other good men helped me get started, 46 years ago. Addison also helped to build it in his time.

I'll be interested in learning how your book company comes along. Please keep in touch. Remember me to my old friends and colleagues, as you meet up with them. Take good care of yourself.

As ever, sincerely,

Charles Stevenson

3. It was in September of 1951, when Dr. Prince and Dr. Stevenson met. Dr. Prince, a 1944 graduate of Wayne Univ., had spent the intervening years in an internship, two years in the military and sundry other goal-less medical endeavors in Detroit and New York. His appointment to the obg. residency in 1951, by Dr. Stevenson, came four years after Branch Rickey, manager of the Brooklyn Dodgers, appointed Jackie Robinson to play for the Brooklyn in 1947. Jackie proved himself worthy of Mr. Rickey's trust by winning the National League's Rookie of the Year Award, the first year; its "Most Valuable Player" award his third year; and becoming the first African American to enter Baseball's Hall of Fame, in 1962.

Likewise Dr. Prince fulfilled his promise by becoming a certified specialist in obg. in 1958, taking a graduate degree in public health and providing outstanding medical care to thousands of women for nearly 50 years. Thanks to the Branch Rickeys and Charlie Stevensons of the world, who have the courage and the urge for fairness sufficient to challenge the racists. Thereby, these two men were able to reach their true potential in the service of their fellow human beings. We salute them all!

4. Benjamin Quarles, *The Negro in the Making of America* (New York: McMillan Publishing Co., 1987) p.220.

5. William Loren Katz, *Eyewitness: The Negro in American History*. (New York: Pittman Publishing, 1972) p. 447-448.

6. A social event that honors a naval officer who is promoted from one rank to another.

7. John C. Dancy, *Sands Against the Wind*. (Detroit: Wayne State Univ. Press, 1966) pp. 145-147.

8. *Michigan Chronicle,* July 21, 1993.

325

Detroit's Man and Wife Medical Teams

1. **Darnita Anderson**, D.O., certified g.p. (Mich. State Univ. 1989) to **Gard R. Hill**, D.O., (Philadelphia, 1985) bd. elig., internal medicine.

2. **Charles Baker**, M.D. (Colorado, 1976) board elig., internal med. and oncology) to **Dolores Baker**, M.D. (Colorado) cert. ob-gyn, 1983.

3. **Margaret Betts**, M.D. (Univ. College of Ohio-Toledo, 1977) cert. int. med., 1981 to **Dexter Fields**, M.D. (Wayne State Univ., 1972) cert. in psych., 1977.

4. The Drs. Boddie, M.D. (Meharry, 1906) were the parents of **Arthur Boddie**, M.D. (Meharry, 1935) and **Lewis Boddie**, M.D. (Meharry, 1938). They both began practices in Georgia; she in Augusta, and he in Forsyth. The father died in 1941, The mother moved to Detroit in 1955 and practiced with her son for several years before she died. Both of their sons, Arthur and Lewis, became physicians and practiced medicine in Detroit.

5. **Waldo Cain**, M.D. (Meharry, 1945) to **Natalie Tanner**, M.D. (Meharry, 1945).

6. **James A.U. Carter**, M.D. (Meharry, 1956) to **Carol Pearson**, M.D. (Univ. of Mich., 1956).

7. **Silas D. Cardwell, Jr.**, M.D. (Wayne State Univ.) to **Karen D. Thompson**, M.D. (Wayne State Univ., 1981).

8. **Steven L. Causey**, M.D. (Wayne State Univ., 1986) to **Michelle Hardaway**, M.D.

9. **Ethelene Crockett Jones**, M.D. (Wayne State Univ., 1966) was married to **Sampson Kpadenou**, M.D. (Wayne State Univ., 1972).

10. **Gloria R. Davis**, M.D. (cert. urology) to **Rodney Davis** (Tulane, 1982) cert. urol. 1989.

11. **Peter Dews III**, M.D. (Wayne State Univ., 1986) to **Vivian D. Jones**, M.D. (Wayne State Univ., 1987.)

12. **Iwok S. Essien**, M.D. (Univ. of London, at Ibadan, Nigeria, 1965) cert. obg., 1974; to **Joyce Kirkland**, M.D. (Wayne State Univ. 1971) cert clinical and gross pathol.

13. **Otis B. Ferguson, III**, M.D. (Wayne State Univ., 1988) to **Patricia Brown**, M.D. (Wayne State Univ., 1988).

14. **William R. Ford**, M.D. (Wayne State Univ., 1984) to **Rosemary Donaldson**, M.D. (Wayne State Univ., 1983).

15. **Linda Harris**, M.D. (Univ. of Ill., 1980) cert. in derm. to **William Higginbothan III**, M.D. (Univ. of Ill., 1979).

16. **Karen Heidelberg**, M.D. (Howard Univ., 1993) to **John Maclin Barnwell**, M.D. (Howard Univ., 1989).

17. **Daniel Holloway**, M.D., (surgeon) to **Marsha Johnson**, M.D. (Mich. State) res. in dermatology.

18. **Barbara Jenkins Anderson**, M.D., (Wayne State Univ., 1957) was married to **Sidney Jenkins**, M.D., (Howard Univ., 1951).

19. **Lonnie Joe**, M.D. (Univ. of Mich.) to **Annette Ingram**, M.D., (Univ. of Mich., 1978).

20. **Linda Jones**, M.D. (Mich. State Univ.) to **Percy C. Helem**, M.D.

21. **Lawrence S. Lackey, Jr.**, M.D. (Wayne State Univ., 1987) to **Sandra A. Jones**, M.D., (Wayne State Univ., 1987).

22. **Curtis Longs**, M.D. (Wayne State Univ., 1992) to **Anita Cain**, M.D. (Wayne State Univ., 1991).

23. **Isaure Loomis**, M.D. (Howard Univ., 1988) to **William Yates**, M.D. (Northwestern, 1987).

24. **Veronica Mallett**, M.D. (Mich. State Univ.) cert. obg. 1989; urol., 1992; to **Raymond Jackson**, M.D. (Wayne State Univ., 1979).

25. **Ernest Martin**, M.D. (Mich. State Univ., 1986) to **Susan K. Thrasher**, M.D. (Wayne State Univ., 1986).

26. **Karleton B. Merritt**, M.D. (Wayne State Univ., 1989) to **Karen D. Whitney**, M.D. (Wayne State Univ., 1988).

27. **Anthony A. Miller**, M.D. (Wayne State Univ., 1983) to **Marsha Armstrong**, M.D. (Wayne State Univ., 1983).

28. **Samuel Byron Milton**, M.D. (Howard Univ., 1987) cert. physiatry, 1992; to **Allison Ventura**, M.D. (Howard Univ., 1989) cert. family prac., 1992.

29. **Paul G. Mitchell**, M.D. (Wayne State Univ., 1973) to **Alicia Matthews**, M.D. (Univ. of Mich.) both cert. in med.

30. **Angela D. Mosley**, M.D. (Wayne State Univ., 1987) to **Carl Allen Williams**.

31. **Logan A.Oney**, M.D. (Wayne State Univ., 1975) to **Stephanie M. Lucas**, M.D. (Wayne State Univ., 1972).

32. **David Portee**, M.D. (Univ. of Mich. 1982) cert. in physiatry; to **Virginia Y. Mesa**, M.D. (Univ. Ill., 1982)., cert. public health.

33. **Elliot Roberts**, M.D. (LSU, 1983) cert. obg. 1990; to **Adale Walters**, M.D. (Univ. of Mich. 1983) cert. psychiatry, gen. & chi., both in 1990.

34. **Ronald A. Romear**, M.D. (1986) to **Debra A. Jones**, M.D. (1986).

35. **Neal Ryan**, M.D. to **Barbara Johnson**, M.D. (Univ. of Mich.).

36. **Eugene K. Sawyer**, M.D. (Wayne State Univ., 1978) to **Laura J. Flanagan**, M.D. (Wayne State Univ., 1978).

37 **Franklyn Seabrooks II**, M.D. (Univ. of California, 1988) to **Donna Hinman**, M.D. (Univ. of California, 1991).

38. **Dexter Shurney**, M.D. (Howard Univ., 1983) to **Wanda Whitten, M.D.** (Howard Univ., 1983).

39. **Lydia Sims**, M.D. (Pa., 1985) to **Daryl Peterson**, M.D., (Hanhemann, 1986).

40. **Ernest Singleton**, M.D. (Wayne State Univ., 1973) was married to **Mildred Purifoy**, M.D. (Wayne State Univ., 1975). Ernest, founder of Black Medication Associaton (BMA) died in 1979.

41. **Lynn Smitherman**, M.D. (Cincinnati)to **Herbert Smitherman**, M.D. (Cincinnati 1987).

42. **Frank Jackson**, M.D. (Meharry) to **Alma Rose George** (Meharry).

43. **Joseph C. Verdun**, M.D. (Wayne State Univ., 1985) to **Hariette D. Green**, M.D. (1985).

The Medical Progeny of Detroit's African American Physicians

This centennial report on the stewardship of African American physician provides an opportunity to review their activities since 1895, and assess their contributions to the growth and development of this nation. In this section, special attention is given to physicians and their medical progeny in the Detroit area.

The first African American father and son team to begin this series was Joseph Ferguson, M.D., a member of Detroit College of Medicine's first class, in 1868, and also the father of Joseph Cyrus Ferguson, M.D. (Detroit College of Medicine, 1875). This event did not reoccur until 51 years later, when Chester Ames, M.D., the son of James Ames, M.D. (Howard, 1894) graduated from Wayne Univ. in 1926.

For the years 1927, 1928, 1930, 1931, 1934, 1935, 1936, 1837, 1938, 1942, 1949, 1952, 1953, and 1954, Wayne University produced no African American physicians. In 1926, 1932, 1939, 1941, 1944, 1945, 1948, 1955, 1956, 1960, and 1964, only one African American physician graduated each year.

The African American enrollment began increasing in 1972, with six African American medical graduates, and reached a peak in 1983 when Wayne University awarded 23 African Americans M.D. degrees—thanks in large part to Dr. Whitten's post-baccalaureate program.

Although Wayne's record for training African American physicians has been abominable, it is better than that of the other two state universities; University of Michigan and Michigan State. All three have done even less to assist Native Americans.

According to Dr. Georgia Johnson,[1] black medical graduate of the University of Michigan, the University of

Michigan's Medical School produced approximately 105 African American physicians between 1872 and 1960, an average of less than one each year. Michigan's most productive output was in 1924, 1931, 1941, 1956, 1957, and 1959, with four African American graduates each year. There was none between 1880-1885, 1885-1888, 1917-1921, 1962-1965 and 1977-1984.[2] Despite these impediments, our medical progeny have done rather well.

My original goal was to look at all of the physicians' children in this group. When that goal proved far too ambitious for one person to undertake, I lowered my sights to include only the offspring who chose medicine as a profession. Occasionally, a child, whose profession is closely related to medicine, is also included. Despite my best efforts, a few may have escaped my probe. As you can surmise, the search has not been easy.

Although the medical parent or relative is the person of reference in the accompanying commentary, full recognition and appreciation of the contributions of the other parent can be safely assumed. Another weakness of this study is that it involves a very small portion of the total product. While I have no doubt that the findings are representative of the whole, an expanded sampling will be most welcome.

For those who depend on the news media for information on what is happening in the African American community, this group will seem like strangers; but not anymore. They have been here all the time and, as you will see, taking care of business.

James Ames, M.D. (Howard, 1894) gen. prac., was the father of:
> 1. Chester Ames, M.D., (Wayne State Univ., 1926); first African American intern in Detroit, 1926; first African American resident (urology), 1927-29; and first member of a medical faculty (urology); all at Wayne Univ. Medical College.[3]

Barbara Jenkins Anderson, M.D. (Wayne State, 1957) cert. gross and clinical pathology, 1966; Alpha Omega Alphga, Hon. Society; and Sidney Jenkins, M.D., (Howard, 1951) cert. psych., 1957; are the parents of:

1. Judith Jenkins Kelly, M.D., (Wayne State Univ., 1983) cert. anesth., 1988

William G. Anderson, D.O. (Des Moines, 1956) cert. surg., 1967; is the father of:
1. William G. Anderson II, D.O., (Mich. State) cert. obg.
2. Darnita Anderson-Hill, D.O., (Mich. State) cert. family practice

Robyn J. Arrington, Sr. M.D. (Meharry, 1939) was the father of:
1. Robyn J. Jr., M.D., (Howard Univ., 1972) bd. elig. obg.
2. Harold, M.D. (Univ. of Mich, 1972) cert. obg., 1978[4]

Ovid Bledsoe, Sr., M.D. (Meharry, 1912) was the father of:
1. Ovid Bledsoe, Jr., M.D. (Meharry, 1945)

Ovid Bledsoe, Jr. M.D. (Meharry, 1945) was the father of:
1. Karen Letta Bledsoe, M.D. (Cincinnati, 1987) int. med.

William F. Boddie, M.D., and Luetta Boddie, M.D. (both Meharry, 1906), were the parents of:
1. Arthur W. Boddie, Sr., M.D. (Meharry, 1935)
    1.1 Arthur Boddie Jr., M.D. (Yale, 1967) cert. surgical oncology, 1974, practicing in Chicago.
2. Lewis Boddie, M.D. (Meharry, 1938) cert. in obg. 1949; is the father of:
    2.1 Kenneth W. Boddie, M.D. (UCLA, 1978) cert. physiat. 1985.
    2.2 Bernice Boddie Jackson, M.D. (UCLA, 1978). Although she completed two-years of residency in orthopedic surgery, she is no longer in active practice.

Horace Bradfield, M.D. (Wayne Univ., 1948) cert. family practice 1977. He was the nephew of:
1. John Cyrus Bradfield M.D. (Starling Medical College; Lima, Ohio). He is also the uncle of:
2. Steven Davenport, M.D. (Yale, 1980) cert. orthop. sur., 1990[5]

James Brown, M.D. (Meharry, 1962) is the father of:
1. Dana Brown, M.D. (Meharry, 1990) res. psych., 1991

Samuel A. Brown, M.D. (Howard) was the father of:
1. Kenneth Brown, M.D. (Case Western, 1958) cert. urol., 1967; and also the grandfather of:
    1.1. Leslie A. Brown, M.D. (Stanford, 1987) cert. ophth., 1992

D.T. Burton, M.D. (Meharry, 1921) was the father of:
1. Gail Burton, M.D. (N.Y.U., 1961) bd. elig. in. psychiatry; was also the grandfather of:
    1.1. Cal Dudley, M.D. (Meharry 1980) cert. psych. 1992
2. Alicia Heron, M.D. (Univ. of Mich., 1974) gen. prac.
3. Alva Heron, M.D. (Meharry, 1976) gen. prac.[6]

John Butler, M.D. (Meharry, 1937) bd. elig. in derm. is the father of:
1. David Napier Butler, M.D. (Wayne 1990) Now a teaching fellow, in gastroent. at Chicago Med. School; and also the uncle of:
2. James Butler, M.D. (Meharry, 1958) cert. ophthal. 1965

James A. Carter, M.D. (Meharry, 1956) and Carol Pearson, M.D. (Univ. of Mich.) cert. psych., 1964 and child psychiatry, 1967; are parents of:
1. Lynne Carter, M.D. (Mich. State Univ., 1994)

Joseph Rush Tanner M.D. (Meharry Med. Coll., 1921) was the father of:
1. Natalia Tanner Cain, M.D. (Meharry, 1945) cert. ped. 1951.

Waldo Cain, M.D. (Meharry, 1945) cert. surg, 1952; and Natalia Tanner Cain, M.D. (1945) cert. ped., 1951; are the parents of:
1. Anita Cain Longs, M.D. (Wayne State Univ., 1991) res. int. med., 1991

Albert B. Cleage, M.D. (Indiana, 1910) was the father of:
1. Louis J. Cleage, M.D. (Wayne Univ., 1940);[7] and also the grandfather of:

     1.1 Ernest Just Martin, M.D. (Mich. State, 1986) cert. gen. psych. and forensic psych.

     1.2 Marie Shreve Nicolai, M.D. (Univ. of Mich. 1987) cert. FP.

Volna Clermont, M.D (Port Au Prince Med. School, Haiti, 1949) cert. ped., 1966; is the father of:

     1. Kimberly Jean Clermont, M.D. (Howard, 1983) cert. int. med., 1989; emerg. med., 1994

James Collins, Sr. M.D. (Univ. of Mich. 1953) cert. ped., 1958; is the father of:

     1. James Collins, Jr., M.D. (Univ. of Mich. 1983) cert. ped.; sub spec. neonat., 1986.[8]

Ethelene Crockett, M.D. (Howard Univ., 1945) cert. obg. 1955; was the mother of:

     1. Ethelene Crockett Jones, M.D. (Wayne State Univ., 1966) cert. in obg., 1974[9]

David Danley, M.D. (Meharry, 1960) is the father of:

     1. Leslie Danley, M.D. (Wayne State Univ., 1998)

Leonard Ellison, Sr., M.D. (Univ. of Mich., 1962) cert. psychiatry is the father of:

     1. Leonard Ellison, Jr., M.D. (Wayne State Univ., 1997.)

Muriel J. Espy, M.D. (Meharry) cert. obg. 1982, is daughter of:

     1. Theodore Espy, M.D. (Meharry, 1940); and the sister of:

     2. Francis Espy Rankin, M.D. (Howard 1969) cert. psychiatry, 1977

Joseph Ferguson, M.D. (Det. College of Med., 1868) was father of:

     1. John Cyrus Ferguson, M.D. (Det. College of Med., 1875); and also great, great, grandfather of:

       1.2. Lorna Lacen Thomas, M.D. (Univ. of Mich., 1983) cert. dermat. 1988

Thomas M. Flake, Sr., M.D. (Wayne Univ., 1951) cert. surg., 1958; is the father of:

1. Thomas M. Flake, Jr., M.D. (Wayne State Univ., 1979) cert. surg., 1988[10]

John Earl Franklin, Sr., M.D. (Univ. of Mich., 1953) bd. elig. in surgery; is father of:
1. John Earl, Jr., M.D. ((Univ. of Mich., 1980) cert. gen. and drug abuse psychiatry, 1985
2. Paula Dawn, M.D. (Univ. of Mich., 1992) in training

Alma Rose George, M.D. (Meharry, 1960), is the daughter of:
1. Phillip Moiser George M.D. (Meharry, 1926). She was the third woman to become president of NMA, 1991.

George Gibson, D.O. (Philadelphia, 1972) bd. elig. in obg. is the father of:
1. Cheryl Gibson, M.D. (Univ. of Vt., 1985) cert. obg., 1991

Donald Givens Sr., M.D. (Indiana, 1924) was the father of:
1. Donald Givens, Jr., M.D. (Univ. of Mich. 1961) bd. elig. int. med.

Alegro Godley, M.D. (Univ. of Mich., 1948) cert. int med. 1955; recert., 1979; is the father of:
1. Jo Ann Godley, M.D. (Yale, 1977) cert. int med., 1980, with sub-spec., gastroent., 1989
2. Paul Godley, M.D. and masters in public policy (both at Harvard, 1984) bd. elig. hematol. oncol., Ph.D. "Epidemiology of Prostate Cancer" and assoc. prof. pub. health, at Univ. of N.C., Chapel Hill.
3. Bernard Godley, Ph.D. (M.I.T. 1987) neuro-endocrine physiology, M.D. (Harvard, 1989) bd. elig. ophthal.

William Goins, M.D. (Wayne State Univ., 1941) cert. obg. 1950; was the grandfather of:
1. Kim Fletcher, M.D. (M.L. King-U.C.L.A.) res. emerg. med., 1991
2. Candice Kumasi, M.D. (Univ. of Mich., 1993)
3. Lisa Thompson, M.D. (Case Western, 1994)

Herman Gray Sr., M.D. (Boston) was the father of:
1. Herman Gray, Jr., M.D. (Univ. of Mich., 1976) cert. pediatrics, 1981

William Goodwin, M.D. (Howard, 1943) cert. X-ray, 1958; is the father of:
1. William Goodwin, Jr., M.D. (Meharry, 1975) cert. family practice
2. Jimmy Goodwin, M.D. (Howard) cert. X-ray

Thomas Green II, M.D. (Meharry, 1954) was the father of:
1. Jennifer Green Stevens, M.D. (Howard)
2. Thomas Green, III, M.D. (Howard) cert. cardiac anesth, 1991

Arthur Drayton Harris, Sr., M.D. (Wayne, 1946) cert. obg. 1952; was the father of:
1. Arthur Drayton, Jr., M.D. (Wayne State Univ., 1980) anesth. Los Angeles.
2. Edmund D., M.D. (Wayne State Univ., 1980) cert. radiol., 1986, Laredo, Tx.
3. Brian W. M.D. (Wayne State Univ., 1987) fp., Monterey, Calif.)

Robert Heidelberg, M.D. (Howard 1965) cert. 1972 dermat.; is the father of:
1. Karen Heidelberg Barnwell, M.D. (Howard, 1993) res., derm., Mayo Clinic, 1994

Laurence Hicks, M.D. (Meharry, 1950) G.P.; was the father of:
1. Lauren Barton, M.D. (Meharry, 1980) cert. general practice

Horace Holloway, M.D. (Meharry, 1944) is the father of:
1. Diedre Holloway Waterman, M.D. (Meharry, 1970) cert. ophthal. 1976
2. Daniel Holloway, M.D. (Mich State) bd. elig., in surgery
3. Linda Holloway Helem, M.D. (Meharry) bd. elig. in pathology. She is no longer in active practice.

Melvin L. Hollowell, M.D. (Meharry, 1959) cert. urol.; is the father of:
1. Christopher Hollowell, M.D. (Wayne State Univ., 1993) urol. res., Univ. of Miami.

2. Courtney Hollowell, M.D. (Illinois) senior, Markle (honorary) scholar at the Univ. of Ill., in a combined DPH-M.D. program; and

3. Sylvia K. Hollowell, M.D. (Wayne State Univ., 1996)

Garnet Ice, M.D. (Wayne State Univ., 1943) cert. surg. 1957; was the father of:

1. Anne-Marie Ice, M.D. (Howard, 1970) cert. ped. 1975

Georgia Johnson, M.D. (Univ. of Mich., 1955) is the mother of:

1. Barbara, M.D. (Univ. of Mich, 1985) cert. child psych. 1990

2. Mary, M.D. (Univ. of Mich.) cert. internal medicine)

Georgia A. Lewis Johnson, M.D. (Univ. of Mich., 1955) is the mother of:

1. Mary Margaret, M.D. (Univ. of Mich., 1984) cert. internal medicine, 1988

2. Barbara Ann, M.D. (Univ. of Mich., 1985) cert. adult & child psychology

Levi Johnson, M.D. (Univ. Heidelberg, Germany) was the father of:

1. Albert Henry, M.D. (Det. College of Med., 1893), and also the great, grandfather of (twins):
    - 1.1. Kelly A. Colden, M.D.
    - 1.2. Kimberly Colden, M.D. (Wayne, 1993) obg. residents in Wayne State Univ. program. They graduated from Wayne 100 years after their grandfather, Albert.

Arnold Jones M.D. (Meharry, 1954) cert. surg., 1962; is the father of:

1. Camille A. Jones, M.D. (Case Western Reserve, 1982) cert int. med., 1985, masters public health, Johns Hopkins, 1987, cert. preventive medicine, 1991. Current employment: director, epidemiology program, division of kidney, urologic and hematologic diseases at the National Institute of Diabetes and Digestive and Kidney Diseases, July 1991-present

2. Camara Phyllis Jones, M.D. (Stanford, 1981) M.S. in Pub. Health), cert. FP. 1986. Ph.D in 1994. She joined

the Harvard Medical Faculty of the School of Public Health, in 1994; and

    3. Clara Yvonne Jones, M.D. (Harvard, 1981) cert. IM (1984) med. dir. Samaritan Village, Inc. N.Y., April 1993-present. faculty, internal medicine track of the residency programs in social medicine, Montefiore Medical Center, July 1984-present.

William Kyle, M.D. (Meharry, 1952) cert. surg., 1965; is the father of:

    1. Kevin Kyle, M.D. (Wayne, 1987) cert. IM and pul. med.

Lawrence Lackey, Sr., M.D. (Kansas, 1952) geriat. was the father of:

    1. Lawrence Lackey Jr., M.D. (Wayne State Univ., 1987) bd. elig. int med.[11]

George Lightbourn, M.D. (Meharry, 1963) cert. urol. 1972; is father of:

    1. Andrea Lightbourn, M.D. (Wayne, 1983) cert. obg.

Ronald Little, M.D. (cert. orth.) is the father of:

    1. Brian Little, M.D. (Wayne State Univ., 1998)

John Loomis, M.D. (Univ. of Mich., 1957) cert. surg., 1966; is the father of:

    1. Isaure Loomis Yates, M.D. (Howard. 1987) cert. g.p., 1992

    2. John Loomis, Jr., M.D. (Univ. of Mich., 1994)[12]

Thomas Love, Sr., M.D. (Univ. of Mich., 1930); was father of:

    1. Thomas A. Love, Jr., M.D. (Univ. of Mich., 1972) bd. elig. psych.

Hayward C. Maben, Sr., M.D. (Meharry, 1945) cert. gen. surg. and thoracic surg, 1975; is the father of:

    1. Hayward Maben, II, M.D. (Meharry, 1986) bd. elig. in anes.

H. G. McCall, Sr., M.D. (Univ. of Mich., 1921) was the father of:

    1. H. G. McCall, Jr., M.D. (Univ. of Mich., 1959) cert. ophth. 1968.

339

Samuel B. Milton III, M.D. (Howard, 1987) cert. physiatry. 1992; is the son of:

1. Samuel B. Milton, Jr., hospital adm., (Univ. of Mich., 1963), and grandson of Sam B. Milton Sr., M.D. (Univ. of Chicago) and Dr. Hollis.

Silas Norman, Jr., M.D. (Wayne State Univ., 1976) Cert IM., 1983; med dir. of Wayne County Jail; is the father of:

1. Silas P. Norman, M.D. (Wayne State Univ., 1996), Alpha Omega Alpha Hon. Society, and
2. Joseph W. Norman, M.D. (Stanford, 1996) M.D-Ph.D. program.

David Northcross, Sr., M.D. and Daisy Northcross, M.D. (Meharry 1906) were the parents of:

1. David Northcross, Jr., M.D. (Meharry 1945), and the grandparents of:
   1.2. Gale Northcross, M.D. (Uniform Armed Services Med. School)

Elihu Potts, M.D. (Howard, 1950) cert. obg. 1963; is father of:

1. Elihue Jr., DDS, (Howard, 1982)
2. Michael Peter, M.D. (Howard, 1984), cert. IM. 1991
3. Kevin Elihue (Howard, 1997).

Maurice Potts, M.D. (Meharry, 1964) bd. elig., obg.; is brother of Elihue Potts, M.D. and the father of:

1. Maurice Potts, Jr., M.D. (Guadalahara, Mex. 1988)
2. Eric K. Potts, medical student at Guadalahara, Mex.

Addison Prince, M.D. (Wayne State Univ., 1944) cert. obg. 1958, M.P.H., 1974; was the father of:

1. Christopher Prince, M.D. (Wayne State Univ., 1982) EM

Frank Raiford, Sr., M.D. (Univ. of Mich., 1917) was the father of:

1. Frank Raiford, III, M.D. (Univ. of Mich., 1943) cert. FP, 1974-1978, recert.

Joseph Rucker, Sr., M.D. (Meharry) is the father of:

1. Joseph Rucker, Jr., M.D. (Mich. State Univ., 1979) cert. PIS, 1986
2. Kenneth Rucker, M.D. (Mich. State Univ.)

Benjamin Franklyn Seabrooks, M.D. (Meharry, 1929) was the father of:

    1. Franklyn Seabrooks, M.D. (Meharry 1962) cert. obg., 1969, and also the grandfather of:

        1.1. Franklyn II, M.D. (Univ. of California, San Francisco, 1988) bd. elig. orthos.

Robert Sims, D.O. (Des Moines, Iowa 1964) is the father of:

    1. Lydia Sims Peterson, M.D. (Penn., 1985) cert. obg, 1990

    2. Leslie Sims, M.D. (Yale 1989) bd. elig. ophthal.

Alf Thomas, Sr., M.D. (Meharry, 1904) served as president of the Allied/Detroit Medical Society for 10 years and was the founder of at least four hospitals. He was the father of:

    1. Alf Thomas, Jr., M.D. (Meharry, 1937)[13]

Joseph T. Thomas, Sr., M.D. (Meharry) was the father of:

    1. Joseph T. Thomas, Jr., M.D. (Meharry) and was closely related to the Thomas' Lorna Thomas, M.D. (Univ. of Mich, 1981) cert. derm. is the great, great, granddaughter of Joseph Ferguson, M.D. (Det. College of Med., 1868), the school's first class

W.A. Thompson, M.D. (Meharry, 1912) was the father of:

    1. Arthur L. Thompson, M.D. (Meharry, 1942) cert. ped., 1956.

Clarence Vaughn, M.D (Meharry) is the father of:

    1. Steven B. Vaughn, M.D. (Wayne State Univ., 1981) cert. IM. 1986

    2. Annette C. Vaughn, M.D. (Wayne State Univ., 1984)

Charles Vincent, M.D. (Wayne State Univ., 1958) cert. obg. 1966. cert. gen. surg. 1971, is the father of:

    1. Charles H. Vincent III, M.D. (Boston Univ., 1986) cert. otolar., 1992. He is also the uncle of;

    2. Gilford S. Vincent, M.D. (Wayne State Univ., 1979) cert. gen. surg and vas. surg., 1986, and is also the cousin of;

    3. James W. Stubbs, Jr., M.D. (Wayne State Univ., 1980) cert. obg, 1988. Also the cousin of;

    4. Richard Arnold Roy, M.D. (Buffalo, 1980, cert. ped. 1987.

Charles Whitten, M.D. (Meharry, 1945) cert. ped., is the father of:
    1. Wanda Whitten-Shurney, M.D. (Howard 1983) cert. pediatrics, 1987.

Delford G. Williams, Jr., M.D. (Howard, 1945) FP., is the father of:
    1. Delford III, M.D. (Univ. of Mich., 1977) cert. vas. surg., 1983
    2. David, M.D. (Meharry, 1980) bd. elig. int med.
    3. Donna L., D.V.M., private practice in Mobile, Al.

W.A. Williamson, M.D. (Howard, 1954) was the father of:
    1. Ronald Williamson, M.D. (Mich. State, 1982) cert. FP.
    2. Cheryl W. Basden, D.O., (Mich. State, 1985) cert. F.P. 89
    3. Derrick Williamson, D.O., (Mich State, 1985) cert. FP.

Charles H. Wright, M.D. (Meharry, 1943) cert. obg. 1955, is the father of:
    1. Carla Wright, M.D. (Univ. of Mich., 1982) cert. physiat., 1988
    2. Stephanie Wright Griggs, MHA, Geo. Wash. U. Mem,. A.C.H.E., Cook County Hosp., Chicago.

Rudolph Wyatt, M.D. (Kansas 1953) cert. obg. 1961, is the father of:
    1. Rhonda Ann Wyatt, M.D. (Uniform Med. Service, 1982) cert. radiol., 1986 and nuclear med, 1992

Watson Young, M.D. (Univ. of Mich., 1942) is the father of:
    1. Aundree Noretee Young, M.D. (Univ. of Mich. 1973) cert. ped. 1989

---

1. Georgia A. Johnson, *Black Medical Graduates of the University of Michigan (1872-1960)*. (Lansing: Georgia A. Lewis Johnson Publication Co., 1994) P.O. Box 4796, Lansing, MI 48826.

2. Insofar as I have been able to ascertain, neither the University of Michigan nor Michigan State's Medical School has now or has ever had an African American physician as a tenured professor on its staff.

3. James W. Ames, a native of New Orleans, attended Straight University before entering Howard Univ. Medical School. After setting up an medical office in Detroit, he married the daughter of

Detroit businessman, James Cole, who bore him four children, one of whom, Chester, also became a physician.

Active in Republican politics, Dr. Ames became a precinct delegate, was elected to the House of Representatives of the Michigan Legislature in 1900, and was on the medical staff of Detroit Board of Health for 10 years. His influence in medical circles was a boost for Chester to become the first African American intern, resident and member of Wayne's medical faculty.

(John M. Green, *Michigan Manual of Freedmen's Progress,* Freedmen's Progress Commission. Detroit: 1915) p. 85.

4. Both doctors selected the Army National Guard rather than the regular army draft, after graduation from medical school. After nearly a quarter of a century of military training, their bearing and demeanor reflect that experience. Both are full colonels, Robyn is state surgeon and Harold is the commander of the Michigan National Guard Hospital, a mobile unit that can be flown to any place on earth and made operable in 48 hours. He was in command of such a unit during the Gulf War when the Iraqi bomb exploded that caused the largest number of allied casualties of that entire war. They are on alert at all times. (Personal interview)

5. John Cyrus Bradfield was named for John Cyrus Ferguson, the son of Joseph Ferguson, M.D., Michigan's first certified African American physician, to whom he was related. Dr. C. Bradfield was remembered in Lima, Oh., with a recreational facility named in his honor.

6. The D.T. and Alice Burton families were dominant figures in African American medicine, locally and nationally, during most of the 20th century. During our interview, Mrs. Burton estimated that the number, from both sides, approaches 100. When she began naming them, I assured her that the number was not in question but my time was.

7. Dr. Louis J. Cleage died in 1994 in Anderson, S.C., at the age of 81.

8. James Collins, Sr., was the token pediatrician appointed to the staff of Harper Hospital to prevent work stoppage on the Detroit Medical Center, in 1962.

9. Dr. Ethelene Crockett, unable to find a residency in obg. after her internship, entered general practice in Detroit in 1946, until a residency became available in New York's Sydenham Hospital in 1952. She closed her office, made special arrangements to accommodate her lawyer husband, George, and their three children and took a three-year leave.

The Sydenham Hospital residency was supplemented by additional training at Detroit's Herman Kiefer Hospital before certification in 1955. Despite a brilliant career, professionally, and otherwise, Ethelene was never able to overcome, fully, the impediments of race and a patchwork residency; sex, the first African American woman obg. in Detroit; and politics, the name Crockett has dogged the steps of the entire family, since George opposed President Truman's cold war policies, 1947.

10. Dr. Thomas Flake Sr. was the first African American to be completely trained as a certified surgeon in Detroit's University system. Although the professors who certified him as a surgeon at the end of his residency accepted his European American classmates on the staff at Harper, they rejected Dr. Flake's application for staff membership in 1957, because of his color. In 1961, forced by a federal government threat to stop the Medical Center development by the Federal Government, Harper's officials accepted a token of four African American physicians. Dr. Flake was chosen in surgery.

    Besides Dr. Flake, the three others who sneaked in under the Medical Center dispensation were: Drs Addison Prince (obg.) who had graduated from Wayne Univ. in 1944; James Collins (Ped) who had graduated from Univ. of Mich. in 1953; and, Dr. William Gibson (Med) who earned his M.D. degree at Howard Univ. in 1949. This was followed by a four-year residency in medicine at Harvard University and an additional year in a cardiac subspecialty at Beth Israel Hospital in New York. (personal interviews with Drs Flake and Collins.)

11. Lawrence Lackey, Sr., M.D., was a pioneer in the budding field of geriatrics, before it became a fully certifiable specialty. Although his sphere of private hospital practice was confined to Sumby and Outer Drive Hospitals, as president of the DMS during the height of the Civil Rights Movement, Lackey's uncompromising opposition to hospital segregation was respected throughout the Detroit Medical Center. One of the many beneficiaries from his efforts is his son, Dr. Lawrence Lackey, Jr., M.D. (Wayne State Univ., 1987). Following his residency in int. med., Dr. Lackey, Jr. was appointed asst. clinical prof. of int. medicine at Wayne State University Medical School and Asst. Program Director of the medical department at Grace Hospital. Sandra Jones Lackey, M.D. (Wayne, 1987), Dr. Lawrence Lackey Jr's wife, is a full-time contract physician in the medical department at Grace Hospital. These positions were offered by the medical institutions, not sought by the individuals.

12. Loomis was first African American intern at Harper Hospital (1957-58). He received a surgical residency in 1958. Harper officials referred to him often in their efforts to prevent the stoppage of the

Medical Center development. Later, his surgical residency was interrupted by a military draft, and he was unable to resume it after the war. He completed his training at Receiving Hospital.

13. After serving an internship at Eloise Hospital in Eloise, Mi., Alf Jr. took over the operation of the Thomas Hospitals. It was the younger Alf's impatient plea, "come on fellas, let's raise some real money" after the brutal murder of Dr. Tom Brewer in Columbus, Ga., in 1956 that gave birth to the NAACP's Freedom Fund dinners in Detroit that same year.

The first Freedom Fund Dinner earned $27,007.64. The 1994 dinner took in more than $1,178,578. During that 38-year span, the total gross amount raised through NAACP Freedom Fund Dinners was $14.3 million.

Epilogue

This has been a most troubling story to write about as it has been to live through. Our first century has been beset by impediments that must be removed or avoided, at all costs, during NMA's second century and the nation's twenty-first.

It seems quite clear that "business as usual" is not serving our, nor the nation's needs, and we must change our way of doing things. One place to begin such changes is within ourselves. We must ask, "What can I do to make a difference to the people I serve? How can I become more accountable?" A diligent search for meaningful answers to such questions leaves little time for finger-pointing and scapegoating. "We must keep our hands on the plow, and hold on, Hold On!"

After a careful review of my options to try to make a difference, I have decided to make a $5.00 rebate to the alumni organizations of the four African American medical schools (Howard, King-Drew, Meharry or Morehouse) for each alumnus, of that school, who buys a copy of my book. This offer is good for the remainder of NMA's anniversary year.

Chronic underfunding of these institutions can be a factor in poor pupil performance, declining prestige of the schools and many other such debilitating influences.

At the turn of the century, when other medical schools were faced with similar problems, the American Medical Association entered into a unilateral agreement with Abraham Flexner (see The Gospel, According to Abraham, page 87) who investigated, evaluated, and, ultimately, closed those institutions which he decided were "unsalvageable."

Little or no effort was exerted to improve the quality of those, much maligned, medical schools, nor was there any significant effort to alter the discriminatory policies of the "approved" medical schools to encourage them to continue the training of the best qualified students, and there were many, from Flexner's "unsalvageable" medical schools.

While there remains sufficient time to prevent a repetition of a similar catastrophe already in the making, remedial measures are urgently needed if we are ever to bring our physician/patient ratio closer to the national average. This rebate offer is my effort to make a difference in this area of acute financial need.

The presence of thousands of Cubans refugees, in the Greater Miami area, is creating acute economic, political, and social problems with explosive potential for many Miamians, immigrant and native-born. An earlier section of this book "The Cuban Physicians," provides some background information on the growth and development of cold war issues in that region that have worsened with the passage of time. [1]

An alarm was sounded by a Public Radio alert, early in 1995. It offered food for thought and cause for action, before it is too late for remedial measures.

The radio reporter disclosed that in some sections of Miami, the primary language is Spanish. The first and foremost requirement for securing a job, in that region, is a working knowledge of Spanish, no matter what other skills are offered. The Cuban issue is being raised, here, because it remains a bone of contention in our struggles for equal opportunity in the medical market place.

Since 1960, the AMA has played a major role in creating this hemispheric crisis. Now, it must devote some of those same resources to finding a solution, while there is yet time.

Since, mid-May, the fuse that was already ignited and fueled by memories, police, military mistreatment of African Americans and Haitians, the snubbing of Mr. Nelson Mandela, in 1992 and a shameless, preferential treatment for Cubans has become more threatening.

According to several articles in the *Wall Street Journal*, during the summer of 1995, many of Miami's "Anglos" have fled to Fort Lauderdale. The *Miami Herald*, in its reach for balanced, objective reporting is becoming the object of increasing immigrant frustration. As has already been the case in Guatemala, Grenada, Nicaragua, Vietnam, Zaire, and many other scenes of U.S., cold war misadventures, the chickens, in Little

Havana, Fla. seem headed home to roost.[2] Time may not be on the AMA's side.

A review of the South African phase of this international drama reveals that Dr. Wendy Orr, a graduate of a medical school of the South African Medical Association, is of British lineage. The daughter of Rev. Robert Orr, a Presbyterian minister, she practices a unique pattern of fearless courage that her father preaches, "the Fatherhood of God and the brotherhood on man."

After graduation from medical school, she was assigned to work as a junior district surgeon, treating African activists who had been assaulted by the South African security police.

Infuriated when her complaints about their mistreatment to her superior officers, Drs. Lang and Tucker, Steve Biko's former doctors were ignored, she turned up the valve by joining protest demonstrations with the relatives of her African patients.[3]

Her next move was to complain to South Africa's Supreme Court, the first South African to protest against security police brutality. She was criticized by the SAMA's Secretary-General and the AMA's choice for membership on the WMA's Ethics Committee, Dr. Viljoen. He raised the question of perjury, if she gave the Supreme Court false testimony.

Undaunted, Dr. Orr persisted and prevailed. The Supreme Court issued its first restraining order against the security police, but Dr. Orr was, promptly, transferred from patient care to supervising old age homes. Evidence that the Court's restraint order was obeyed was not evident.[4]

Some South African physicians, including Dr. B.T. Naidoo, of Indian descent, came to her support by resigning from membership in the South African Medical Association. A South African Psychiatric Association cited her for her courage.

Dr. Naidoo expressed displeasure that the Medical and Dental Council had exonerated all of the doctors who had been involved in Steve Biko's murder. "That cast a slur on the entire South African medical profession." The Association hoped that others "would follow her example."

The outlook for the NMA's second century and the well-being of this entire nation would be improved by a meaningful apology from the AMA for their aggressive actions, for the past century and a half, at home and abroad. A radical reorganization of that body will require considerably more than the election of their first African American, Dr. Peter Marshall Murray, to their House of Delegates in 1949,[5] and Dr. Lonnie Bristow, as their first African American president in 1995, the 148th year since they came on line, in 1847.[6]

Mr. Mandela would do well to consider Dr. Orr for a position in South Africa's Justice Department. She has earned the right and demonstrated the courage that she will help to establish a future policy of justice and fair play in a country where these issues have also, until quite recently, been in short supply.

1. U.S. Policy on Cuba Has Exiles in Miami Hungry for Change, *Wall Street Journal,* June 2, 1995.

2. *Ibid.*

3. *The Sowetonian,* October 6, 1985, and The Associated Press.

4. Benson, Mary. (1986). *Nelson Mandela,* Penguin Books, 242.

5. Dr. Peter Marshall Murray had been president of the NMA in 1932 and was chairman of the department of gynecology at New York's Harlem Hospital when he was elected to the AMA's House of Delegates. One of his first duties that year was to attend Detroit's NMA convention and try to get their membership to support AMA's opposition to Medicare. His efforts were opposed, and defeated, by Dr. W. Montague Cobb, who approved the NMA's support of the measure.

6. *The Detroit Free Press,* June 20, 1995.

Bibliography

Allen, James, *Reconstruction. The Battle for Democracy, 1865-1876.*

Black Americans in Congress, 1870-1989

Boggs, James. *The American Revolution: Pages from A Negro Worker's Notebook.* New York: Monthly Review Press, 1963

Bordley III, M.D., J. & Harvey, A.M., M.D. *Two Centuries of American Medicine, 1776-1976.* Philadelphia: W.B. Saunders Co. 1976.

Blaustein, Albert P. & Zangrando, Robert. *Civil Rights and the American Negro. A Documentary History.* Washington Square Press, New York, 1968.

Boykin, Ulysses. *A Handbook on the Detroit Negro.* Detroit; Minority Study Associates.

Catlin, George. *The Story of Detroit, The Evening News Association, Detroit, Michigan,* 1926. Chicago: The Lakeside Press.

Cobb, William Montague. *The First Negro Medical Society, 1939.*

Comejo, Peter. *Racism, Revolution, Reaction 1861-1877, The Rise and Fall of Radical Reconstruction.* Monad Press, New York, 1976.

Congressional Research Service. *The U.S. Government and the Vietnam War, Part 1, 1845-1963.* April 19 U.S. Government Printing Office

Dancy, John. *Stand Against the Wind.* Detroit: Wayne State University Press.

Davis, David B. *The Problem of Slavery in the Age of the Revolution: 1770-1823.* Ithaca and London: Cornell University Press, 1975.

Detroit in Perspective, A Journal of Regional History. Vol. 1, No. 2, 1973, The Detroit Historical Society.

Detroit in Perspective, A Journal of Regional History, Vol 2 No. 3, 1976, p 189. The Detroit Historical Society.

Dubois, W.E.B. *Against Racism: Unpublished Essays, Papers Addresses, 1887-1961.* Amherst, Mass: The University of Massachussets Press, 1985.

Dubois, W.E.B., *A Reader.* New York: Meyer Weinberg Harper Wow, Publishers, 1970.

Dubois W.E.B. *Black Reconstruction in America 1860 -1880.* West Hanover, Mass: Athenaeum Press, 1935

Dumond, Dwight L. *Antislavery-The Crusade for Freedom in America.* Ann Arbor: The University of Michigan Press, 1961

Editors of Ebony Magazine. *The Ebony Handbook.* Chicago: Johnson Publishing Company, Inc., 1974.

Fleming, C. James & Burchel, Christian E., *Who's Who in Colored America.* 7th Edition, Yonkers-on-Hudson, N.Y.: Christian E. Burckel & Associates 1950.

Franklin, John Hope, and Moss Jr. Alfred A. *From Slavery to Freedom,* Alfred A Knopf, 1987.

Genovese, Eugene D. *The World the Slaveholders Made.* New York: Vintage Books, 1971.

Guzman, Jessie P. *Negro Year Book. A Review on Events Affecting Negro Life 1941-1946.* The Department of Records and Research Tuskegee Institute, Alabama.

Higginbotham Jr., A. Leon. *In a Matter of Color.* New York: Oxford University Press, 1978

Hill, Daniel G. *The Freedom-Seekers: Blacks in Early Canada.* Agincourt, Canada: The Book Society, 1981.

Katz, William Loren. *Eyewitness; The Negro in American History.* New York: Pittman Publishing Corporation, 1967.

Katzman, David M. *Before the Ghetto.* Urbana, Ill: Univ. of Ill. Press, 1973

Keemer, Edgar B. *Confessions of a Pro-life Abortionist.* Vinco Press.

King, Lester B.. *American Medicine Comes of Age, 1840-1920.*

King, Martin Luther, *Why We Can't Wait.* New York: Signet, 1964.

Krouse, An W. *Who's Who Among Black Americans 1977-1978,* 2nd Edition 1977-1978 Vol. 1, Northbrook, Ill.: Publishing Co.

Larrie, Reginald R. *Makin' Free: African-Americans in the Northwest Territory.* Blaine-Ethridge Books, 1981.

Littlejohn, Edward J., and Hobson Donald L. *Black Lawyers, Law Practice, and Bar Associations - 1844 to 1970.* A Michigan History

The Wolverine Bar Association, 1987.

Locke, Hubert. *The Detroit of 1967.* Detroit: Wayne State University Press, 1969.

Logan, Reyford W. *The Betrayal of the Negro.* New York and London: Collier Macmillan Ltd.

McLean, Franklyn C., *Negroes in Medicine.* Chicago: National Medical Fellowships, Inc. Vol.11, 1964-1965.

McRae, Norman. *Negroes in Michigan During the Civil War.* Edited by Sidney Glazer. Lansing: Michigan Civil War Centennial Observance Commission, 1966.

McRae, Norman, *The American Negro,* Impact Enterprises, Inc. 1965.

Meharry Medical College - Alumni Directory, 1986. White Plains New York: Bernard C Harris Publishing Co. Inc., 1986.

Medical History of Michigan. Minneapolis- St Paul, Minn: Bruce Publishing Co., under the auspices of the Michigan State Medical Society, 1930.

Miller, Loren. *The Petitioners - The Story of the Supreme Court of the United States and the Negro.* New York: Pantheon Books, 1966.

Motley, Mary Penick, ed. *Invisible Soldier: The Experience of the Black Soldier, World War II.* Detroit: Wayne State University Press.

Norris, Harold. *Education for Popular Sovereignty Through Implementing the Constitution and the Bill of Rights.* Detroit: The Detroit College of Law, 1991.

Olmstead, Frederick Law. *The Slave States.* New York: Capricorn Books, 1959.

Patterson, William L. *The Man Who Cried Genocide. An Autobiography.* New York: International Publishers, 1971.

Perry, Marvin. *A History of the World.* Boston: Houghton Mifflin Co., 1985

Quarles, Benjamin. *The Negro in the Making of America.* New York: McMillan Publishing Co., 1987.

Ragsdale, Bruce A., and Treesew, Joel D. *Black Americans in Congress, 1970-1989.* Washington, DC: U.S. Government Printing Office, 1990.

Rich, Wilbur. *Coleman Young and Detroit Politics: From Social Activist to Power Broker.* Detroit: Wayne State University Press

Smedley, Audrey. *Race in North America, Origin and Evolution of a Worldview.*

Stamp, Kenneth M. *The Peculiar Institution.* New York: Vantage Books, 1956.

Sumerville, James. *Educating Black Doctors: A History of Meharry Medical College.* The University of Alabama Press, University of Alabama, 1983.

The Michigan Historical Review. Vol 12, No. 1, Clarke Historical Library, Mt Pleasant. MI: Central Michigan University, 1986.

Washington, Booker T. *Up from Slavery.* New York.

Washington, Forrester. *The Negro in Detroit; A Survey of the Conditions of a Negro Group.*

Williams, Harry T. Current, Richard N., and Freidel, Frank. *A History of the United States.* Alfred A. Knopf, 1963.

Wilson, Joseph T. *The Black Phalanx. A History of the Negro Soldier in the Wars of 1775, 1812 and 1861-1865.* Hartford, Conn: The American Publishing Co, 1888.

Woods, Esmo. Pontiac: *The Making of a U.S.Automobile Capital 1918-1958.* 1991.

Wright, Charles H. *Robeson: Labor's Forgotten Champion.* Detroit: Balamp Publishing, 1975.

Yenser, Thomas. *Who's Who in Colored America,* (fifth edition). Brooklyn, N.Y.: 1940.

Index

A

African American firsts in medicine in Michigan, 269-296
African National Congress, 221
Alexander, Charles R., xvi
Allen, Blythe, 56
Allied Medical Society, 50, 101
AMA adopts a pro-apartheid foreign policy, 226-227
AMA and the Cuban Physicians, 209
AMA and the Hungarian Uprising, 205-207
AMA Council on Medical Education, 8
AMA Officials Visit South Africa, 225
AMA rejoins WMA, 226
AMA Withdraws Membership in WMA, 225
American Association of Medical Colleges, 8
American Bar Association, 104
American Dental Association, 186
American Hospital Association, 186
American Medical Association, 7, 103, 186
      1948 House of Delegates' Meeting, 106
      Founding, 13
      Opposition to Medicare, 121
      Council on Medical Education, 92
      Southern membership, 106
"American Medicine Comes of Age," 7
Ames, Dr. Chester, xiv, 75, 53
Ames, Dr. James, 53
Anderson, Dr. William G., 45
Anderson, Dr. William G., pres. of American Osteopathic Association, 296-300
Angola, 215
Anti-Haitian Foreign Policy, 216
Aquadilla, Puerto Rico, 1
Arawok Indians, 1
Argosy Newspaper Ltd, 60
Armstrong, Dr. Wiley, 183, 195
Art
      Dr. Walter Evans' art collection, 252-254
      Leroy Foster's "Kaleidoscope," 77
Articles Against Discrimination, 178-180
Atlanta Compromise, 31, 34
Atlanta Graduate Assembly, NMA delegates to the, 44

B

Babcock, Dr. James, 52
Bailer, Dr. Lloyd, 279
Bailer, Kermit, 158
Balduf, Carl, 72
Ball, George, 216
Barbie, Klaus, 210

Barclay, Robin, 78
Batchelor, Dr. Thomas, xvi, 72, 154, 173, 300-316
Battle Creek Sanitarium, 61
Battle of the Alamo, 3
Bay of Pigs, 209
Bear Flag Revolt, 4
Bell, Dr. R.E., 45
Belle Isle Casino, 102
Bentley, Dr. William, xvi, 159, 177-178
Berea v. Kentucky, 93
Berry, Leonidas, 119, 195, 198
Bethel AME Church, 18
Bevan, Dr. Arthur Dean, 49
Bicknell, Dr. Frank, xiv, 56
Bilko, Steve, 221-223
Billings, Dr. Frank, 8, 88
Billingslea, Dr. Thomas, 118
Billups, Dr. J.T., 122
Blasingame, Dr. F.J.L., 196
Blockson, Charles, xvi
Blue Cross/Blue Shield, 71
Boddie, Dr. Lewis F., 272
Boggs, Dr. Robert, 211
Boland, Dr. Robert, 11, 19
Bounten, Dr. W. Andrew, 196
Bousfield, Midian O., 112
Bowles, Dr. Alvin, 316
Boyd, Dr. Robert F., 35
Boyd's Infirmary, 35
Bradfield, Dr. Horace, 148
Brewer, Sr., Dr. Thomas, 44
British Guiana, 58
Brown, Dr. Richard O., 220
Brown, Harley, 78
Brown, John, 14
Brown v. Board of Education, 18, 24
Bryant, Faris, 211
Bulletin of the Medico-Chirrurgical Society, 40
Bundy, Dr. George, 54
Bureau of Indian Affairs, 2
Burney, Dr. W.A., 24
Burton, Dr. DeWitt T., 75-76, 162
Burton, Dr. Gail, 76
Burton, Dr. John, 280
Burton, Senator Harold, 110-111
Butler, Dr. R., 35-36
Butzel, Fred, 52

C

Cain, Dr. Natalia Tanner, 280
Cain, Dr. Waldo, 146, 160, 172
Caldwell, Dr. Charles, 6
Calloway, Augustus, 77
Camp Kilmer, N.J., 206

Canady, Dr. Alexis, 293
Caraco Pharmaceutical Laboratories, Ltd., 251
Caribbean, 1
Carnegie Foundation, 34, 87, 92
Caroff, Atty. Julia, 79
Carpenter, Dr. William, 160
Carrington, Ethyl Bert, 121
Cartmill, George, 166
Castro, Fidel, 209
Cavanagh, Jerome, 157
Celebrezze, Anthony, 186, 188
Centurion, Dr. Jose J., 211
Chapman, Dr. Paul, 154
Chapman, Dr. Roland, 154
Charles Drew University, 193
Charleston Medical Journal, 6
Chicago Medical College, 36
Christopher Columbus, 1
Clark, Septima, 45
Clay, Henry, 4
Cleage, Dr. Albert B., 54
Clement, Dr. Kenneth W., 135
Cobb, Dr. W. Montague, xi, 40, 106, 121, 163
Cole, Florence, 53
Cole, James, 53
Collins, Dr. James, xvi
Colored Physicians of Georgia, 36
Comprehensive Health Service of Detroit, xvi, 308
Constitution, U.S., 5
Constitutional Acts
        Civil Rights Act of 1866, 16
        Civil Rights Act of 1957, 18
        Civil Rights Act of 1964, 40, 186
        Fugitive Slave Act of 1793, 13
        Fugitive Slave Act of 1850, 14
        Mutual Security Act, 212
        Voting Rights Act of 1965, 17
Constitutional Amendments
5th Amendment, 45
        13th Amendment of 1865, 32
        14th Amendment of 1867, 32
        15th Amendment of 1870, 17, 36
Continental Congress of 1787, 12
Cooley, Chief Justice Tom, 17
Cotillion Club, 152, 154
Cotton States International Exposition, 30
Cotton, Dorothy F., 45
Council Hearings on Medical Center, 164
Council on Medical Education, 8
Couzens Community Affairs Committee, 52
Couzens, Senator James, 52
Crittenton Home, 63-64
Crockett, Dr. Ethelene, 157, 172, 173, 273
Crockett, Judge George, 157

Cuban Emergency Center, 210
Cuban Medical Association (CMAE), in exile, 210
Cuban National Medical Association, 209
Cuban physicians and the Cold War, 215
Cuban physicians in Angola, 215
Cuban physicians in Granada, BWI, 215
Cuban physicians, 200
Cupitt, Pam, xv
Curry, Dr. C. Arnold, xvi, 251-252
Curtis, Dr. Austin, 39
Curtis, Dr. James, xvi

D

Dailey, Dr. Ulysses Grant, 40
Dancy, John, 52, 63
Dancy, Dr. Joseph, 69
Davenport, Mrs. Elvin, 77
Davis, Dr. Albert M., 44
Dawson, Dr. Robert, 220
deBaptist, John D., 14
DeBusk, Dr. Roger, 172-173
Delaney, Dr. Martin R., 13
Dellus, Allen, 209
Detroit's Disciples; Drs. Waldo Cain, Garnett Ice & Hayward Maben, 258-268
Detroit's first HMO, 300-316
Detroit's husband & wife medical teams, 327-330
Detroit Board of Education, 16
Detroit Board of Health, 53
Detroit Book Cadillac Hotel, 103
Detroit College of Medicine, 16, 20
Detroit Community Union, 63
Detroit Free Press, xiv, 14
Detroit Hospital Authority, 163
Detroit Hospital Study Committee, 141
Detroit Medical Center, 16
Detroit Medical Society, 139-181
Detroit Memorial Park Association, 68
Detroit Receiving Hospital, 49
Detroit Urban League, 63, 141
Diaz Antonio Rodrigez, 212
Diggs, Jr., Hon. Charles, xiv, 56, 154
Dodge, Percival, 63
Douglass, Frederick, 14
Drew, Dr. Charles, 103-104
Drew Medical School, 8
DuBois, W.E.B., 13, 31
Dudley, Dr. Cal, 76
Dumas, Sr., Dr. Albert, xv, 35
Dunbar Hospital, 52, 102, 219
Dunbar Medical Museum, 72

E

Eastern High School, 102
Eastside Medical Laboratory, 68

Eaton, Dr. Chester Arthur, 94
Eaton, Dr. Hubert, 94-95, 183
Edward, Dr. Gloria, xvi
Ellison, Dr. James P., 44
Emerson, Dr. John, 6
Emory University Medical School, 46
Emrich, Bishop Richard, 166
Eppert, Ray, 165
Evans, Dr. Franklin, 210
Evans, Dr. Tommy, 178
Evans, Dr. Walter, 252-254

F

Falk, Dr. Henry, 121
Falling, Katherine, 175
Farmer, Judge Charles S., 158
Fascell, Dante B., 212
Faulkner, William, 15
Feemster, Dr. John, 219
Ferguson, Dr. Joseph, xv, 11, 18
Ferguson, William W., 17
First Negro medical society, 40
Firsts in the several medical specialties, 269-294
Fishbein, Dr. Morris, 104, 106
Fisher, Dr. George, 173
Fitzbutler, Jr., Dr. William Henry, 11, 21, 23, 89
Flake, Sr., Dr. Thomas, 168
Flanders, Nurse Ann, xv
Flexner, Abraham, 8
Flexner Commission Report; Gospel according to Abraham, 23, 87, 92
Flint Medical College, 88
Florence Crittenton Home, 63-64
Ford Hospital, 49
Foster, Leroy, 77
Fourth Circuit Court of Appeal, 185
Fowler, Dr. Melvin, 173
Fugitive Slave Act of 1793, 13
Fulton County Criminal Court, 44
Fulton County Medical Society, 44
Fulton Dekalb Hospital Authority, 43

G

Gamble, Dr. Parker G., 55
Garrett, Joyce, 77
George, Dr. Alma Rose, 71, 316-317
George, Senator Walter, 110-111
Georgia Dental Association, 45
Georgia State Medical Society, 43
Gibson, Dr. Ralph, xv
Gill, Jr., Dr. John T., 44
Gillium, Dr. Linda, xv-xvi
Glass, Herman, 154
Glidden, George R., 6
Gluckman accuses security police of brutality, Jonnathon, 28

Godley, Alegro, 172
Goins, Dr. William, 273
Gotham Hotel, 117
Grace Hospital, 49
Grady, Henry, 36
Grady Hospital, 46
Grady School of Nursing, 45
Gray, Dr. Howard, 294
Gray, Jr., Dr. Herman B., xvi
Graystone Ballroom, 102
Great Lakes Mutual Life Insurance Company, 68
Greaves, Angelina, 59
Green, Roy, 211
Greenberg, Atty. Jack, 186
Greenidge, Dr. Robert, xiv, 55-57, 62, 101
Greenidge, Isaac Theopolis, 59
Greer, Dr. Pedro J., 214
Grimes, Grover, 157
Guinyard, Freddie, xiv
Gundersen, Dr. Gunnar, 210
Gurdjian, Dr. E.S., 173

H

Hall, Dr. Jeffrey, 293
Harlan, Justice John, 37
Harpers Ferry Raid, 15
Harris, Dr. Arthur D., 172, 273
Hart, (D-Mich.)Senator Phillip A., 162, 176
Heart of Atlanta Hotel, 44
Heidelberg, Dr. Robert, 270
Henderson, Dr. Allison B., 270
Heron, Dr. Alicia, 76
Heron, Dr. Alva, 76
Heustis, Dr. Albert E., 176
Hill, Dr. Luther, 110
Hill, Senator Lister, 110-111
Hill-Burton Act, 43, 109-111, 113, 191
Hirsch, Dr. Bernard L., 196
Holloman, Dr. John, 195
Holt, Dr. Willard, 270
Home Federal Savings, 68
Hood, M. Louise, 63
Hopper, Jodge Frank, 46
Hospitals
     Bethesda Hospital, 69
     Boulevard General Hospital, 74
     Burton Mercy Hospital, 74
     Children's Hospital of Detroit, 142
     Delray Hospital, 70, 74
     Dunbar Hospital of Detroit, 52, 102, 219
     Edith K. Thomas Hospital, 69
     Fairview Hospital, 69
     Freedman's Hospital, 41
     Good Samaritan Hospital, 69

Grady Hospital, 45
Harlem Hospital, 175
Harper Hospital, 16, 49
Haynes Memorial Hospital, 69
Herman Kiefer Hospital, 49, 69
James Walker Memorial Hospital, 183
Kirwood Hospital, 70
Lincoln Hospital of the Bronx, 38
Mercy General Hospital of Detroit, 49-50, 102
Moses Cope Hospital, 186
Mount Carmel Hospital, 160
Mt. Lebanon Hospital, 73
Parkside Hospital of Detroit, 69
Provident Hospital of Chicago, 36
Resthaven Hospital, 74
Southwest Detroit Hospital, 74, 77-78, 83
St. Mary's Hospital, 16
Taborian Hospital, 256
Trinity Hospital, 73
Trumbull General Hospital, 74
United Community Hospital, 83
Wayne Diagnostic Hospital, 75
Women's (Hutzel) Hospital of Detroit, 56
Howard, Dr. Ernest B., 196
Howard, Dr. T.M., 256
Howard University, 88
Howard University Medical School, 23
Howard University School of Medical Technology, 41
Howell, Dr. Joel, xvi
Huertes, Enrique, 212
Hungarian physicians, 207
Hungarian relief, 205
Hunter, John E., 39
Hurley, Mark K., 165
Hutzel Hospital, 56
Hutzel Hospital Library, xv

I

Ice, Dr. Garnet, 261
Imhotep Conferences, 123-127, 160
Imprisonment & murder of Steve Biko, 221
Imprisonment of ANC leadership, 221
Ingram, Dr. Alvin J., 196

J

Jackson Prison, 15
Jackson, Dr. Roosevelt P., 44
Javits, Senator Jacob, 110
Jenkins, Dr. Sidney Bernard, 286
John A. Andrews Medical Clinic of Tuskegee, 39
Johnson, Atty. William, xv
Johnson, Dr. Georgia A. Lewis, 317
Johnson, Rev. Louis, 159
Johnston, Dr. George A., 96

Jones, Dr. Ralph, 211
Jones, Dr. Sophia Bethena, 11, 24
Journal of the National Medical Association, 39
      Cobb, Dr. W. Montague, 40
      Dailey, Dr. Ulysses Grant, 40
      Roman, Dr. Charles V., 39
      Sampson, Dr. Calvin, 41
      The Index Medicus, 41
      The National Library of Medicine, 41
Judd, Dr. Charles Hollister, xiv, 56
Just, Ernest E., 95

K

Kadar, Janus, 205
Keemer, Jr. confessions, Dr. Edgar B., 243-245
Keith, Hon. Damon, 154
Kellogg, Dr. Henry, 61
Kellogg Sanitarium, 61, 63
Kenney, Jr., Dr. John, 39, 132, 195
Kenney, Sr., Dr. John, 94, 132, 139
Kentucky Medical Liscensing Board, 23
Kerr Photo Studio, 60
King, Dr. Lester B., 6
King, Jr., Rev. Dr. Martin Luther, 190
King-Anderson Act (Medicaid), 121
Kirk, Atty. Stanley, xv
Kline, Dr. M. Author, 205
Knights and Daughters of Tabor, 255
Ku Klux Klan, 11

L

Lackey, Clarice, xi
Lackey, Dr. Lawrence, xi, 160, 167, 272
Lander, Charles, 15
Larson, Leonard W., 210
Lawrence, David, xiv
Lawrence, Dr. George C., 44
Leader, Dr. Luther, 148
Lee, Andre, 79
Lee, Atty. James, 158
Lefall, Dr. LaSalle, 220
Leonard Medical School, 39, 88
Levagood, Dr. Floyd, 173
Liaison Committee Final Report, 198-203
Liaison Committees, 131-138, 195-204
Liel, Dr. George, 104
Life Choice Quality Health Plan, 78
Lillie, Dr. Frank Rattray, 95
Littlejohn, Dr. Edward, xvi
Loeb, Dr. Jacques, 95
Long, Dr. Wesley W., 196
Louisville Medical School, 23, 88, 90
Love, Dr. Thomas A., 317
Lovett, Louise, 120

Lumumba, Patrice, 210
Lundy, Dr. William C., 22
Lyle, Dr. John, 52
Lynk, Dr. Myles V., 29, 35-36

M

Maben, Dr. Hayward, 219
Madras Medical School, 178
Malloy, Catherine, 170, 175
Markoe, Dr. Rupert, 153-154
Marks, Richard, 154
Marshall, C. Herbert, 119
Marshall, Chief Justice Thurgood, 129
Marshall-Murray, Dr. Peter, 121-122
Martin, Dr. D.L., 36
Mason, Dr. Vaughn, 120
Matney, William T., 154
Matthew's Disciples, 255-268
Matthew's Disciples are organized, 257-258
Mazique, Dr. Edward, 129
McCabe, Dr. W. Peter, 234
McCarthy, Glen, 122
McClean, Dr. Don, 172
McClean, Dr. Franklin C., 121
McClendon, Dr. Earle, 44
McClendon, Dr. James, 153, 170
McCollough, Dr. John, 280
McCook, Dr. George, 12
McCurdy, Sarah, 21
McDuffie, Gov. George, 5
McGraw, Dr. Theodore, 16
McGraw-Hill Book Co., 72
McKinnon, Dr. Irville H., 212
McKlown, Dr. Raymond, 196
McNamara, Secretary James, 115, 239
Mcquire Air Force Base, 206
Medical Committee for Human Rights, 190
Medical Facilities Amendment, 191
Medical Gospel According to Abraham, 8
Medical Trailblazers, 11
Medico Chirrurigical Society, 29
Meharry Medical College, 8, 88
Memphis Medical School, 88
Menendez, Aristedes, 213
Mesa, Dr. Virginia, 286
Meyers, Dr. Don, 172-173
Meyers, Dr. Marjorie Peebles, 271
Miami Herald, xiv
Michigan Chronicle, 75, 177
Michigan College of Medicine, 20
Middleton, John, 45
Miller, Dorie, 282
Miriani, Mayor Louis, 156, 167, 170
Mji, Dr. Dilza, 236

Molner, Dr. Joseph, 154
Monroe, Rev. William, 14
Morris, Atty. John, 195
Morris, Dr. Marva Jenkins, 269
Morrison, Dr. George W., 279
Morton, Dr. Sameul G., 6
mouthpiece, 193
Murray, Dr. Peter Marshall, 39, 121
Murray, Senator, 111
Museum of African American History, 72

N

NAACP, 40, 115, 134, 141, 151, 161, 170, 184
Nagy, Imy, 205
Naidoo, Dr. B.T., 349
National Association of Colored Physicians, Dentists and Pharmacists, 35
National Medical Association
        1895 founding, 29
        1896 second meeting, 38
        1927 Detroit meeting, 101
        1949 Detroit meeting, 117
        1959 Detroit meeting, 129-130
        1979 Detroit meeting, 220
        1986 Nashville meeting, 38
        Auxiliary, 193
        original Mission Statement, 37
Native Americans, 1
Nelson, Dr. Lorenzo, 121
New Treaty of Eschota, 2
New York County Medical Society, 106
New York Times, 112
Niagera Movement, 105
Non-medical firsts, 296
Norris, Atty. Harold, xv, 104
Northcross Sanitarium, 50
Northcross, Drs. Daisy & David, 50
Northcross, Mrs. Ophelia, 51
Northcross, Jr., Dr. David, 51
Northern District Dental Society, 45
Northwest Territory, 12
Nott, Dr. Josiah, 6
Nuttall, Dr. Harry Montgomery, 318-319

O

Old North State Medical Society, 184
Omega Mason Scholarships, 194
opinions of pro-Castro physicians, 214
opposition to Cape Town convention, 229-237
Orr, Dr. Wendy, 228
Osby, William C., 52
Oscela, Seminole Chief, 2
Osius, Dr. Eugene, 168
Osterberg, Armaine, xv
Osterberg, Bert, xv

P

Patton, James, 307
Perry, Dr. Harold, 286
Phillips, Dr. Burton, 280
Plummer, Dr. Jon O., 98
Presidents, Mexican
   Antonio Lopez de Sante Anna, 3
Presidents, U.S.
   Clinton, Bill, 217
   Eisenhower, Dwight, 18, 206
   Fillmore, Millard, 14
   Johnson, Andrew, 17
   Johnson, Lyndon B., 152
   Lincoln, Abraham, 19
   Nixon, Richard M., 190
   Polk, James K., 4
   Reagan, Ronald, 215
   Roosevelt, Franklin D., 53
   Roosevelt, Theodore, 42
   Truman, Harry S., 110, 112
   Tyler, John, 10
   VanBuren, Martin, 4
Prince, Dr. Addison, 274
Progeny; The keepers of the flame, Detroit's African American, 31-344
Price, Atty. William, xv
Phillips, Hikanius, xv
Phillips, Wilburn, xvi, 71
Ponce deLeon, 1, 2
Plessy v. Ferguson, 24, 32
Plessy, Homer S., 33, 37
Penn, I. Garland, 35
Palmer, Dr. James, 46
Providence Hospital, 49
Parke-Davis Pharmaceutical Plant, 103
Powell, U.S. Rep. Adam Clayton, 115
Patrick, Atty. William, 151, 161, 173
Pendleton, Cassius, 154
Proctor, Leonard, 154
Pinkie, Dr. Miller, 173
Pearson, Dr. Homer L., 196
Purchase and conversion of Dunbar Hospital into museum, 219

Q

Queen Victoria, 58
Quarker, Dorothy, 154

R

Raiford, Sr., Dr. Frank, 55
Raikes, Dr. James A., 285
Raines, Capt. Gabriel J., 3
Rangarajan, Dr. N.S., xvi, 177
Reed, Dr. Barbara Ross, 299
Rivers, Dr. Emanuel, 270
Robinson, Sr., Remus, 288

Robinson, Dr. Remus, 143, 161, 288
Roman, Dr. Charles V., 37, 39
Rose, Marcella, xv
Rucker, Gloria, xv
Richards, John D., 14
Reconstruction failure, 18
Reese, Dr. Louis F., 44
Rutledge, Phil, 157
Robinson, Dr. James, 160
Rahn, 195
Rouse, Dr. Milford, 196
Ribicoff, Abraham, 213
Recent developments in U.S.-Cuban foreign relations, 216

S

Sampson, Dr. Calvin, 41
Savimbi, Dr. Jonas, 3
Scott, Dred, 5
Scott, Dr. D.N.C., 36
Sickle Cell Anemia, 70
Smith, Dr. C. Miles, 44
Smith, Dr. James McCune, 8
South Africa Medical Association, 223-225
South Africa Medical Journal, 222
Southwest Detroit Hospital, 79
Spanish language, 181
Stevenson, Dr. Charles Summers, 274-279
Stith, Dr. Dwight E., 77
Swan, Dr. Lionel, 151-152, 160
Sweet, Dr. Ossian, 102
Simmons, Julia, xiv
Shifman Library, xv
Saulsberry, Dr. Guy O., 70
Saulsberry, Essell, xvi
Seminole casualties, 2
Siddell, Rep. John, 4
Spanish American War, 5
St. Matthews Episcopal, 14
Second Baptist Church, 14
St. Mary's Hospital, 16
Stone, Alice, 52
Selma to Montgomery March, 17
Storr School for Children, 19
Sherman, Gen. William T., 30
Speer, Judge Emory, 35
Spaulding Pavilion, 43
Smith, Edwina, 45
Stewart, Dr. William, 46
Scott, General Winfield, 2
Sisters of Charity, 49
Seears family, 59-60
Sharples School, 59
Stanislaw School & College, 59
Seven Day Adventist Church, 61

Stearns, Wayland S., 63
Storey, Atty. Morefield, 105
Salchow, Dr. Paul, 154
Schaffer, Dr. Dorothy, 154
Saltstein, Harry, 166
Scott, Dean Gordon, 177
Small, Dr. Bessie B., 193
Simenstad, Dr. L.O., 196
Storm cloud gathering over Miami, 217
Spock, Dr. Benjamin, 230
Sensenich, R.L., 111

T

Taft, Senator Robert, 111
Taney, Justice Roger B., 5
Taylor, Dr. Amos, 270
Taylor, Hobart, 158
Terry, Dr. Luther, 188
Texas, Republic of, 3
Texas & New NMexico Act, 4
Texas annexation, 3-4
Texas sovereignty, 3
Thomas, Sr., Drs. Alfred, Jr. and Alfred, 69
Thompson, Dr. Arthur, 282
Trail of Tears, 3
Trenholm, Pres. H. Council, xvi
Trianos Indians, 1
Tribulations in central Georgia, 245-251
Truman Doctrine of 1946, 114
Tucker, Dr. Benjamin, 237-239
Turner, Dr. Alexander Loudin, 53-54, 101, 287
Turner, Dr. John P., 98
Tutu, Bishop Desmond, 221

U

U.S. Agency for International Development & Project Hope, 216
Union troops withdrawal, 17
University of Glascow, 9
University of Miami, 210
University of Michigan Medical School, xv, 178

V

VanBuren, President Martin, 4
VanDyke, Prof. Henry Louis, xvi
Victoria University-Toronto, 22
Victory Loan Assn., 68
Viljoen, Dr. C.E.M., 226, 349
Vincent, Dr. Charles, 160, 294-295

W

Wagner, Senator, 111
Walker, Dr. Matthew, 256-258
Walton, Jr., Dr. Tracy, xii
Ward, Dr. Donovan F., 196

Warner, Dr. Clinton, 44-45
Warren, Charles W., 52
Warsaw Pact, 205
Washington, Booker T., 30
Watson, Dr. Carl Webber, 24
Watts, Dr. Charles, 183
Wayne State University, xv, 168, 177
Wayne University Medical College, 26
Webb, Charles, 52
Webb, Judge James, 44
Webb, Martha Ann, 12
Webb, William & Agnes, 12
Welch, Atty. Edward M., 165
Wellness Plan (The), 300
Wells, Alma, 193
White supremacy, 2
Whitten, Dr. Charles F., xvi, 70, 319-323
Whittier, Dr. C. Austin, 118
Wickersham, Atty. George W., 105
Wilkins; NAACP, Roy, 162
Williams, Dr. Daniel Hale, 36
Williams, Dr. Joshua, 45, 245
Williams, Hon. G. Mennen, 162
Williams, John, xvi
Williams, Sr., Dr. Delford, xvi, 77
Wilson, William, 14
Windsor, Canada, 102
Wise, Blanche Parent, 165
Wolverine State Medical Society, 220
Workman, Joseph, 16
World Medical Association, 228, 230
Wright, Dr. Charles H., 173-178

Y

Yancey, Dr. Asa, 46
Yeakey, Dr. Lamont, xvi

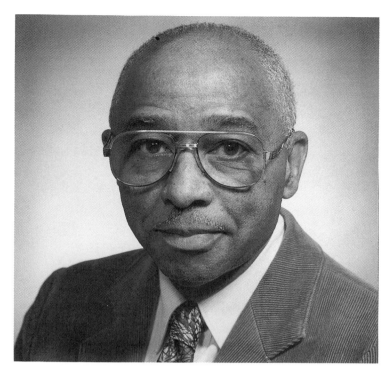

About the Author

Charles H. Wright was born in Dothan, Ala., on September 20, 1918. After his secondary education, in the heart of the Wiregrass (southeastern) section of Alabama, he entered Alabama State College in 1935, and earned a B.S. degree in 1939 that prepared him for a career as a teacher.

His application to Meharry Medical College was denied, but with their blessing, he took qualifying pre-medical courses during the summer at Alabama State, was accepted in Meharry's freshman class in the fall of 1939, and graduated in 6th place in 1943. After an internship and a year of pathology at New York's Harlem Hospital, he spent another year in pathology at the Cleveland City Hospital.

In 1946, Dr. Wright, unable to gain acceptance to a residency program, began a four-year tour as a private practitioner in Detroit, Mich. In 1950, Dr. Wright married Louise Lovett, of Chicago. Luckily, he found an opening and returned to Harlem Hospital for a three-year residency in obg. In 1953, he resumed private practice as a specialist in Detroit.

Certification as a specialist in obg., followed in 1955, and fellowship in the American College of Surgeons, thereafter. He was appointed to the clinical faculty of medicine at Wayne State University and to the staffs of Burton Mercy, Grace, Highland Park, Hutzel (also, trustee) and Sinai hospitals.

In 1960, Dr. Wright helped to organize the African Medical Education Fund that provided financial assistance for the medical education of fifty Africans from 13 different countries. In 1965, Dr. Wright founded the Museum of African American History and served as the chairman of the board of trustees until he resigned in 1990.

Dr. Wright's other trusteeships have included Hutzel Hospital, Channel 56 (public TV), the University of Detroit, and, currently, Penn Center Inc., where he served as a trustee, and its Michigan Support Group, where he still serves as president.

His publications include four books, two plays, two films and many papers about a variety of subjects. His community efforts have attracted a treasure-trove of citations and awards.

Dr. and Mrs. Wright had two daughters: Stephanie, deputy director of Cook County Hospital, and Dr. Carla, a physiatrist in Milwaukee. Following Louise's death in 1985, Dr. Wright married Roberta Greenidge Hughes, Ph.D., an attorney and writer, in 1989.

Roberta, also has two children: Wilbur III, general manager and member of the board of directors of Detroit Memorial Park; and Dr. Barbara Finch, dept. head, counseling, at Golightly Education & Career Center.

Your purchase of *The National Medical Association Demands Equal Opportunity: Nothing More, Nothing Less* entitles you to a five dollar credit to one of the medical institutions listed below. Please fill out this form and return it to us for immediate attention.

YES! I want to support one of the Black Medical Schools listed below:

☐ Meharry Medical College, Nashville, Tenn.

☐ Howard University College of Medicine, Washington, D.C.

☐ Morehouse School of Medicine, Atlanta, Ga.

☐ Charles R. Drew Medical School, Los Angeles, Calif.

☐ Ohio University School of Osteopathic, Athens, Ohio

Optional:

Name _____

Address _____

City _____ State _____ Zip _____

May we include you on our mailing list?

☐ Yes   ☐ No

☐ I purchased this book for myself.

☐ I purchased this book as a gift.

☐ I received this book as a gift.

☐ I plan to pursue a medical career.

☐ I am currently in a pre-med program.

☐ I am currently in med. school.

☐ I am currently in the field of medicine.

What field of medicine do you practice? _____

☐ I have retired from medicine.

What medicine did you practice? _____

☐ I have a family member who is in the medical field.

☐ I am not in medicine.

☐ I have no intentions of pursuing medicine.

I purchased this book because: _____

_____

_____

See other side for address, ordering information,
and additional titles available from Charro Book Co., Inc.

TO ORDER additional copies of *The National Medical Association Demands Equal Opportunity: Nothing More, Nothing Less* or any of the other books available from Charro Book Co., Inc., please fill out this order form and return it to us for quick shipment.

	Quantity	Price	Total
The National Medical Association Demands Equal Opportunity: Nothing More, Nothing Less	_____	x $33.68	= $_____
The Peace Advocacy of Paul Robeson	_____	x $ 4.00	= $_____
Paul Robeson's 80th Birthday Salute, 1978	_____	x $ 8.00	= $_____
The Birth of the Montgomery Bus Boycott	_____	x $13.00	= $_____
An Annotated Bibliography of the Sea Islands of Georgia and South Carolina	_____	x $13.00	= $_____
A Tribute to Charlotte Forten, 1837-1914	_____	x $13.00	= $_____
		Total	= $_____

(Note: Above price list includes shipping and handling)

Name _____

Address _____

City _____ State _____ Zip _____

Daytime Phone _____

_____ Payment enclosed (check or money order; no cash please)

Please mail to:

Charro Book Co., Inc., 29777 Telegraph Rd., Suite 2500, Southfield, MI 48034

810/356-0950

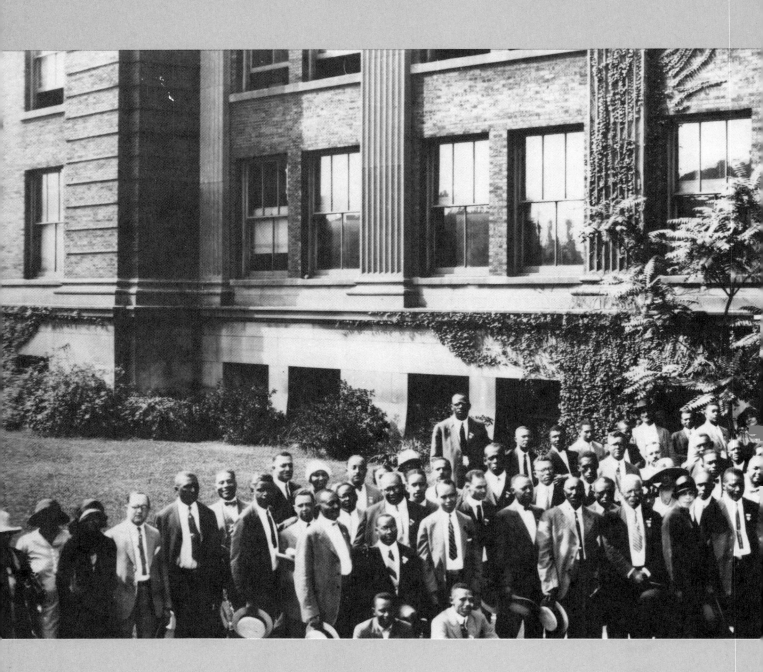